PROGRESS IN PEDIATRIC NEUROLOGY

Editor

J. GORDON MILLICHAP, M.D., F.R.C.P.

Professor of Pediatrics and Neurology,
Northwestern University Medical School,
Children's Memorial Hospital,
Chicago, Illinois

Visiting Professor, Chief of Pediatric Neurology,
Southern Illinois University School of Medicine

Formerly, Pediatric Neurology Consultant,
Mayo Clinic

P N B • Pediatric Neurology Briefs • Publisher
Chicago • London

Published and Distributed Throughout the World by
P N B • P u b l i s h e r s
Pediatric Neurology Briefs
P.O. Box 11391
Chicago, Illinois 60611, U.S.A.

Printed In U.S.A.

ISBN 0-9629115-0-X
Library of Congress Catalog Card Number: 91-90076

To my wife, Nancy,
without whose encouragement and
assistance, this book would not have
been published.

PREFACE

The material included in this book is based on a review of the literature which began in June 1987 and was continued through December 1990. The abstracts and editorial comments have appeared in monthly issues of PEDIATRIC NEUROLOGY BRIEFS, Volumes I-IV. They have been compiled under subject heading and in chronological order of appearance in order to provide an update and overview of current PROGRESS IN PEDIATRIC NEUROLOGY. A comprehensive index is supplied so that the reader may have ready access to the material reviewed and the subject matter included in the editorial comments.

Epilepsy, headache, attention deficit and learning disorders, neuromuscular disorders, neurocutaneous syndromes, brain neoplasms, congenital and degenerative diseases, including Rett syndrome, are some of the topics covered. The specialty of pediatric neurology bridges not only pediatrics and neurology but also psychology and the education of learning disabled children. Original articles have been selected from the medical world literature and journals of pediatrics, neurology, developmental medicine, neurosurgery, psychology, psychiatry, epilepsy and other specialities. The editorial comments draw on both recent and past publications on each subject. The institutions and country of origin of the reports are provided in addition to full references.

PROGRESS IN PEDIATRIC NEUROLOGY is intended to provide pediatric neurologists, pediatricians, neurologists, neurosurgeons, psychiatrists, psychologists, educators and other interested professionals with an update of the diagnosis, etiology, pathology, treatment and prognosis of nervous diseases of infants, children, and adolescents.

J. GORDON MILLICHAP, M.D., F.R.C.P.

TABLE OF CONTENTS

Page

CHAPTER 1

EPILEPSY AND RELATED DISORDERS

INTRODUCTION

Current research in pediatric epilepsy emphasizes the toxic effects of anticonvulsant drugs. Of 115 articles published and reviewed in the years 1987 through 1990, 18 (16%) pertained to the adverse effects of commonly prescribed antiepileptics, whereas 14 (12%) were concerned with drug efficacy and 7 (6%) with alternative neurosurgical treatments for epilepsies in infants and children.

The cognitive deficits attending the use of phenobarbital and other established medications and the serious, sometimes fatal, adverse effects of newer drugs such as valproic acid have prompted a change in attitudes toward long-term anticonvulsant therapies and a greater reliance on alternative methods of treatment. Intermittent prophylactic or therapeutic, rectal diazepam is recommended by some authorities in preference to chronic phenobarbital therapy of febrile seizures, but efficacy is unproven and poor compliance may limit its value in practice. Withdrawal of anticonvulsant therapy is attempted earlier than previously recommended, and monotherapy has taken precedence over polytherapy in an attempt to lessen the risk of adverse drug reactions and interactions.

Neurosurgeons have responded to the neurologist's increasing dissatisfaction with anticonvulsant drugs by adopting a more heroic approach to the surgery of epilepsy. Surgery once limited to temporal lobectomy for refractory complex partial seizures in adults has now been extended to children and even neonates with partial seizures and hemispherectomy is regaining some popularity. The prevention of intellectual deterioration that may attend chronically recurrent seizures is proposed as a compelling reason for early surgical intervention, and psychological testing pre- and post-operatively has become an integral part of the neurosurgical approach to epilepsy treatment.

The future of the neurologist's role in epilepsy management should involve a greater emphasis on seizure etiology and prevention, the use of specific therapies, and the investigation and development of new and different classes of antiepileptic compounds based on recent advances in seizure mechanisms.

SEIZURE CLASSIFICATIONS

Revised Classification Of Epilepsies

The proposals for a revised classification of epilepsy and epileptic syndromes (1981-1985) have again been revised by the Commission on Classification and Terminology of the International League Against Epilepsy. The major classes are I. generalized epilepsy, and II. localization related, partial or focal epilepsies. Epilepsies of known etiology (symptomatic or secondary "epilepsies") are separated from idiopathic (primary) and cryptogenic. Idiopathic epilepsies are defined by age related onset, clinical and electroencephalographic characteristics and a presumed genetic etiology. Cryptogenic epilepsies are presumed to be symptomatic and the etiology is unknown; they are age related but often do not have well defined electroclinic characteristics. In addition to the localization related and generalized epilepsies and syndromes there are III. unclassified epilepsies, and IV. special syndromes, e.g. febrile convulsions. There are two appendices to the revised classification. 1. Symptomatic generalized epilepsies of special etiologies including malformations and inborn errors of metabolism and Appendix 2 precipitated seizures, e.g. reflex epilepsies, startle epilepsy, and primary reading epilepsy. (Commission on Classification and Terminology of the International League Against Epilepsy. Proposal for revised classification of epilepsies and epileptic syndromes. *Epilepsia* July/August 1989; *30*:389-400).

COMMENT. The Commission recognizes that the revised classification is not totally satisfactory. Patients may move from one syndrome to another during the evolution of the epilepsy, e.g. a child in West syndrome may later satisfy the criteria for the Lennox-Gastaut syndrome. It is of interest that the Commission is reverting to the older traditional concept of an idiopathic "primary" epilepsy of presumed genetic etiology as separate from the cryptogenic epilepsies presumed to be symptomatic. Criticisms of the new classification not stressed by the Commission are as follows: 1) The grouping of seizure patterns proposed are at variance with therapeutic correlations, e.g. absence and tonic-clonic seizures grouped together as generalized epilepsies require different types of medication for their control, and 2) The oversimplification and emphasis of syndromes might lead to a decreased awareness of etiologies and misdiagnoses of underlying pathologies. - Editor. *Ped Neur Briefs* Aug 1989.

Variability of Seizure Classification

One senior neurologist (JBB) from the Department of Neurology and Pediatrics, West Virginia University,

Morgantown, W.Va., USA, and three neurology residents from the University of Oklahoma, Harvard University, and W.Va. University reviewed descriptions of seizures transcribed from medical records and classified them according to the International League Against Epilepsy (ILAE) Classification system, 1981. The overall agreement in classifying seizure types by the ILAE system was relatively poor and only slightly better than would have been expected by chance. Agreement was particularly weak for atypical absence, partial seizures with secondary generalization, and generalized motor seizures. It was better for simple and complex partial, simple absence and infantile spasms. Approximately 22% of descriptions were insufficient for classification by the ILAE system. The authors conclude that the development and testing of more explicit criteria for the diagnosis of specific seizure types may be especially useful in improving the reliability of seizure classification. (Bodensteiner JB et al. Interobserver variability in the ILAE classification of seizures in childhood. *Epilepsia* March/April 1988; *29*: 123-128).

COMMENT. A classification of seizure types is of little value without assessment of its reproducibility in practice. Surprisingly, this study appears to be the first test of the reliability of the ILAE system of seizure classification, first proposed in 1970 and generally employed in statistical trials of anticonvulsant drugs. The relatively low level of concordance among observers using the ILAE system in the present study is disturbing, and the substitution of a more specific seizure classification should be entertained especially in therapeutic trials. - Editor. *Ped Neur Briefs* Apr 1988.

NEONATAL SEIZURES

Neonatal Seizure Classification

Investigators in the sections of Neurophysiology and Pediatric Neurology, Baylor College of Medicine, Houston, TX, have characterized and classified 415 clinical seizures recorded in

71 neonates and 11 with EEG seizure activity without clinical accompaniments. A cribside EEG/polygraphic/video monitoring system was employed. Seizures with a close association to EEG seizure discharges were focal clonic (58 in 14 patients), myoclonic (38 in 4 patients), focal tonic (8 in 2 patients), and apneic (4 in 1 patient). Seizures with an inconsistent or no relationship to EEG seizure discharges were motor automatisms ("subtle seizures") involving mouth, eyes, limb pedaling and swimming (140 in 22 patients), generalized tonic (90 in 13 patients), and myoclonic (66 in 13 patients). Only 2 neonates had infantile spasms. Clonic seizures with focal EEG seizure activity correlated with focal brain lesions such as infarction or intracerebral hemorrhage and a favorable short-term outcome. Seizures with no or inconsistent relationship to the EEG were correlated with diffuse hypoxic-ischemic encephalopathy and a poor prognosis (50% with abnormal neurologic exams at discharge, and 20% died). Those with myoclonic seizures had high morbidity (35%) and mortality (29%) compared to those with clonic seizures (71% normal at discharge). The authors question the use of potentially neurotoxic anticonvulsant drugs in neonates with nonepileptic seizures or "behaviorisms" not accompanied by EEG seizure activity. (Mizrahi EM, Kellaway P. Characterization and classification of neonatal seizures. *Neurology* 1987; *37*:1837-1844).

COMMENT. I contacted Dr. Gerald Fenichel at Vanderbilt Univ Sch of Med, an authority on neonatal seizures, for his opinion regarding the use of anticonvulsants in the treatment of "subtle" seizures. Unless the motor automatisms or tonic posturings can be correlated with a simultaneous recording of EEG seizure activity, he considers these subtle seizures as non-epileptic and advises against treatment with anticonvulsants. Patients with epileptiform seizures associated with acute hypoxic-ischemic encephalopathy are given IV phenobarbital in a loading dose of 20-30 mg/kg to provide a serum level of 40 mcg/ml. If the patient is free from seizures on recovery from the acute illness and at the time of discharge from hospital, anticonvulsants are discontinued (personal communication). Despite the enthusiastic promotion of newer antiepileptics, there is a growing and greater awareness of the potential toxicity of anticonvulsants in general. Any practical, less hazardous alternative or safe means of withholding medication must be considered seriously, especially in the neonate and young child. See Brent et al (*Pediatrics* 1987; *80* (Dec):909). re phenobarbital-induced depression and suicidal behavior in epileptic children, another area for concern in the long-term use of anticonvulsant drugs. - Editor. *Ped Neur Briefs* Dec 1987.

Neonatal Seizure Patterns and Etiologies

The clinical patterns, etiologies and times of onset of seizures were determined in a retrospective study of 150 newborns with seizures evaluated between 1982-87 in the neonatal intensive care unit at Washington University School of Medicine, Children's Hospital, St. Louis, MO. Subtle seizures in 97 (65%) infants were characterized by eye movements, sucking, lip-smacking, chewing, tonic posturing, pedaling or rowing movements, and/or apneic spells. Other seizures patterns were multifocal clonic (54%), focal clonic, generalized tonic and myoclonic. Of 78% patients with at least one EEG, only 11% had ictal tracings. Hypoxic ischemic encephalopathy (HIE) in 65% of the total was the most common cause of seizures in both preterm and term infants and 90% occurred in the first two days. Intracranial hemorrhage accounted for 10% of seizures. Other less common causes were metabolic, developmental defect, infection and drug withdrawal. In those with developmental defects, the onset of seizures was after 7 days of age. (Calciolari G, Perlman JM, Volpe JJ. Seizures in the neonatal intensive care unit of the 1980's. *Clinical Pediatrics* March 1988; *27*:119-23).

COMMENT. The authors admit that the absence of simultaneous video-EEG monitoring may lead to misinterpretation of the nature of some clinical phenomena regarded as seizures. Subtle seizures reported in more than half of the patients and associated with HIE have an inconsistent or no relationship to EEG seizure discharges (Mizrahi EM, Kellaway P. *Neurology* 1987; 37:1837), and some authorities advise against anticonvulsant therapy unless EEG epileptiform confirmation is obtained (*Ped Neur Briefs* 1987; 11:47-8). Self-resolution of "seizures" cannot be ruled out in a proportion of those apparently responding to anticonvulsant drugs, a therapy not without potential toxicity. - Editor. *Ped Neur Briefs* March 1988.

Neonatal Seizure Revised Classification

The current concepts and revised classification of neonatal seizures are the subject of a special article from the Division of Pediatric Neurology, Washington University School of Medicine, St. Louis, MO. The clinical classification includes the following: 1) subtle, 2) clonic (focal, multifocal), 3) tonic (focal, generalized), and 4) myoclonic (focal, multifocal, generalized). The focal and multifocal clonic, focal tonic, and generalized myoclonic seizures are commonly associated with simultaneous electrographic seizures. Some varieties of subtle seizures have simultaneous EEG seizure discharges. Neonatal seizures not usually accompanied by EEG seizure activity include: certain subtle seizures, most generalized tonic seizures, and the focal and multifocal myoclonic seizures. These may represent "brain stem release phenomena" and may occur in infants with hydranencephaly and anencephaly. The absence of EEG seizure activity does not rule out an epileptic origin for a clinical seizure. Clinical characteristics can be used to distinguish epileptic and nonepileptic phenomena. Epileptic seizures are not stimulus sensitive, not suppressible by restraint and are likely to be accompanied by autonomic phenomena. If nonepileptic the behavior is 1) stimulus sensitive, 2) may be suppressed by gentle passive restraint, and 3) is not accompanied by autonomic changes such as tachycardia and an increase in blood pressure. Epileptic seizures should be treated because of the threat of brain injury from the seizures per se. Nonepileptic events, e.g.

generalized tonic posturing or subtle clinical phenomena without autonomic accompaniments and EEG seizure activity, should not be treated with anticonvulsant drugs. Nonepileptic events rarely interfere with respiration or circulation, they are not harmful to the brain, and unusually high blood levels of phenobarbital are needed to suppress this clinical activity. More data are needed to resolve the issue of a danger of electrical seizure activity to the brain of the newborn in the absence of clinical activity suppressed by anticonvulsant drugs. The author does not attempt to eliminate all electrographic seizure activity because the high doses of medication needed may impair ventilation and/or cardiac function. He discontinues all drugs except phenobarbital as soon as the acute illness is completed (usually when intravenous lines are discontinued) and if the neurologic examination is normal. The etiology of the seizures is important: the risk of recurrence of seizures is 100% with cerebral cortical dysgeneses and 30% with hypoxic ischemic injury and nil with transient metabolic disturbances. He believes that infants should be maintained with phenobarbital for as brief a period as possible. (Volpe, JJ. Neonatal seizures: Current concepts and revised classification. *Pediatrics* September 1989; *84*:422-428).

COMMENT. Brain damage as a result of seizures per se in the neonate is controversial. The present author believes that there is strong indirect evidence that repeated neonatal convulsions may result in brain injury whereas Lombrozzo and Freeman hold that there is no proof that neonatal seizures can induce brain damage. The degree of emergency in the treatment of neonatal convulsions and the best therapeutic techniques remain in dispute. It seems reasonable to treat all recurring seizures, maintaining the phenobarbital at nontoxic levels. (For a review of this subject see Aicardi J. Epilepsy in Children. Raven Press, New York. 1986). Although anticonvulsant treatment is often the only therapeutic option available, care must be taken to exclude causes amenable to specific therapy, e.g. hypocalcemia, hypomagnesemia, pyridoxine dependency, biotin deficiency or some cases of hypoglycemia. The use of nasopharyngeal electrodes in electroencephalographic studies of neonatal seizures is potentially hazardous and should be discouraged. The clinical manifestations are usually sufficient to distinguish epileptic and nonepileptic phenomena. In the absence of routine electrographic confirmation, electrodes placed on the facial zygoma may be sufficient to record from the temporal lobe of an infant. In doubtful and persistent cases a trial of anticonvulsant medication would be justified. - Editor. *Ped Neur Briefs* Sept 1989.

Abstinence-Associated Neonatal Seizures (AANS)

The neurodevelopment of 14 infants with AANS was assessed during the first year of life in the Division of Neonatology (Dr. Kandall), Beth Israel Medical Center, First Ave at 16th St, New York, NY. Bayley developmental scores remained normal and most early EEG and neurological abnormalities, including hypertonia, hyperreflexia, tremors and irritability, became normal during follow-up. Seizures, mainly myoclonic, were controlled initially with phenobarbital I.V. and then oral phenobarb or paregoric. Medications were gradually discontinued if EEG's reverted to normal. Of 9 original abnormal EEG's, 4 were normal by 8 weeks of age and only one remained abnormal at 6 months. Clinical improvement paralleled EEG improvement. Prognosis for AANS was good and different from that of neonatal seizures due to other causes. (Doberczak TM et al. One-year follow-up of infants with abstinence-associated seizures. *Arch Neurol* June 1988; 45:649-653).

COMMENT. Infants born to methadone and heroin-dependent mothers have a reported risk of 20% and 4%, respectively, of developing seizures. Fortunately, these neonatal seizures appear to be transient and unassociated with persistent neurological deficits, whereas infants with neonatal seizures from other causes have a mortality rate of 35% and two-thirds of survivors suffer from cerebral palsy, epilepsy or retardation. (Holden KR et al. *Pediatrics* 1982; *70*:165). - Editor. *Ped Neur Briefs* June 1988.

Treatment Of Neonatal Seizures

The rapid sequential phenobarbital treatment of neonatal seizures was examined in 120 newborns and the efficacy of high dose monotherapy was compared with the addition of a second anticonvulsant for persistent seizure activity. Patients were examined in three participating neonatal intensive care units: Comprehensive Epilepsy Center, Pharmacokinetics Laboratory, Miami; Greensboro Area Health Education Center; and Department of Neonatal Medicine, Moses H. Cone Memorial Hospital, Greensboro, North Carolina. A single loading dose of phenobarbital 15-20 mg/kg was administered initially and non-responders received sequential bolus doses of 5-10 mg/kg until seizures ceased or a serum concentration of 40 mcg/mL was obtained. Infants with refractory seizures received additional phenobarbital to a maximum serum concentration of 100 mcg/mL. The majority of neonates with recurrent seizure activity (77%) responded to phenobarbital monotherapy administered in a rapid sequential dosing schedule that achieved a serum concentration of 40 mcg/mL. In 40%, seizures were controlled with a single 15-20 mg/kg initial loading dose and a serum concentration in the range of 10-30 mcg/mL. Of 28 subjects refractory to phenobarbital, 13 (46%) were controlled by a second anticonvulsant (phenytoin or lorazepam) and four were controlled by three or more agents. Eleven were resistant to medication and ten died. There was no significant difference in drug responsiveness among patients with different seizure patterns and seizure etiology was not a significant determinant of phenobarbital responsiveness. Subjects less than 32 weeks gestational age responded better than those 32 weeks or greater in gestation. (Gilman JT et al. Rapid sequential phenobarbital treatment of neonatal seizures. *Pediatrics* May 1989; *83*:674-678).

COMMENT. The therapeutic effect of phenobarbital monotherapy in the treatment of neonatal seizures is dose dependent but the effect plateaus at 40 mcg/mL and further increases only induce sedation and compromise neurologic assessment. A second anticonvulsant should be given promptly if seizures persist when phenobarbital serum concentrations are 40 mcg/mL or above. The availability of rapid serum determinations of drug levels is important because delays in additional drug therapy were thought to predispose to further seizures and risks of serious neurologic sequelae. The authors emphasize that adequate patient monitoring and slow infusion rates of phenobarbital should always be used to avoid possible cardiovascular toxicity.

In our own experience of 63 newborns with seizures admitted January 1985 to December 1987 in the high risk nursery at SIU School of Medicine, monotherapy with phenobarbital was used in 70% and polytherapy in 30%. The mean serum phenobarbital levels after loading doses of 10 and 20 mg/kg were 20 and 40 mcg/mL, respectively. Factors predictive of a poor prognosis included 1) polytherapy, 2) Apgar score less than 5 at five minutes, 3) abnormal EEG, and 4) abnormal brain ultrasound. Normal EEG and ultrasound were predictive of a normal follow-up examination. The addition of phenytoin or other polytherapy did not appreciably increase the degree of seizure control or improve prognosis (unpublished observations). - Editor. *Ped Neur Briefs* March 1989.

Neonatal Intractable Seizures And Valproic Acid Therapy

Seizures resistant to phenobarbital were controlled in four of six neonates by valproic acid (VPA) monotherapy and in one with polytherapy at the Moses H. Cone Memorial Hospital, Greensboro, NC. The pharmacokinetics of VPA showed a prolonged half-life in neonates in contrast to the short half-life in older children and adults. A loading dose of 20 mg/kg followed by a maintenance dose of 10 mg/kg every 12 hrs was recommended until VPA clearance and serum levels are determined.

VPA-induced hyperammonemia in all six patients was reason to discontinue VPA in three. One patient with meningitis whose seizures were unresponsive to VPA died shortly after the drug was discontinued; a serum ammonia elevation to 990 umol/1 after 5 days of treatment returned to normal within 24-48 hrs after discontinuing the drug. (Gal P, Weaver R et al. Valproic acid efficacy, toxicity, and pharmacokinetics in neonates with intractable seizures. *Neurology* March 1988; *38*:467-71).

COMMENT. VPA toxicity, particularly hepatotoxicity, in infants and young children may be reduced in frequency by elimination of concurrent anticonvulsants, but serum ammonia must be closely monitored even with monotherapy. Cerebral edema, increased intracranial pressure, cytotoxic changes in the brain and coma are reported with hyperammonemia exceeding 500 umol/1 in neonates, and intellectual retardation and brain damage are correlated with duration of hyperammonemia and coma (Msall M et al. *N Engl J Med* 1984; *310*:1500). Animal experiments show that VPA-induced hyperammonemia is caused primarily by impairment of hepatic intramitochondrial citrullinogenesis, and the renal contribution to systemic hyperammonemia is small. (Marini AM et al. *Neurology* March 1988; *38*:365).

Brown JK, at the Royal Hospital for Sick Children, Edinburgh, writing on valproate toxicity in Developmental Medicine and Child Neurology (Feb 1988; 30:121), cautions that any congenital inborn error of metabolism that affects mitochondrial function or any acquired mitochondriopathy might be expected to increase the risk of serious valproate toxicity in the neonate, and VPA is not generally recommended in the newborn period. He stresses the need for detailed investigation of cases of hepatopathy, including a full screen of mitochondrial enzyme function, as well as histology for possibly Reye-type changes, before accepting a diagnosis of VPA-induced hepatotoxicity. - Editor. *Ped Neur Briefs* March 1988.

Outcome Of Neonatal Convulsions

The risk factors, causes, and prognosis of convulsions in 156 neonates are reviewed at the Mater Misericordiae Mothers Hospital, South Brisbane, Queensland, Australia. The incidence of early neonatal convulsions was 3/1000 live births. Compared to infants who did not convulse, the leading risk factors for convulsions were prematurity, intrauterine growth retardation, low 5 min Apgar score, preeclampsia, antepartum hemorrhage, twin pregnancy, and breech presentation. The cause was hypoxic-ischemic encephalopathy (HIE) in 40%, intracranial hemorrhage (30%), metabolic (12%), infection (8%), malformation (3%), misc (7%). Mortality (31%) was related to etiology: 57% for intracranial hemorrhage, 33% infection, 27% HIE. Of the 107 infants who survived, long-term disability occurred in 43%; severe in 25 infants, moderate in 8 and mild in 10. The highest mortality and morbidity are associated with prolonged convulsions, tonic and multifocal clonic convulsions, convulsions due to asphyxia and intracranial hemorrhage, and an abnormal neurologic examination at discharge. (Tudehope DI et al. Clinical spectrum and outcome of neonatal convulsions. *Aust Paediatr J* August 1988; *24*:249-253).

COMMENT. The outcome of neonatal convulsions in this study is similar to that reported in a Dublin Collaborative Study of neonatal asphyxial seizures in which 43% had a poor outcome (Curtis PD et al. *Arch Dis Childh* September 1988; *63*:1065-8). In the Dublin study, asphyxial seizures occurring within 48 hours of birth in 0.87/1000 live births were correlated with antenatal complications, primiparity, and prolonged pregnancy. The incidence of seizures ranged from 0.55-1.2/1000 in the 3 participating maternity hospitals, reflecting differences in management policies in regard to frequency of cesarean section, induced labor, and forceps delivery. The mortality rate was

18% and of those who survived, 28% were handicapped at 1 year. Outcome was correlated with the infants' feeding habits at 1-2 weeks, those requiring tube feeding for more than 14 days being handicapped at follow-up. - Editor. *Ped Neur Briefs* August 1988.

Prognosis Of Neonatal Seizures: Value Of EEG

The value of standard and ambulatory electro-encephalography in the prediction of continuing neonatal seizures was investigated in the Department of Neurology, State University of New York, Buffalo, NY. Thirteen neonates with seizures occurring after 7 days of age were evaluated with standard short-term electroencephalography (SEEG) during the initial seizures and with ambulatory EEG (AEEG) when each infant was within 37-44 weeks corrected age (i.e., gestational age plus chronologic age). The etiology of the seizures was hypoxia in 7, infectious in 3, and idiopathic in the remainder. The occurrence of seizures at 3-4 months corrected age was accurately predicted by SEEGs in 8 of 13 cases, by AEEGs in 10 to 13, and with the combined use of SEEG and AEEG in 12 of 13. The combined analysis of SEEG and AEEG provided the best prediction of continued seizure activity in infants with neonatal seizures. (Kerr SL et al. Sequential use of standard and ambulatory EEG in neonatal seizures. *Pediatr Neurol* May-June 1990; 6:159-162).

COMMENT The identification of high risk infants who require antiepileptic drugs beyond the neonatal period should be facilitated by using this technique. Neonatal seizures become recurrent in approximately 25% of cases. - Editor. *Ped Neur Briefs* August 1990.

FEBRILE SEIZURES

Immunogenetic Aspects Of Febrile Convulsions

Investigators in Genetics, Pediatrics, Neurology, and Immunology, at Mansoura UN., Mansoura, Egypt found a gene frequency of 0.284 (c.f. 0.093 in controls) and a highly significant association between HLA-B5 antigen and febrile convulsions in 39 patients compared to 380 healthy controls. The high frequency of HLA-B5 antigen (48.7 in patients c.f., 17.6 in controls) reflected a significantly high relative risk and indicated that children having antigen B5 are 4.4 times more susceptible to febrile convulsions than those without that antigen. The means of IgA (89 mg%) and E-rosette (54%) were significantly low c.f. controls (151 and 64, respectively). The authors suggest that the genetic control of febrile convulsions is in linkage disequilibrium with HLA-B5, low IgA and low total T-cells and that this altered immune function may predispose to acute infections and high fever which precipitate the febrile convulsions. (Hafez M, Nagaty M, El-Shennawy F, El-Ziny M. *J Neurogenetics* 1987; *4*:267-274).

COMMENT. Ehrengut W and Ehrengut J (*Deutsch Med Wschr* 1964; *89*:166) found a lack of immunoglobulins beta-2A and beta-2M and a reduction of gamma globulin in 4 of 6 patients and postulated a weakness of defense mechanisms against infection as a possible cause of febrile convulsions. This report was the first and only reference to hypoimmunoglobulinemia cited in the monograph *Febrile Convulsions* 1968 Macmillan, N.Y., which included a review of world literature published in English and foreign languages. Isaac et al (*Arch Dis Child* 1984; *59*:367) reported low serum IgA in children with febrile convulsions and Grob and Herold (*Br Med* J 1972; *2*:561) and others have found IgA deficiency among epileptics receiving anticonvulsants, especially hydantoins (see Hafez et al).

The multifactorial inheritance of febrile seizures is alluded to in the 6th annual Merritt-Putnam Symposium (Bird TD. *Epilepsia* 1987; *28* (Suppl 1):S71-81). Siblings have approximately a 8-12% risk of also having febrile seizures. If the index child and one parent are affected, the risks to siblings are 30-40% (50% if both parents are affected). A high proportion of probands and their siblings develop EEG abnormalities 3-5 years after the febrile seizure, including generalized spike-and-wave and a photo-convulsive response (Hauser et al 1985; Millichap, 1968). - Editor. *Ped Neur Briefs* September 1987.

Phenobarbital And Valproate For Febrile Convulsions

Data from 6 British trials of phenobarbital and 4 trials of valproate for the prophylactic treatment of febrile convulsions were polled and analyzed on an intention to treat basis at the Dept of Neurology, Royal Manchester and Booth Hall Children's Hospitals, Manchester. The risk of recurrence in the treatment groups compared to controls expressed as an overall odds ratio was as follows: for phenobarbital, 66 of 296 (22%) of treated children had recurrence compared to 58 of 236 (25%) of controls (overall odds ratio or relative risk of 0.8, nonsignificant difference); for valproate, 49 of 145 (34%) treated children had recurrence compared with 36 of 136 (25%) controls (overall odds ratio of 1.42, nonsignificant result). The follow-up period ranged from 6 months to a mean of 30 months. An odds ratio of less than 1 suggests benefit; greater than 1 suggests no benefit from treatment. (Newton RW. Randomized controlled trials of phenobarbitone and valproate in febrile convulsions. *Arch Dis Child* Oct 1988; *63*:1189-91).

> COMMENT. Pooled analysis of the British trials data failed to show any overall value in the prophylactic treatment of febrile convulsions with either phenobarbital or valproate. With side-effects reported in up to 40% of the treated group, continuous anticonvulsant therapy in the prophylaxis of simple febrile convulsions cannot be recommended. The same conclusion was reached in comparing the relative value of phenobarbital administered intermittently, at the time of fever, or continuously in a group of 40 patients (Millichap JG. *Febrile Convulsions*. Macmillan, NY, 1967). Long-term phenobarbital was recommended only in children with complex febrile convulsions (those

whose seizures are prolonged 20 min, complicated by EEG seizure discharges, or having neurological abnormalities). Alternative methods of treatment such as rectal diazepam are advised in those at risk of recurrence, and parents must be counseled in the first aid management of seizures. - Editor. *Ped Neur Briefs* October 1988.

Fever And Recurrent Febrile Seizures

The relation of the height of the fever to the recurrence rate of febrile convulsions was studied in 154 children admitted to the Paediatric Department, Ahmadi Hospital, Kuwait. The children were divided into three groups according to the height of the fever recorded on presentation. Group 1, temperature greater than 40°C, group 2, 39-39.9°C, and group 3, 38-38.9°C. The children were followed at three month intervals for a mean of 40 months and recurrences occurred between one and 22 months after the original first febrile seizure. The recurrence rates of febrile convulsions were significantly greater in infants aged 6 to 18 months in whom the initial febrile convulsions had been associated with a lower temperature. The rate of recurrence was over nine times higher in infants who had the lowest fever, 38-38.9°C and over seven times higher in infants with temperatures of 39-39.9°C. Repeated convulsions with each febrile episode occurred in only four children (3%). (El-Radhi AS and Banajeh S. Effect of fever on recurrence rate of febrile convulsions. *Arch Dis Child* June 1989; 64:869-870).

COMMENT. These findings are confirmation of a febrile seizure threshold dependent on the height of the fever first proposed 30 years ago (Millichap JG. Studies in febrile seizures I. Height of body temperature as a measure of the febrile seizure threshold. *Pediatrics* 1959; 23:76). It is not surprising that children who convulse with a relatively low fever have a poorer prognosis than those convulsing only with high fevers. Another factor noted in many studies to increase the risk of recurrence of febrile seizures is an early age at the first febrile seizure. Frantzen et al (1968) found that children who experienced their first seizure at less than 13 months of age had a 2.3:1 chance for developing further febrile seizures compared to a 1:2 chance when the seizure occurred between 14 and 32 months of age and a 1:5 risk when the onset was after 32 months of age. Nelson and Ellenberg (1978) found a 50% recurrence rate with the onset in the first year of life compared to a 28% recurrence rate when the onset was after the first year. The height of the fever is a most important determinant of the occurrence of febrile seizures in the infant and young child. - Editor. *Ped Neur Briefs* June 1989.

Treatment Of Febrile Seizures

The risk of febrile seizure recurrence was studied in 186 consecutive children aged between 6 and 72 months admitted to the Booth Hall and Royal Manchester Children's Hospitals, Pendlebury, Manchester, England. Patients were allocated randomly to one of three study groups if they had a febrile convulsion in the first year of life, a complicated febrile convulsion (defined as more than five minutes in a child with a positive family history, two or more febrile convulsions in one day, duration more than 15 minutes, or a focal convulsion), or more than one febrile convulsion within two years. The three study groups were: 1) A controlled group receiving no regular anticonvulsant treatment (a convulsion lasting longer than five minutes was treated with diazepam 0.5 mg/kg rectally); 2) a group given sodium valproate 30 mg/kg divided into twice daily doses; 3) a group given phenobarbital 5 mg/kg once daily at night. Follow-up was at three to six month intervals and medication was withdrawn after freedom from convulsions for two years. Serum anticonvulsant levels were measured after treatment was established, following a seizure recurrence or if side effects occurred. One hundred twenty-seven patients who completed the study were followed further by mail questionnaires. The overall risk of recurrence was 30% and the risk of a prolonged seizure was 2%, even in patients with adequate drug levels. Prophylactic treatment with sodium valproate or phenobarbital did not significantly lessen the risk of febrile seizure recurrence. Side effects occurred in 24% of the valproate group and in 61% of the phenobarbital group. Comparative data for infants with onset of febrile seizures at less than 12 months were not available. The authors do not recommend the use of sodium valproate or phenobarbital prophylaxis for children with febrile convulsions even in those considered high risk categories. They endorse the key role of family counseling and education of those who care for young children with febrile convulsions and they recommend that rectal diazepam be made available to the families of children with high recurrence risks. (McKinlay I, Newton R. Intention to treat febrile convulsions with rectal diazepam, valproate or phenobarbitone. *Dev Med Child Neurol* October 1989; *31*:617-625).

COMMENT. To treat or not to treat the febrile convulsion is a question that remains controversial. The results of this study are of interest but drug-level monitoring was performed infrequently; in children with recurrences the levels of valproate and phenobarbital were subtherapeutic in 40-60% of cases.

In a more recent article concerning the use of long-term phenobarbital for febrile seizures (Farwell JR et al. *N Engl J Med* Feb 8, 1990; *322*:364-9) the authors concluded that "phenobarbital depresses cognitive performance in children and that this disadvantage is not offset by the benefit of seizure prevention". The statistical design and analysis of this study are complicated, requiring explanations for patient dropout rate and poor compliance. In those with seizure recurrence, blood phenobarbital levels were unavailable and parents had discontinued phenobarbital in one-third of cases.

Phenobarbital is the safest drug available and is prescribed for complex febrile seizures by 90% of pediatricians and family practitioners in Illinois. (Millichap JG et al.

Ann Neurol (abstract) Sept 1989; *26*:473). Significant reductions in seizure recurrence have been reported by several investigators when compliance is carefully controlled. Until new approaches to the management of febrile seizures can be defined by well controlled studies, the following recommendations are suggested: 1) Emphasis on parental counseling and education in the management of fever and convulsions. 2) Intermittent prophylactic therapy with oral diazepam, 0.5 mg/kg/daily in divided doses, at times of subsequent fever, as an alternative to long-term phenobarbital. 3) An approved rectal preparation of diazepam for the treatment of the acute febrile seizure in the home for use by selected parents in high risk patients. 4) Phenobarbital, when indicated in selected patients, should be limited to 6-12 months seizure free periods and monitored by blood levels (15 mcg/ml) at six weeks to three month intervals and by behavioral and psychological evaluations before and during therapy. Editor. *Ped Neur Briefs* January 1990.

Diazepam For Febrile Seizures

The efficacy and side effects of intermittent oral diazepam for the prevention of febrile seizure recurrence were investigated in the Departments of Clinical Pharmacology, Neurosurgery, and Biostatistics, University of Tours, France. Between May 1985 and June 1988, 185 children, eight months to three years of age, with a first febrile seizure and normal neurological development were randomly assigned in a double-blind fashion to receive oral diazepam (0.5 mg/kg, then 0.2 mg/kg every 12 hours) or placebo, whenever the rectal temperature was more than 38°C. The duration of the study was three years and eight different centers in France participated. There were 462 febrile episodes and 1000 days with prophylactic treatment. The seizure recurrence rate in the diazepam group was 16% and in the placebo group 19.5% and the difference was not significant. Those with recurrent seizures were aged 17 ± 6.9 months and those with no recurrence were 21 ± 8.5 months at the time of the first seizure. In children with seizure recurrence, diazepam had been correctly administered in only one of 15 children and the placebo had been given in seven of 18 children with recurrences. Poor compliance with the intermittent treatment was explained by 1) seizure as the first manifestation of the fever in seven cases in each group, 2) noncompliance by parents in nine cases, and 3) patient refusal to take treatment in two. Hyperactivity was more frequent as a side effect in the diazepam than in the placebo group. The findings reflect a lack of efficacy of the intermittent method of treatment rather than the diazepam itself. (Autret E et al. Double-blind, randomized trial of diazepam versus placebo for prevention of recurrence of febrile seizures. *J Pediatr* September 1990; *117*:490-494).

COMMENT. The poor compliance rate which might explain the lack of efficacy of the intermittent diazepam prophylaxis in this study is disappointing and dampens the growing enthusiasm for this form of therapy as a substitute for continuous phenobarbital prophylaxis. The conclusion of Dr. Rosman's controlled study of oral diazepam is eagerly awaited.

In a recent national survey of pediatric neurologists, 22% recommended the use of intermittent prophylactic therapy with diazepam in an average dose of 0.46 mg/kg/day; oral diazepam was preferred by 8% and rectal administration was used by 16%. An alternate drug, lorazepam or clonazepam, was preferred by 2%. (Millichap JG et al. *Ann Neurol* September 1990; *28*:444). - Editor. *Ped Neur Briefs* October 1990.

Antecedents Of Febrile Seizures

Prenatal and perinatal characteristics as possible risk factors for febrile seizures were reviewed by analysis of the data from the collaborative perinatal project of the National Institute of Neurological Disorders and Stroke at the Neuroepidemiology Branch, Bethesda, MD. Family history was the major factor identified as contributory to febrile seizure vulnerability. Both febrile and nonfebrile seizures in the mother were related to an increased tendency to febrile seizures in the child. Glomerulonephritis during the pregnancy was also associated with a risk exceeding 10%. The number of hospitalizations and the number of cigarettes smoked during pregnancy showed a trend but less than twofold increase in risk of febrile seizures in the child. Socioeconomic status was inversely related to risk of febrile seizures in white children. Respiratory distress syndrome and degree of respiratory difficulty showed odds ratios greater than 2; sepsis and errors of metabolism had odds ratios exceeding 4; breech delivery, cesarean section, low Apgar scores, birth weight 2500 grams or less, and feeding problems had odds ratios higher than 1. The authors considered that no complication of labor or delivery was an important risk factor for febrile seizures. (Nelson KB, Ellenberg JH. Prenatal and perinatal antecedents of febrile seizures. *Ann Neurol* Feb 1990; *27*:127-131).

COMMENT. The authors indicate that several earlier reports have shown that abnormalities in perinatal histories were relatively frequent in children with febrile seizures but the studies were not controlled. Of a total of 3427 patients reported in 19 studies between 1933-1963 17% showed evidence of possible brain injury caused by trauma or anoxia as an antecedent of febrile seizures. The evidence for brain injury at birth was often presumptive and equivocal, but the agreement among figures quoted in the 19 series of patients was remarkable. (Millichap JG. *Febrile convulsions.* New York: Macmillan, 1968).In reports that analyzed complicated cases compared to those having febrile seizures alone the incidence of birth injury was not significantly changed by this arbitrary division of patients. Trauma or anoxia at birth was a frequent finding in the history of the febrile convulsive disorder and was implicated with equal frequency in patients with simple febrile seizures and those with complex febrile seizures. In the present NIH study the antecedents of complex febrile seizures were not distinguished from those of simple febrile seizures. The authors indicate that some relationships not uncovered in the study of the total cohort of febrile seizures might emerge in an analysis of clinically defined subsets. - Editor. *Ped Neur Briefs* March 1990.

Predictors Of Recurrent Febrile Seizures

The results of 14 published reports were analyzed to evaluate the strength of association between proposed risk factors and recurrence of febrile seizures in a metaanalytic review from the Departments of Pediatrics and Epidemiology and Public Health, Yale University School of Medicine, New Haven, CT; Montefiore Medical Center, The Albert Einstein College of Medicine, Bronx, New York; and Columbia University College of Physicians and Surgeons, New York, NY. Young age at onset (less than one year) and a family history of febrile seizures each distinguished between groups with approximately a 30% versus a 50% risk of recurrence. Family history of afebrile seizures, focal, prolonged, and multiple seizures were associated with an inconsistent or only a small increment in risk of recurrence. Only one of five indications for anticonvulsant prophylaxis as defined by the 1980 NIH Consensus Developmental Conference was consistently predictive of a recurrence of febrile seizures. (Berg AT et al. Predictors of recurrent febrile seizures: A metaanalytic review. *J Pediatr* March 1990; *116*:329-337).

COMMENT. The risk factors and indications for long term phenobarbital prophylaxis of febrile seizures need to be reconsidered. Therapeutic guidelines may be helpful but the decision to treat must be made on an individual basis. Greater reliance on parental education and intermittent therapy should lessen the necessity for long term therapy with potentially toxic medications. - Editor. *Ped Neur Briefs* March 1990

Shigella-Associated Recurrent Seizures

The risk of subsequent febrile or nonfebrile seizures following Shigella-associated convulsions was investigated in 55 children in a ten year follow-up study at the Assaf Harofeh Medical Center and the Sackler School of Medicine, Tel Aviv University, Israel. Only two children (3%) had recurrent episodes of febrile convulsions and none had nonfebrile seizures. The incidence of recurrent seizures in this group of patients was similar to that observed in the general population and significantly different from the average estimated recurrence rate of febrile seizures (33%). (Lahat E et al. Recurrent seizures in children with Shigella-associated convulsions. *Ann Neurol* September 1990; *28*:393-395).

COMMENT. Among 1292 patients with convulsions associated with Shigellosis in nine publications in the literature, the incidence of seizures varied from 4% to as high as 45% with an average of 13%. Among 2241 patients in two studies of Shigella negative diarrheas the incidence of convulsions was only 1.7%. The higher incidence of febrile seizures with shigellosis in comparison with Shigella negative diarrheas was unexplained by neurotoxin formation and could be related to differences in severity of the infections, the height of the fever, and complications of water and electrolyte imbalance. (Millichap JG. *Febrile convulsions.* Macmillan Company, New York, 1968). The present study suggests that Shigella-associated convulsions are benign and not associated with an increased incidence of either febrile or nonfebrile seizures. An hereditary factor to explain an increased incidence of convulsions with Shigella infections was not supported by this study. - Editor. *Ped Neur Briefs* October 1990.

INFANTILE SPASMS

Tuberous Sclerosis And Infantile Spasms

Forehead plaques, smooth patches of slightly raised skin with a reddish or yellowish discoloration, can be the earliest skin manifestation of tuberous sclerosis (TS) according to the authors who describe 2 patients seen at Bath and Bristol, UK., presenting with infantile spasms at 3 and 5 months of age. (Fryer AE et al. *Arch Dis Child* 1987; *62*:292-293).

> COMMENT. Early diagnosis of tuberous sclerosis (TS) is important for genetic counseling and prognostic predictions. The prevalence of TS in patients with infantile spasms has been estimated at 25% or higher in some series. A Wood's light examination of the skin for hypopigmented maculae, a more frequent characteristic dermatologic manifestation of TS, is important in all infants with myoclonic spasms and hypsarrhythmia. - Editor. *Ped Neur Briefs* June 1987.

Tuberous Sclerosis And Infantile Spasms: Prognosis

The short- and long-term outcome of 24 children with infantile spasms and tuberous sclerosis was studied at the Department of Pediatrics, University of Turku, Finland and at the Children's Hospital, University of Helsinki. They comprised 10% of all cases of infantile spasms treated in the two hospitals between 1964 and 1985. CT showed brain calcifications in 20 patients examined at an early age. Three of 14 patients tested by renal ultrasound had large polycystic kidneys and severe arterial hypertension. Early diagnosis and the avoidance of ACTH therapy could have prevented hypertensive crises secondary to ACTH injections. One child developed severe myocardial hypertrophy during ACTH therapy and two had rhabdomyomas demonstrated by cardiac ultrasound and angiography at age one week. Short-term outcome was good but relapses were frequent and the long term outcome was disappointing. All were mentally retarded, only 4% were seizure free at follow-up and 42% had behavioral problems. When examined at 2-1/2 to 19 years of age, 58% had partial or focal, often secondary generalized seizures, and 37% had myoclonic astatic or Lennox-Gastaut syndrome. The dose of ACTH was 20-40 IU daily for six weeks in eight children and 80-140 IU daily in 14 children. Arterial hypertension occurred in ten, two developed cardiac failure, three had fluid retention in the cysts of polycystic kidneys and developed hypertensive crises during therapy. Infections (otitis, gastroenteritis, pneumonia) occurred in four. (Riikonen R, Simell O. Tuberous sclerosis and infantile spasms. *Dev Med Child Neurol* March 1990; *32*:203-209).

> COMMENT. The demonstration of cerebral calcifications by CT in all patients with tuberous sclerosis at an early age is of interest. The necessity for abdominal ultrasound in diagnosis and before ACTH therapy is indicated by the study. The dosage of ACTH used was exceptionally large and would have accounted for the unusually high incidence of side effects and frequency of arterial hypertension. Many authorities are content with much smaller doses, 10 and at the most 20 IU of ACTH daily given for shorter periods (three weeks) and repeated at intervals when necessary. Early treatment with ACTH is important in terms of the response of infantile spasms to therapy and possibly in relation to subsequent development (Gordon N. *Dev Med Child Neurol* April 1990, *32*:363). In the present study of patients with tuberous sclerosis and infantile spasms, early treatment with large doses of ACTH provided an initial good response but the long-term outcome was poor despite prolonged administration. - Editor. Ped Neur Briefs April 1990.

Cortical Dysgenesis And Infantile Spasms: PET Studies

The identification of focal cortical dysgenesis by positron emission tomography (PET) in 5 of 13 children with cryptogenic infantile spasms is reported from the Departments of Neurology and Pediatrics and Division of Neurosurgery, UCLA

School of Medicine, Los Angeles, CA. There was unilateral hypometabolism of cerebral glucose involving the parieto-occipito-temporal region. Neuropathological examination of resected tissue in four infants showed microscopic cortical dysplasia. The CT was normal in all infants and the MRI showed a subtle abnormality only in one. The EEG showed hypsarrhythmia and at times, a localized abnormality corresponding to areas of PET hypometabolism. PET may identify unsuspected focal cortical dysplasia in infants with cryptogenic spasms and resective surgery offers improved prognosis. (Chugani HT, Shields WD et al. Infantile spasms: I. PET identifies focal cortical dysgenesis in cryptogenic cases for surgical treatment. *Ann Neurol* April 1990; *27*:406-413).

COMMENT. Early studies showed that infantile spasms were cryptogenic in about 40% of patients (Millichap et al. *Epilepsia* 1962; *3*:188) whereas more recent studies have demonstrated that this figure has diminished to 9-14%. The PET studies have uncovered further symptomatic cases previously not identified by CT and MRI. The same authors report lenticular nuclei hypermetabolism in 12 of 25 infants with spasms of cryptogenic or symptomatic types. They suggest that the lenticular nuclei may contribute to the pathogenesis of infantile spasms. (Chugani HT et al. *Neurology* April 1990; *40*:suppl 1:407). - Editor. *Ped Neur Briefs* April 1990.

Infantile Spasms And Partial Seizures

Four infants with partial seizures evolving to infantile spasms were investigated using simultaneous EEG-video-Telemetry recording in the Dept of Pediatrics, Nagoya University, Nagoya, and Division of Pediatric Neurology, Central Hospital, Aichi Prefectural Colony, Kasugai, Japan. Partial seizures were characterized by cessation of activity, staring, flushing, automatisms, increased tone and laughter. (Yamamoto N, Watanabe K et al. Partial seizures evolving to infantile spasms. *Epilepsia* Jan/Feb 1988; *29*:34-40).

COMMENT. A cry or scream is the most common ictal element in infantile spasms, and laughter and a frightened or confused expression, manifestations of partial seizures, are frequently described (Jeavons PM, Bower BD. *Clinics in Developmental Medicine No 15*, 1964, London, Spastics Society and Heinemann). The above report appears to be the first in which infantile spasms were preceded by partial seizures confirmed by EEG-VT. However, one of the above authors, in a previous study of the evolution of EEG abnormalities accompanying infantile spasms, reported hypsarrhythmia preceded by focal sharp wave patterns, compatible with partial seizures (Watanabe K et al. *Dev Med Child Neurol* 1973; *15*:584). - Editor. *Ped Neur Briefs* March 1988.

Infantile Spasms, Hypsarrhythmia, And Adrenoleukodystrophy (ALD)

An 8-1/2 month-old girl with seizures beginning at 5 days, hypsarrhythmia in the EEG, severe retardation, and a clinical diagnosis of infantile spasms was discovered to have biochemical and pathological features of adrenoleukodystrophy, as reported from the John F. Kennedy Institute, Johns Hopkins University, Baltimore, Maryland. Laboratory studies showed elevated plasma levels of very long chain fatty acids, and postmortem examination at 14 months reveals cerebral destructive lesions and adrenal cortex atrophy. Seizure frequency had diminished initially with Prednisone 20 mg/daily, but improvement was not maintained. The biochemical changes resembled the abnormalities observed in X-linked ALD and differed from those in the neonatal form. Comparison with other known peroxisomal disorders suggested a unique example of this category of disease. (Naidu S et al. Neonatal seizures and retardation in a girl with biochemical features of X-linked adrenoleukodystrophy: a possible new peroxisomal disease entity. *Neurology* July 1988; *38*:1100-7).

COMMENT. For an excellent review of the various entities now classified as generalized peroxisomal disorders, please refer to Naidu, Moser, Moser. *Pediatr Neurol* 1988; 4:5 (reviewed in *Ped Neur Briefs* 1988; 2:30). Immunopathological factors have been postulated in the pathogenesis of CNS lesions in X-linked adrenoleukodystrophy. Cyclophosphamide administered to 4 boys between 6 and 11 years of age with proven ALD failed to slow the rate of neurological progression. (Naidu S et al. *Arch Neurol* August 1988; 45:846. Also, Stumpf et al. *Arch Neurol* 1981; 38:48. - Editor. *Ped Neur Briefs* August 1988.

TREATMENT OF INFANTILE SPASMS

Thyroptropin-Releasing Hormone (TRH): An Alternative Therapy For Infantile Spasms

Pediatric neurologists at the Central Hospital, Aichi Prefectural Colony, Kasugai, Aichi 480-03, Japan, compared the effects of TRH in 31 children and ACTH in 33 with severe epilepsy. Approximately half the cases had infantile spasms and the remainder had Lennox-Gastaut syndrome. In the TRH group, complete control of infantile spasms occurred in 7 of 13 (53.7%) and marked improvement of the EEG's was observed in 8 (61.5%). In the ACTH group, infantile spasms were controlled in 75%. TRH treated patients had no serious side-effects whereas 66.7% of the ACTH group had complications, including pneumonia, hypokalemia, cataracts, and brain shrinkage.

TRH-tartrate (TRH-t), 0.5-1.0 mg, was administered intravenously to determine immediate effects on seizures and EEG and then intramuscularly once daily for 1-4 weeks. TRH was effective in controlling infantile spasms within 4-16 days of its initiation. Three of the 7 responders remainder seizure-free for greater than 6 months. (Matsumoto a, Kumagai T, Takenchi T, Miyazaki S, Watanabe K. *Epilepsia* 1987; 28:49-55).

COMMENT. ACTH is effective in the control of infantile spasms and hypsarrhythmia in 50% of cases. The response rate is higher in infants treated early and under one year of age than in those diagnosed later. Hypertension, cushingoid obesity, congestive heart failure, infection, and cerebral atrophy are some of the more serious side-effects of ACTH therapy. The significant response of infantile spasms to TRH without serious toxicity offers a promising alternative therapy to ACTH. The anticonvulsant action of TRH appears to be central and unrelated to its endocrine action through the pituitary-thyroid axis. - Editor. *Ped Neur Briefs* June 1987.

Infantile Spasms And ACTH Dosage

Results of corticotropin treatment of 33 patients with infantile spasms are reported from the Instituto Clinica Pediatrica, Universita di Siena, Italy. The etiology was undetermined in 8 and secondary in 25 (pre- or perinatal distress in 17 and tuberous sclerosis in 2). Pyridoxine 300 mg IV tried in all cases initially with EEG monitoring was without effect. ACTH 2 units/kg daily for 10 days followed by alternate day treatment for 10 days with a repeat course in some resulted in improvement in all idiopathic cases (complete in 6) and in 15 secondary cases (complete only in 2). The authors advocate low doses and short courses of ACTH, claiming results comparable with larger amounts (up to 10-12 u/kg/day) for longer periods (3 mos) employed by some. (Fois A et al. Further observations on the treatment of infantile spasms with corticotropin. *Brain Dev* 1987; *9*:82-84. Ibid, *Eur J Pediatr* 1983; *42*:51.

COMMENT. The mechanism of the anticonvulsant action of ACTH in infantile spasms is unknown. It is probably independent of the adrenal (Neurology 1965; 15:1136) and a possible direct CNS effect is a reason proposed for the use of high dosage schedules. In agreement with the present study, my own results with smaller, 10-20 units daily irrespective of body weight for 20 days, have equalled those reported with higher doses and longer courses, and serious side effects have been avoided. - Editor. *Ped Neur Briefs* November 1987.

High Dose ACTH For Infantile Spasms: Cortisol Levels

The efficacy and plasma levels of ACTH and Cortisol were studied in 15 children with infantile spasms and hypsarrhythmia using a high dose (150 IU/M2/D ACTH) and are reported from the Department of Pediatrics, University of Alabama at Birmingham School of Medicine, and the Comprehensive Epilepsy Center, the Alabama Children's Hospital, Birmingham, AL. An endocrinologic evaluation before and after initiation of the ACTH showed that all patients had normal prolactin, insulin, cortisol and ACTH levels in plasma and normal thyroid function before treatment, and plasma cortisol rose rapidly within one hour after ACTH administration and continued a slower rise from 12-24 hours after the ACTH dose. Spasms were controlled and the EEG became normal in 14 of the 15 children. The initial dose was 75 IU/M2 intramuscularly twice daily for one week, 75 IU/M2/D for one week, followed by 75 IU/M2 every other day for one week and followed by a nine week taper. All patients developed cushingoid features and hyperirritability and one became hypertensive. One child with tuberous sclerosis developed a cardiac arrhythmia and was found to have an atrial myxoma. (Snead OC. Benton JW et al. Treatment of infantile spasms with high dose ACTH: Efficacy and plasma levels of ACTH and cortisol. *Neurology* August 1989; *39*:1027-31).

COMMENT. The use of high dose ACTH regimen for infantile spasms and hypsarrhythmia is contrary to the recommendations of many pediatric neurologists in the U.S. but favored also by my colleagues at the Hospital for Sick Children, Great Ormond Street, London. The clinical response to the high dose ACTH in the present study and the relative paucity of serious adverse effects were remarkable. The authors suggest that a sustained high level of plasma cortisol may be more effective in controlling infantile spasms than the pulse effect expected with oral steroids or low doses of ACTH. However, it is admitted that the ACTH may exert its anticonvulsant effect independently of cortisol and by a direct effect on the brain. Personally, I would be concerned about the potential risks of the high dose of ACTH therapy (e.g. cortical atrophy, gastrointestinal bleeding) and the reevaluation of CT scans following treatment would have been of interest in this study. The group of children reported was unusual in that one-half had other kinds of seizures that preceded the onset of infantile spasms. This might account for the need for high dose ACTH treatment to effect control. Smaller doses of 10-20 IU daily for a period of three or four weeks are usually advised and are generally effective in 50-80% of patients under one year of age. With the smaller dose schedules a lower incidence of serious side effects would be expected. - Editor. *Ped Neur Briefs* August 1989.

ACTH Treatment Of Infantile Spasms Reviewed

The rationale, dosage, and side effects of ACTH treatment of infantile spasms are reviewed from the Department of Neurology, University of Southern California School of Medicine, and Children's Hospital of Los Angeles, CA. Admission to hospital is recommended for the initiation of ACTH therapy so that baseline laboratory tests can be obtained and response to treatment can be supervised for the first three days. The author recommends an initial dose of ACTH 150 units/m²/day (Acthar gel), 80 units/ml intramuscularly in two divided doses for one week. In the second week the dose recommended is 75 units/m²/day in one daily dose for one week. In the third week the dose is 75 units/m² every other day for one week. ACTH is gradually withdrawn over the next nine weeks. A change in the lot number of ACTH gel is indicated when no response occurs in two weeks. The author admits controversy concerning the dose, duration of therapy, and effectiveness of ACTH relative to oral steroids as well as the long-term benefit of either of these therapies. (Snead OC III. Treatment of infantile spasms. *Pediatr Neurol* May/June 1990; 6: 147-150).

> COMMENT. Exceptionally large doses of ACTH recommended in this report were also used by Riikonen R and Simell O in the treatment of infantile spasms associated with tuberous sclerosis. (See *Ped Neur Briefs* April 1990; 4:30-31). There was an unusually high incidence of side effects, including arterial hypertension, with two patients developing cardiac failure and three with fluid retention in polycystic kidneys. My own preference is for smaller doses (10-20 units of Acthar gel daily by intramuscular injection for three weeks) with the avoidance of cushingoid complications and a lesser incidence of other side effects. Early treatment is important in terms of the response to therapy and possibly in relation to subsequent development. - Editor. *Ped Neur Briefs* June 1990

ACTH In Infantile Spasms: Low Dose Regimen

The relationship between dose of ACTH and the initial effect and long-term prognosis was investigated in 41 children with infantile spasms at the Department of Pediatrics, Kyoto University, Kyoto, Japan. ACTH therapy began at 2-13 months of age (mean: 11.8 months) and the average treatment lag was 4.5 months. All patients were treated with Vitamin B6, valproate, and other anticonvulsants without benefit before ACTH therapy was begun. All patients had hypsarrhythmia on the EEG. The cause was acquired in 30 patients, unknown in 8 and associated with developmental delay, and idiopathic in 3 patients whose development was normal. The doses in 16 patients was 0.5 mg (20 IU) for those older than one year of age and 0.25 mg (10 IU) for those less than one year; daily injections were given for two weeks, every other day for two weeks, and twice weekly for a total of 30 injections. One-half of these doses were used in 14 patients and doses were calculated on the basis of body weight (0.01-0.015 mg) (0.4-0.6 IU)/kg in 11 patients. More than 0.015 mg (0.6 IU)/kg/day of ACTH was needed for a good initial response of seizures and EEG abnormalities. Doses lower than 0.015 mg/kg/day provided less seizure control at the end of treatment and less EEG improvement. ACTH in a dose of 1.6-2.4 IU/kg/day and a total dose of 44-60 IU/kg resulted in better mental development than smaller doses, but side effects increased with larger daily doses or larger total doses. Seizures were controlled in 71-89% with doses above 0.6 IU/kg/day. ACTH-induced cerebral atrophy increased with the total dose of ACTH but was not seen when daily doses were 2.4 IU/kg/day or less and total dose was 60 IU/kg. (Ito M et al. ACTH therapy in infantile spasms: Relationship between dose of ACTH and initial effect or long-term prognosis. *Pediatr Neurol* July/Aug 1990; *6*:240-244).

COMMENT. The authors recommend that ACTH doses based on body weight or body surface area should be used in future studies to compare the results obtained at different institutions. The doses used in this study from Japan were relatively small and ranged from 7.3-47.6 IU/m²/day whereas those recommended in some recent publications have been much higher and usually 150 U/m²/day. Snead OC (*Pediatr Neurol* May/June 1990; *6*:147) advocated 150 U/m²/day for one week, 75 U/m²/day in the second week, and 75 U/m² on alternate days for the third week. Bobele GB, Bodensteiner JB from the University of Oklahoma and Morgantown, West Virginia University, (*Neurologic Clinics* August 1990, W. B. Saunders, Philadelphia) recommend 150 U/m²/day for a total of 6-8 weeks and the same dosage on alternate days for a further 6-8 weeks followed by tapering for a total treatment period of 4-6 months. These larger doses are associated with an increased frequency of serious side effects from ACTH. My own preference has favored the more conservative treatment with smaller doses and the experience in Japan tends to support the recommendation of doses of 1-2 IU/kg/day and a total ACTH dose of approximately 50 IU/kg. - Editor. *Ped Neur Briefs* September 1990.

Methysergide And Infantile Spasms

A trial of antiadrenergic and antiserotonergic drugs in the treatment of 24 newly diagnosed and previously untreated infantile spasm patients is reported from the Epilepsy Research Center, Section of Neurophysiology, Department of Neurology, Baylor College of Medicine; the Methodist Hospital; and Texas Children's Hospital; Houston, TX. Response to therapy was determined with 24 hour polygraphic/video monitoring techniques and was defined as complete control of spasms and disappearance of the hypsarrhythmic EEG pattern. Two of 12 patients treated with alpha-methylparatyrasene and one of 12 treated with methysergide showed a response. (Hrachovy RA et al. Treatment of infantile spasms with methysergide and alpha-methylparatyrasene. *Epilepsia* October 1989; *30*:607-610).

> COMMENT. The hypothesis that infantile spasms may result from a dysfunction of monoaminergic neurotransmitter systems is not exactly confirmed by the results of this study. However, the authors were impressed that the patients responding to treatment were not in spontaneous remission. Methysergide cannot displace ACTH as the treatment of choice in infantile spasms. - Editor. *Ped Neur Briefs* November 1989.

Prognosis Of Infantile Spasms (West Syndrome)

Investigators at the Instituto di Neuropsychiatria Infantile, University of Rome, Italy, followed 58 cases of West syndrome for 3 years or more (mean 5 yr 5 mo). Eight (14%) were classified as idiopathic, and 50 (86%) were symptomatic, of which 17 were secondary to birth asphyxia or cerebral hemorrhage and 11 (19% of total) had tuberous sclerosis. All were treated with ACTH, 25-50 IU daily for 3 weeks and 25 IU daily for further 3 weeks or more if no response.

IQ was normal or borderline (>70) in 5 (8%) and retarded in 53 (92%). A low IQ at final follow-up was correlated with developmental and/or neurological abnormalities before the onset of spasms, symptomatic etiology, and abnormal CT findings (cerebral atrophy 30 (52%), calcifications 11 (19%), callosal agenesis 3 (5%). An IQ above 50 in 13 (23%) was associated with early speech development (first word before 2 years and two-word sentence before 3 years) and an IQ below 50 was found in children with retarded speech development. Motor milestones did not correlate with subsequent mental development even in cases without neuromotor impairment. Whereas clinical and CT evidence of cerebral damage correlated with mental retardation, the absence of cerebral abnormalities was not predictive of a normal mental development. A poor prognosis in WS was predictable but normal development at follow-up was not reliably associated with favorable variables at onset. (Favata I, Leuzzi Y, Curatolo P. Mental outcome in West syndrome: prognostic value of some clinical factors. *J Ment Def Res* 1987; *31*:9-15).

COMMENT. Of 1,558 cases of West syndrome reported in the literature between 1954 and 1973, a 20-year span, 624 (40%) were idiopathic and 934 (60%) were symptomatic (Lacy JR, Penry JK. *Infantile Spasms*. Raven Press, New York, 1976). The unusually high percentage of symptomatic cases in this study could explain the relatively higher incidence of mental retardation. Could the 52% incidence of cerebral atrophy demonstrated by CT be caused in part by ACTH? As the authors point out, their data related to a poor mental outcome cannot strictly be regarded as prognostic factors since they are an expression of the symptomatic character of WS, accounting for 86% of their cases. Among 11 patients with tuberous sclerosis, 4 (36%) had an IQ 50 at follow-up and 7 (64%) were moderately to severely retarded. Unfortunately, the relation of IQ to the age at time of treatment and response to ACTH was not evaluated, a frequently debated question. In a study at the Mayo Clinic (Millichap JG, Bickford RG. *JAMA* 1962; *182*:523), psychomotor retardation was generally more severe in patients with symptomatic infantile spasms than in those with cryptogenic seizures. ACTH was possibly more effective in patients with IQ's of 70 or above than in those with retarded development before treatment. Control of infantile spasms and hypsarrhythmia by ACTH was approximately 50% and equal in cryptogenic and symptomatic groups of patients. - Editor. *Ped Neur Briefs* August 1987.

OCCIPITAL LOBE EPILEPSIES

Epilepsy With Occipital Paroxysms

A 15 year prospective study of 18 children with benign childhood epilepsy with occipital paroxysms was carried out at the Division of Neurology and Clinical Neurophysiology, King Khalid University Hospital, Riyadh, Saudi Arabia. These patients represented one-fifth of all benign age-and localization-related idiopathic epilepsies seen with onset before the age of 13 years. There was a preponderance in females and peak age at onset was five years. The seizures consisted of tonic deviation of the eyes and vomiting, followed by unilateral or generalized convulsions. They were mainly nocturnal. Remission usually occurred one to two years after onset and no seizures occurred after 12 years of age. Two children were exceptional, having frequent diurnal episodes with visual hallucinations, postictal headaches, and occasional nocturnal hemiconvulsions. EEG abnormalities consisted of repetitive spike and slow-wave discharges in the occipital regions, attenuated with eyes open. The EEG abnormalities persisted after clinical remission, sometimes up to age 16. (Panayiotopoulos CP. Benign childhood epilepsy with occipital paroxysms: a 15-year prospect study. *Ann Neurol* July 1989; 26:51-56).

COMMENT. The authors propose a definition of benign childhood epilepsy with occipital paroxysms as follows: A syndrome of brief or prolonged partial seizures marked by deviation of the eyes and vomiting. The seizures are usually nocturnal and frequently evolve to hemiconvulsions and generalized tonic-clonic fits. Onset is between the ages of two and eight years, with a peak occurring at five years and remission before 12 years. There is a preponderance in females and prognosis is excellent. In addition, there is a late onset variant with mainly diurnal seizures consisting of visual symptoms often followed by hemiclonic seizures or automatisms and migraine headache. Prognosis appears relatively good. The EEG in both shows repetitive occipital spikes/sharp and slow waves that are often asymmetrical and which attenuate or disappear when the eyes are open.

This syndrome is related to basilar migraine with epileptiform EEG abnormalities (Camfield PR, Metrakos K, Andermann F. *Neurology* 1978; *28*:58 - Editor. *Ped Neur Briefs* August 1989.

Epilepsy With Occipital Calcifications

Four patients, aged 13-22 yrs, with focal epilepsy, and bilateral occipital corticosubcortical calcifications without facial cutaneous angioma were followed at the Neurological Institute, University of Bologna Medical School, Via Ugo Foscolo, Bologna, Italy, and were found to develop a severe encephalopathy with progressive mental impairment. The age at onset of seizures was 3-8 years and psychomotor function was normal while seizures remained controlled from 1-2 years. Unexpectedly, the seizures recurred and were refractory to medication. Concomitantly, all patients had progressively severe mental impairment, and the EEG's showed progressive slowing of the background activity. During non-REM sleep, fast polyspike bursts, diffuse and with greater prominence in both occipital regions, were observed. CT's showed occipital calcifications and skull X-ray in one patient showed double-contoured curvilinear calcifications. The authors regarded a diagnosis of atypical Sturge-Weber syndrome as questionable. (Gobbi G et al. Epilepsy with bilateral occipital calcifications: A benign onset with progressive severity. *Neurology* June 1988; *38*:913-920).

COMMENT. A case of Sturge-Weber-Dimitri disease without facial nevus (Taly AB et al. *Neurology* 1987; *37*:1063), published after submission of this paper and noted by the authors as an addendum, was found to have bilateral leptomeningeal angioma. Bilateral calcification and bilateral ectodermal angioma in Sturge-Weber syndrome may not have been reported often but they occur in my experience. A progressive epileptic encephalopathy also may occur, particularly as a sequel to status epilepticus with Sturge-Weber disease. In the present cases the cause for the deterioration was unclear. This experience should prompt consideration of early neurosurgical excision in similar cases with unilateral calcified lesions, despite initial responsiveness to anticonvulsant medication. - Editor. *Ped Neur Briefs* May 1988.

MYOCLONIC EPILEPSIES

Progressive Myoclonus Epilepsy (Lafora Type)

The diagnosis of Lafora's syndrome, progressive myoclonus epilepsy and intracytoplasmic periodic acid-Schiff-positive inclusions (Lafora bodies), was made by skin biopsy in a 16-year-old girl at the Depts of Pathology and Dermatology, University of Texas Medical Branch, Galveston, TX. She presented because of refractory generalized convulsions. In good health until 8 months previously, she developed progressive incoordination, slurred speech, weakness, and impaired school performance followed after 2 months by her first generalized tonic-clonic seizure and progressive mental deterioration. The family history was negative. Metabolic, endocrine, and infectious disorders were excluded. CT scan was normal. EEG showed "generalized cerebral dysfunction." Round to oval, intracytoplasmic inclusions, strongly PAS-positive, in eccrine duct cells and peripheral nerve bundles of dermis were demonstrated histologically in cryostat- and paraffin-embedded sections and by electronmicroscopy. Skin biopsy, the least invasive method of identifying the Lafora body, was first proposed by Carpenter S. Karpati G (*Neurology* 1981; *31*:1564). A summary of other disorders and their characteristic inclusions that may be diagnosed by skin biopsy includes neuronal ceroid lipofuscinoses (Bielschowski and Spielmeyer-Vogt), glycogenosis II (Pompe's), metachromatic leukodystrophy and occasionally, globoid leukodystrophy (Krabbe). (Newton GA et al. Lafora's disease. The role of skin biopsy. *Arch Dermatol* 1987; *123*:1667-1669).

COMMENT. A number of syndromes of progressive myoclonus epilepsy, frequently autosomal recessive in inheritance, have been described. The Lafora type is characterized by a rapidly progressive dementia, myoclonus, and intracytoplasmic Lafora body inclusions demonstrated in neurons, especially localized in the substantia nigra and dentate nucleus, in the heart, liver, muscle, retina, nerves and now in skin. The EEG shows discharges of fast spike-waves and polyspike-waves, photosensitivity, deterioration of background activity, and multifocal abnormalities especially posteriorly. The onset occurs between 6 and 19 years of age and the patient dies within an average of 5.5 years after onset. No enzymatic defect has yet been identified.

The Unverricht-Lundborg types have a slower rate of progression than the Lafora myoclonic epilepsy, with onset at about age 10 years, variable severity of myoclonus, associated cerebellar ataxia, and milder mental symptoms, patients surviving for 15 years and more. This variety known as the Finnish or "Baltic" myoclonus epilepsy in which Lafora bodies are absent was exacerbated by phenytoin and benefitted by sodium valproate. (Eldridge R et al. *Lancet* 1983; 2:838). - Editor. *Ped Neur Briefs* January 1988.

Progressive Myoclonus Epilepsies: Classification
Progressive myoclonus epilepsies and related disorders were classified at an international workshop in Marseille, France.

Myoclonus refers to sudden, brief, shock-like involuntary movements. The progressive myoclonus epilepsies (PME) are a group of rare genetic disorders characterized by myoclonus, epileptic seizures and progressive neurological deterioration, particularly dementia and ataxia. Many specific diseases can cause the PME syndrome. Electrophysiological findings share many similarities including generalized spike wave discharges, photosensitivity, focal epileptiform discharges, vertex spikes in rapid eye movement sleep, and giant somatosensory evoked potentials. Slow background activity occurs particularly in PME caused by diffuse neuronal damage or storage diseases. Five disease entities account for most of the cases: 1) Unverricht-Lundborg ("Baltic myoclonus"), 2) LaFora disease, 3) neuronal ceroid-lipofuscinoses, 4) mitochondrial disorders, and 5) the sialidoses. The term Ramsay Hunt syndrome was discarded in favor of two main syndromic categories: 1) Progressive myoclonus epilepsies and 2) progressive myoclonic ataxias (PMA). PMA comprises myoclonus, and progressive cerebellar ataxia with infrequent or absent epileptic seizures and little or no dementia. The causes of PME syndrome are better defined than those of PMA. PMA may be caused by spinal cerebellar degenerations, mitochondrial disease, early cases of Unverricht-Lundborg disease, sialidosis and in association with celiac disease. Progressive myoclonus is distinguished from static myoclonus encephalopathies such as post anoxic myoclonus (Lance-Adams syndrome). Phenytoin may exacerbate myoclonus whereas treatment with benzodiazepines and valproate is most effective. (Andermann E et al. Classification of progressive myoclonus epilepsies and related disorders. Marseille Consensus Group, *Ann Neurol* July 1990; *28*:113-116).

COMMENT. Myoclonus and its relation to monoamine, GABA and other receptors is reviewed from the Departments of Neurology and Pediatrics, University of Southern California School of Medicine, Los Angeles, CA. (Snodgrass SR. *FASEBJ* July 1990; *4*:2775-2788). The term myoclonus was first used in 1881 by Freidreich with reference to a progressive movement disorder of a gradual onset in a middle-aged man. By 1891 Unverricht had written a book on myoclonus, describing a family with myoclonus and progressive deterioration. Snodgrass, in the present article, classifies myoclonus in four categories: a) stimulus-sensitive myoclonus, b) stimulus-insensitive myoclonus, c) sleep myoclonus, and d) asterexis and negative myoclonus. Distinction between epileptic and nonepileptic myoclonus is often difficult. Posthypoxic action myoclonus (Lance-Adams syndrome) is associated with reduced CSF levels of 5-HIAA, the serotonin metabolite, and 50% respond to treatment with 5-HTP. Benzodiazepines and valproic acid are the most useful drugs for patients unresponsive to HTP. Various animal models of myoclonus are described. (Gundlach AL. *FASEB J* July 1990; *4*:2761-2766).

"Severe myoclonic epilepsy of infancy" is discussed by Hurst DL (*Epilepsia* July/August 1990; *31*:397-400) from the Department of Medical and Surgical Neurology, Texas Tech University, Lubbock, Texas. The central features of this syndrome include: 1) normal development before the onset of seizure activity, 2) repeated prolonged febrile seizures, 3) later onset of mixed/myoclonus epilepsy, 4) developmental slowing with onset of seizure activity, and 5) evolving EEG abnormalities. The incidence of the syndrome is estimated at one in 40,000 children. Dravet, who first described the syndrome in 1978, found a 30% prevalence in a group of 142 children with myoclonic epilepsy. A more vigorous, rather than conservative, approach to the management of complex febrile seizures might be suggested by this report. - Editor. *Ped Neur Briefs* August 1990.

Reflex Myoclonic Epilepsy

A case-report from the Dept of Medicine, University of Peradeniya, Sri Lanka, concerns a young adult with myoclonic epilepsy since 15 yrs of age whose attacks were precipitated while playing with the Rubik's Cube, a three-dimensional colored puzzle. The EEG at rest and with photic stimulation was normal; playing the cube produced generalized 3 Hz S/W accompanied by myoclonic jerks and mental blocking. Arithmetic, draughts (checkers), card games, and reading precipitated EEG epileptiform discharges but not jerks. Diazepam prevented the seizures, but made him drowsy. The patient preferred to disengage his mind from the puzzle when he felt a jerk. (Senanayake N. Epileptic seizures evoked by the Rubik's Cube. *J Neurol Neurosurg Psychiatry* 1987; *50*:1553-1559).

> COMMENT. Having played the Rubik's Cube and Rubik's Magic unsuccessfully myself and given up in despair, I can imagine that frustration could be a factor responsible for the patient's seizures as much as "spatial and decision making processes." The same author has described seizures evoked by card games, draughts, and a local game with sea shells called "unchi" (*Epilepsia* 1987; 28:356). Ch'en, Chi'in, and Ch'u were the first to describe Chess and Card epilepsy! (*Chinese Med J* 1965; *84*:470). - Editor. *Ped Neur Briefs* December 1987.

Hot Water Epilepsy (HWE)

Seizures precipitated by very hot water-head baths or showers (40-50°C), a regional religious custom, were seen in 279 patients between 1980-83 in Bangalore, Southern India, and are reported from the Depts of Neurology and Biostatistics, National Institute of Mental Health and Neurosciences, Bangalore, India, and the Neuroepidemiology Branch, National Institute of Neurological Disorders, NIH, Bethesda, MD, USA. The ages ranged from 8 mos to 58 yrs with a childhood preponderance and 28% below 6 years. The male:female ratio was 2.65:1. Only 7% had a history of febrile convulsions. Complex partial seizures were the most frequent manifestation of HWE (67%) and generalized tonic-clonic seizures occurred in 33%. Spontaneous non-reflex epilepsy followed or preceded the onset of HWE in 30%. A positive family history of epilepsy was obtained in 22% and for HWE in only 7%. The avoidance of the hot water stimulus should be supplemented with anticonvulsant medication in therapy. (Satishchandra P et al. Hot-water epilepsy: a variant of reflex epilepsy in Southern India. *Epilepsia* Jan/Feb 1988; *29*:52-6).

> COMMENT. The mechanism of HWE is unclear. A hot-air stimulus to the heads of patients failed to induce attacks. A kindling effect has been induced in rats by repeated exposure of the head to hot water (Klanenberg BJ, Sparber SB. *Epilepsia* 1984; *25*:292). Hot water applied to the abdomen induces fever and changes in cortical electrical activity of cats and kittens (Kashiwase Y. *Brain Nerve (Tokyo)* 1962; *14*:698). The body temperature of patients in the present study is not documented and fever induced by the hot water stimulus may explain some cases, especially in younger children.

> Absence epilepsy evoked by thinking or talking about driving an automobile is an unusual example of reflex epilepsy also reported in the current issue of *Epilepsia* (Bencze KS et al. of the Dept of Neurology, University of South Florida, Tampa, FL). - Editor. *Ped Neur Briefs* March 1988.

Seizures During Exercise

Three children with epileptic seizures occurring during exercise are reported from the Sections of Electroencephalography and Pediatric Neurology, Mayo Clinic, Rochester, MN. Epileptiform paroxysms were noted with exercise but not with hyperventilation during EEG recordings in these patients. The pathophysiologic mechanism was unclear. (Ogunyemi AO et al. Seizures induced by exercise. *Neurology* April 1988; *38*:633-634).

> COMMENT. A cardiac pathogenesis is usually suspected when seizures occur during physical exercise, as noted by

the authors. A full cardiac examination including EKG and echocardiogram is advisable in patients with seizures occurring during physical exertion, even in children. Exercise is an unusual precipitant of seizures and is generally accompanied by a reduction in EEG seizure discharges. A clinical seizure was not induced but a spike and wave discharge occurred in each of these three patients after 5, , 7-1/2 and 27 minutes of pedaling a stationary bicycle. - Editor. *Ped Neur Briefs* April 1988.

Reading Epilepsy

Precipitating stimuli, including eye-movements, reading aloud versus reading silently, linguistic complexity, and concentration, were investigated in a 24 year old young woman with reading epilepsy seen in the Division of Neurology and Clinical Neurophysiology Laboratory, University of Ottawa General Hospital, and Depts of Psychology and Computer Engineering, Carleton University, Ottawa, Ontario, Canada. A viral illness at 19 years of age was followed by episodic jerking of the jaw while reading silently and a single generalized tonic-clonic seizure. After 2 years freedom from symptoms, the jaw jerking returned while reading, and was aggravated by fatigue or stress. Reading material was presented on a microcomputer video display monitor while the patient underwent EEG radiotelemetry video monitoring. Seizures were most readily elicited by reading aloud material of medium or high linguistic complexity. (Christie S et al. Primary reading epilepsy: Investigation of critical-provoking stimuli. *Epilepsia* May/June 1988; *29*:288-293).

COMMENT. Bickford et al., in their original description of reading epilepsy, observed precipitation of seizures by difficult reading matter (*Trans Am Neurol Assoc* 1956; *81*:100), and other authors have stressed the cortical or "lexical" aspects of the reading process in seizure provocation. The results of the present study suggest that a combination of factors involved in reading, including saccadic eye movements, articulation, and difficulty of linguistic content, contribute to epileptogenesis. Seizures were more readily provoked when greater demand was placed on each of the subtasks collectively and no factor acted solely as the critical stimulus.

In an article in the same issue of Epilepsia from the National Centre for Children with Epilepsy, Park Hospital for Children, Headington, Oxford, England, Verduyn et al surveyed mothers' impressions of seizure precipitants in children with epilepsy. Reading was not included in the list of precipitants, but stimuli that are somatic, psychological, and sensory were frequently followed by seizures. Mothers reported a relaxed state, emotional state, anxiety, exercise, and drowsiness as precipitants in 60-75% of the sample of 446 children. Sensory-evoked epilepsy in 2.5% was provoked by loud noise, startle, flashing lights, bright light, diet, touch, television, and pattern. (*Epilepsia* 1988; *29*:251). - Editor. *Ped Neur Briefs* July 1988.

Ictal Vomiting

Paroxysmal vomiting in 9 patients, 3 children (7, 8, and 11 years of age) and 6 young adults, is reported from the Section of Epilepsy and Clinical Neurophysiology, Cleveland Clinic, Cleveland, OH. Amnesia for the episodes occurred in 8 of the 9 patients. Other ictal phenomena prior to the vomiting included staring, automatisms, eye-blinking, grimacing, eye-rolling, chewing, and swallowing. After vomiting, only one patient regained normal alertness immediately. Four patients had temporal lobectomy, the pathology specimens showing mild inflammatory changes, gliosis, and neuronal heterotopia. (Kramer RE et al. Ictus emeticus: an electroclinical analysis. *Neurology* July 1988; *38*:1048-1052).

COMMENT. The authors note that reports of ictal vomiting recorded electrographically are scarce and that 13 of 14 cases published have an onset or lateralization of EEG findings to the right hemisphere. In one case the vomiting was induced by photic stimulation. Another case may be added to this list from the French literature (Giroud M et al. Un symptome critique epileptique rare: le vomissement. *Arch Fr Pediatr* 1987; 44:231-4). In this 9 year old boy, the paroxysmal episode of vomiting was synchronized with an epileptiform discharge in the left frontotemporal area on the EEG. That cyclic vomiting may represent a form of epilepsy in children was proposed in a report of 33 patients, 7 (21%) having a history of grand mal or complex partial seizures in addition, and 25 (76%) with seizure discharges in the EEG, some focal and predominantly in the temporal lobe. (Millichap JG, Lombroso CT, Lennox WG. *Pediatrics* 1955; *15*:705). The EEG was not recorded at the time of the vomiting and, in retrospect, some of our cases may have been more correctly classified as migraine. - Editor. *Ped Neur Briefs* July 1988.

SYMPTOMATIC SEIZURES

Biotinidase Deficiency And Seizures

Authors from La Jolla, USA and Florence, Italy report the case of a boy who was first admitted to hospital at 5 years of age because of acute somnolence, alopecia, keratoconjunctivitis, and perioral stomatitis associated with lactic acidemia. At 6 years of age he had grand mal seizures and ataxia and at 7 years he was admitted in coma. The diagnosis of multiple carboxylase deficiency due to biotinidase deficiency was then suspected and treatment with biotin 10 mg p.o. q.d. was started after urine for organic acid analysis was collected. The clinical response was dramatic. Coma and acidosis resolved within a few days. No further seizures occurred. The skin gradually returned to normal and hair, eyebrows and eyelashes regenerated. Ataxia responded after a few weeks but optic atrophy and nerve deafness persisted.

This patient's history began at 6 months of age with seizures. He had multiple generalized tonic-clonic seizures without fever, apparently unresponsive to medication. His subsequent motor development was slow; he sat at 1 year and walked at 2 years. The EEG showed a diffuse abnormality with poorly localized spike foci. Alopecia, a characteristic sign of biotinidase deficiency, did not develop until after 2 years of age. (Thuy LP et al. *J Neurogenet.* 1986; *3:*357-363).

COMMENT. Biotin-related genetically determined disorders are of two types: 1. young infantile or neonatal disease caused by deficiency of holocarboxylase synthetase and 2. late infantile disease due to biotinidase deficiency. Neurological manifestations are prominent in the late-onset group and seizures may precede the cutaneous eruption and loss of hair.

Having encountered one such patient who presented at the age of 5 years with ataxia and seizures refractory to medications (In *Nutrition, Diet, and your Child's Behavior.* Charles C. Thomas, Springfield, 1986), I now make it a practice to prescribe biotin 10 mg daily as a therapeutic test when this diagnosis is suspected. Treatment reverses the organic aciduria so that a urine collection for analysis should precede administration of the vitamin. A dramatic response to a vitamin in a single daily dose is certainly an improvement over long-term anticonvulsant drug therapy with its attendant potential side-effects. Supplies of biotin from Roche Labs are available only for research at present. (See *Biotin.* Ed. by Dakshinamurti K, Bhagavan HN. *Ann NY Acad Science.* New York, 1985; *447:*222-224, 297-313). - Editor. *Ped Neur Briefs* June 1987.

Rasmussen Encephalitis And Partial Seizures

Immunological abnormalities associated with chronic encephalitis, epilepsy, and progressive hemiplegia in a three-year, nine-month old girl are reported from the University of Utah School of Medicine and the Primary Children's Medical Center, Salt Lake City, Utah. The child developed simple partial seizures refractory to medications and associated with a contralateral hemicerebral atrophy. Immunologic abnormalities were indicated by elevated antinuclear antibody, CSF oligoclonal bands and elevated immunoglobulin G (IgG). A right subtotal hemispherectomy resulted in control of the seizures. Pathological study showed widespread cerebral vasculitis and severe cortical atrophy with marked neuronal loss. (Andrews JM et al. Chronic encephalitis, epilepsy and cerebrovascular immune complex deposits. *Ann Neurol* July 1990; *28*:88-90).

COMMENT. Immunofluorescence microscopy revealed granular accumulation of IgG, IgM, IgA within the cerebral vessels of this patient suggesting an immune complex disease as the basis for Rasmussen's syndrome. - Editor. *Ped Neur Briefs* Aug 1990.

Seizures Following DTP Immunization

The incidence of seizures following the administration of DTP vaccine at the Group Health Cooperative of Puget Sound, Seattle, has been estimated by epidemiologists at the Harvard School of Public Health, Boston, and by the Boston Collaborative Drug Surveillance Program, Waltham, MA. For a population of children born in GHC hospitals, 1972-83, records of hospitalizations for neurologic disease and prescriptions of common anticonvulsant drugs were reviewed to establish the probable nature of the illness, the date of its onset, and the temporal relation to DTP.

Children omitted from the study for various reasons were as follows: 1) those not hospitalized nor treated with drug therapy (e.g., uncomplicated first febrile seizures and children with infantile spasms who received only ACTH and steroids as outpatients); 2) those with seizures and a history of possible predisposition due to trauma, asphyxia, malformation, metabolic defect, premature birth, CNS infection and sepsis; 3) those without a clear date of onset for the seizures or neurologic illness; 4) 8 cases of seizures beginning before immunization in the first 30 days of life; 5) 8 cases with a history of first seizures recorded at a subsequent visit; and 6) 2 cases of infantile spasms and 5 acute encephalopathies with onset recorded 30 days or more after DTP immunization.

Of 231 post-immunization first seizures selected for study without other predisposing cause in children 30 days of age or older, 55 had afebrile seizures, and 176 had febrile seizures. The incidence of recorded febrile seizures in the immediate post-immunization period was 3.7 times that in the period 30 days or more after immunization. One child suffered a prolonged status epilepticus on the evening of her third DTP shot, and neurologic sequelae included focal epilepsy at 6-yr follow-up. Six cases of first seizures occurred within 30 days of immunization, and the expected incidence without immunization in this time interval was calculated at 5.07. The authors conclude that serious neurologic sequelae of DTP immunization are extremely infrequent in otherwise healthy children. (Walker AM et al. Neurologic events following diphtheria-tetanus-pertussis immunization. *Pediatrics* March 1988; *81*:345-9).

COMMENT. The omission of several groups of children from this retrospective epidemiological study detracts from the significance of the conclusions and estimates of incidence of DTP-related febrile and non-febrile seizures. The role of DTP as a precipitating cause in children with a predisposition to seizures and as a possible cause of infantile spasms is neglected. It is unfortunate that the study did not address the risks of DTP in children with prior neurologic disease or predisposition to seizures including positive family history (see *Ped Neur Briefs* Nov 1987; 1:40). - Editor. *Ped Neur Briefs* March 1988.

ADDENDUM. At the annual meeting of the Child Neurology Society, Oct. 1990, a committee with one dissenting vote endorsed a statement that pertussis immunization has no significant correlation with serious neurologic sequelae including infantile spasms. - Editor.

Drug-Induced Seizures

Recreational drug-induced seizures in 47 patients seen at the San Francisco General Hospital between 1975 and 1987 were reported by the Division of Clinical Pharmacy and Department of Neurology, University of California, San Francisco, CA. Over the twelve year study period 49 episodes of seizures followed the use of most of the popular street drugs and were seen after ingestion, snorting, smoking and injection. The average age of the 28 men and 19 women was 27 years (range 19-42 years). The majority of patients experienced a single generalized tonic-clonic seizure but seven had multiple seizures and two developed status epilepticus. The recreational drugs were cocaine (32), amphetamines (11), heroin (7), and phenycyclidine (4). A combination was responsible in 11. Seizures occurred independent of the route of administration and in both first-time and chronic abusers. Ten (21%) had prior seizures, all closely associated with drug abuse. Apart from the patient with status epilepticus, none had permanent neurologic impairment at the time of discharge from hospital. (Alldredge BK et al. Seizures associated with recreational drug abuse. *Neurology* August 1989; *39*:1037-1039).

COMMENT. Although the patients in this study were adults, the possibility of drug abuse should be considered in the evaluation of infants, children and adolescents with seizures. Heroin withdrawal has been associated with seizures in neonates (Herzlinger RA et al. *J Pediatr* 1977; *91*:638) but not in older patients. It is fortunate that seizures due to recreational drug abuse appear to be self-limiting and not associated with neurologic sequelae. Anticonvulsant treatment is usually not required. - Editor. *Ped Neur Briefs* August 1989.

Focal Myoclonus And Cortical Dysplasia

Four patients aged 9 to 19 years with focal myoclonus and intractable focal motor seizures beginning at age 4 to 6 years were treated surgically at the Montreal Neurological Hospital and Institute, McGill University, Montreal, Quebec, Canada. All 4 had a mild progressive hemiparesis, cognitive deficits, focal EEG seizure discharges in the contralateral rolandic areas, 3 showed cortical architectonic abnormalities on MRI, and evidence of focal cortical dysplasia with abnormally wide gyri at operation. All improved following surgery. The authors stress the value of the MRI in visualization and diagnosis of neuronal migration cortical dysplasia whereas other imaging techniques have been unrevealing. (Kuzniecky R, Berkovic S, Andermann F (correspondent) et al. Focal cortical myoclonus and rolandic cortical dysplasia; clarification by magnetic resonance imaging. *Ann Neurol* April 1988; *23*: 317-325).

COMMENT. The authors consider the clinical, MRI and pathological features of these 4 patients sufficiently similar to suggest a clinical entity not previously described. The focal seizure pattern, hemiparesis, focal epileptiform EEG discharges and focal cortical dysplasia all indicated a localized lesion, yet a generalized abnormality of EEG background activity and widespread cognitive defects pointed to a more diffuse cerebral dysfunction as well. The differential diagnosis included tumor, post-traumatic or ischemic lesions, metabolic disorder, and chronic localized encephalitis of Rasmussen T et al. (*Neurology* 1958; *8*:435). The report of macrogyria in 3 of the patients and giant astrocytes in both patients with histological studies is suggestive of a forme fruste tuberous sclerosis that might be entertained in the differential diagnosis. - Editor. *Ped Neur Briefs* April 1988.

Intractable Epilepsy, Pseudobulbar Palsy And Macrogyria

Four patients with medically intractable epilepsy, pseudobulbar palsy and mental retardation and found to have bilateral central macrogyria on CT and MRI are reported from the Department of Neurology and Neurosurgery, McGill University, and the Montreal Neurological Institute and Hospital, Montreal, Canada; and the Department of Neurology, University of Minnesota, St. Paul Ramsey Hospital, St. Paul, MN. The pseudobulbar palsy was associated with oromotor incoordination, developmental delay and mild retardation. Minor seizures developed between the ages of eight and nine years and one patient had infantile spasms at three months of age. Electroencephalographic epileptogenic abnormalities were secondary generalized or multifocal. CT scans revealed symmetrical bilateral sylvian and rolandic macrogyria extending into the parietal regions. The cortex appeared thick and smooth with the underlying white matter diminished. The MRI confirmed the CT findings and showed that the abnormal cortex had a lower signal as compared to normal gray matter of frontal and occipital regions. The thick cortical structures surrounded a large central sulcus reminiscent of a fetal sylvian fissure. Two patients tried on multiple anticonvulsants continued to have frequent seizures whereas two treated by callosotomy had no subsequent drop attacks and improved behavior. The authors suggest that the clinical and imaging features of these patients indicate a distinct and specific syndrome and the malformations appear to result from specific derangement of neuronal migration. (Kuzniecky R, Andermann F et al. Bilateral central macrogyria: Epilepsy, pseudobulbar palsy, and mental retardation — A recognizable neuronal migration disorder. *Ann Neurol* June 1989; 25:547-554).

COMMENT. Neuronal migration disorders, including agyria (or lissencephaly), macrogyria (or pachygyria), polymicrogyria, schizencephaly, and other heterotopias of the gray matter are being recognized more frequently by the use of the magnetic resonance imaging technique. The role of neurosurgical treatment in patients with neuronal migration disorders is being explored. The early recognition and effective surgical management of these cases might improve prognosis and prevent the development of intractable epilepsy and mental deterioration. - Editor. *Ped Neur Briefs* July 1989.

Epilepsy And Hemiparetic Cerebral Palsy

The incidence of epilepsy, the IQ, and laterality of cerebral palsy were investigated in 51 children with hemiparetic CP at the Department of Neurology, Charles University, Katerinska, Praha, Czechoslovakia. Epilepsy had developed in 19; two had partial jacksonian seizures and 17 generalized tonic-clonic seizures. Epileptic paroxysms in the EEG were found in 35 (80%). An IQ of 95 or above was found in 32 and an IQ of 94 or below in 19. No difference in IQ was found between patients with right-sided or left-sided hemiparesis whereas clinical seizures were more common in those with right-sided hemiparesis. Clinical epilepsy was related to impaired intellectual performance. Abnormal paroxysmal EEGs were more frequent with left-sided hemiparesis. Among those with clinical epilepsy a lower IQ was found in almost all with left-sided hemiparesis and almost half of those with right-sided hemiparesis. (Sussova J et al. Hemiparetic forms of cerebral palsy in relation to epilepsy and mental retardation. *Dev Med Child Neurol* Sept 1990; 32:792-795).

COMMENT. A lower IQ may be expected in CP patients with clinical epilepsy, especially in those with left-sided hemiparesis. EEG abnormalities alone are not associated with a lower IQ. - Editor. *Ped Neur Briefs* October 1990.

Posttraumatic Seizures

Factors influencing the occurrence of posttraumatic seizures in 92 of 937 children with head injuries (9.8%) were studied in the Division of Neurosurgery, Children's Memorial Hospital, Chicago, IL. Seizures were generalized in 64% and focal in 28%. They occurred within 24 hours after injury in 95% and within 7 days in 98%. The injury was caused by a fall in 60%. Children with a severe head injury (Glasgow Coma Scale

<8) had a 7 times higher incidence of seizures than those with minor trauma. Those with CT evidence of diffuse cerebral edema or subdural hematoma had the highest incidence of seizures. Prophylactic use of anticonvulsants was recommended in children with diffuse cerebral edema, subdural hematoma, open depressed skull fracture, or severe head injuries. (Hahn YS et al. Factors influencing post-traumatic seizures in children. *Neurosurgery* May 1988; *22*:864-867).

> COMMENT. Unfortunately, the duration of prophylactic anticonvulsant therapy was not addressed in this report, although the follow-up period was 7 months to 6 years. In a previous study at the Mayo Clinic involving 2747 patients of all ages with head injury, early seizures occurred in 2.1%. The risks of posttraumatic seizures after severe injury were 7.1% within 1 year and 11.5% in 5 years, after moderate injury 0.7% and 1.6%, and after mild injury 0.1% and 0.6%. Children were at a greater risk for early seizures after severe trauma than adults, but late seizures in children were less frequent and had no relation to the occurrence of early seizures. Mild head trauma in both children and adults did not cause epilepsy. (Annegers JF et al. *Neurology* 1980; *30*:683). - Editor. *Ped Neur Briefs* June 1988.

Phenytoin For Posttraumatic Seizures

A randomized, double-blind study of phenytoin was conducted in 404 patients with serious head trauma at the Departments of Neurological Surgery, Rehabilitation Medicine and Medicine, University of Washington, Seattle. An intravenous loading dose of phenytoin was given within 24 hours of injury to 208 patients and 196 received placebo for a one year period in a double-blind fashion. Serum levels were maintained in the high therapeutic range (3-6 mcmol/1). Statistical analyses were performed according to the intention to treat and based on efficacy. Between the initial drug loading dose and day seven, 3.6% of patients assigned to phenytoin had seizures compared to 14% of patients assigned to placebo (P<.001). From day eight to the end of year one and the end of year two of the study, there was no significant difference between the seizure incidence in the phenytoin and placebo groups, approximately 1 in 5 having a recurrence. The relapse was not explained by low phenytoin levels. (Temkin NR et al. A randomized, double-blind study of phenytoin for the prevention of post-traumatic seizures. *N Engl J Med* August 23, 1990; *323*:497-502).

COMMENT. The authors concluded that phenytoin exerts a beneficial effect by reducing posttraumatic seizures only during the first week after severe head injury. Dr. Allen Hauser, in an editorial comment, states that early administration of loading doses of IV phenytoin to patients with severe head injury may be warranted to prevent early seizures and their complications, but prolonged therapy after stabilization does not seem justified. Other anticonvulsants such as phenobarbital and benzodiazepines should be considered as alternatives, and treatment with antioxidants which reduce edema and prevent neuronal damage caused by iron salts deposited at the time of injury may be of benefit. - *Editor. Ped Neur Briefs* September 1990.

A neurosurgical colleague recently treated an 8 year old girl prophylactically with phenytoin after surgery to remove an arrow that had pierced an eye and orbit and had penetrated the brain to the occipital lobe. She had no seizures in the first week but she developed Stevens-Johnson's syndrome after 10 days treatment, with blistering and exfoliation of the entire skin surface, necessitating admission to the burn unit. My colleague's decision to withhold anticonvulsants in future brain trauma cases and to treat only when seizures occur appears justified. - Editor.

COMPLEX PARTIAL SEIZURES

Gustatory Hallucinations In Epileptic Seizures

Gustatory hallucinations occurred as a manifestation of parietal, temporal or temporoparietal seizures in 30 (4%) of 718 patients investigated for intractable epilepsy by stereoelectroencephalographic exploration at the Unite de Recherches 97, Inserm, et Service de Neurochirurgie de l'Hopital Sainte-Anne, Paris. The electrically-induced seizures which included a gustatory hallucination in 20 patients were obtained by stimulation of the hippocampus and amygdala. The associated ictal events varied with the origin of the seizures: 1) during parietal seizures, they consisted of staring, clonic facial contractions, deviation of eyes and salivation, 2) during temporal lobe seizures, there were oral movements, autonomic disturbances, purposeless movements and epigastric or other abdominal symptoms. Gustatory hallucinations were related to the disorganization of the parietal and/or rolandic operculum. The seizure onset was at a mean age of 9.7 yrs (2-34 yrs) and the gustatory manifestations appeared at a mean age of 14.5 yrs (2-34 yrs). (Hausser-Hauw C, Bandaud J. *Brain* 1987; *110*:339-359).

COMMENT. Children with drug-resistant temporal lobe epilepsy should be considered for neurosurgical treatment. Deterioration of behavior in a school-age child with complex partial seizures carries a poor prognosis if surgery is delayed. Reversal of social, intellectual, and character deficits associated with temporal lobe epilepsy may be expected after operation. (Lindsay J, Ounsted C, Richards P. *Develop Med Child Neurol* 1984; *26*:25-32).

Gustatory hallucinations elicited by a careful history may be helpful in the cortical localization of the seizure discharge. In my experience, this manifestation of temporal lobe seizures is rare in children but nonetheless important to consider. - Editor. *Ped Neur Briefs* July 1987.

Speech Abnormalities And Temporal Lobe Seizures

The role of speech manifestations in the lateralization of temporal lobe seizures was reviewed at the Section of Epilepsy and Clinical Neurophysiology, Department of Neurology, Cleveland Clinic Foundation, Cleveland, OH, by the review of videotapes of 100 complex seizures in 35 patients who underwent temporal lobectomy for intractable epilepsy. All patients had prolonged EEG video monitoring with scalp and subdural electrodes and their speech dominance was determined with an intracarotid amobarbital test. Speech manifestations were classified as vocalization, normal speech, or abnormal speech. Vocalizations of sound without speech quality occurred during the seizure in 48.5% of patients. Normal speech occurred ictally in 34% of patients. Abnormal speech (speech arrest, dysphasia, and dysarthria) occurred in 51% of patients either during the seizure or postictally. Only postictal dysphasia and ictal identifiable speech had significant lateralizing value: 92% of patients with postictal dysphasia had their seizures originating from the dominant temporal lobe, and 83% of those with ictal identifiable speech had seizures localized to the nondominant side. (Gabr M et al. Speech manifestations in lateralization of temporal lobe seizures. *Ann Neurol* Jan 1989; *25*:82-87).

COMMENT. This study shows that speech manifestations are common in complex partial seizures of temporal lobe origin and can help to lateralize the origin of the seizure. John Hughlings Jackson noted that seizures in the dominant hemisphere could result in speech abnormalities and Penfield found that electrical stimulation of the speech areas in the dominant hemisphere produced dysphasia whereas stimulation of the motor speech area of either hemisphere produced vocalization. - Editor. *Ped Neur Briefs* July 1989.

Verbal Memory, The Hippocampus, And Temporal Lobe Epilepsy

The relationship of memory impairment and hippocampal damage was studied in 35 patients with medically refractory epilepsy localized to the temporal lobe at the Departments of Neurosurgery, Neuropathology, and Neurology and Psychiatry, Yale University School of Medicine, New Haven, CT. The temporal lobe lesion was left-sided in 18 and right-sided in 17. A history of febrile convulsions was obtained in 27. The mean age at which seizures became recurrent was ten years and the mean age at surgery was 29 years. The groups (left foci versus right foci) did not differ significantly with regard to the history of febrile convulsions, age when recurrent seizures developed, and age at surgery. All patients were seizure-free after surgery at a minimum follow-up of six months. Patients completed the Verbal Selective Reminding Test and the WAIS-R before surgery which involved anteromedial temporal lobectomy and radical hippocampectomy. Contrasted with normative standards for the verbal memory test, the means of patients with left temporal seizure foci (78.9) and right temporal seizure foci (101) were less than that achieved by healthy adults (115). Left temporal seizure foci were associated with significantly greater preoperative verbal memory impairment than right temporal seizure foci. Volumetric cell densities of hippocampal subfields (CA3 and the hilar area) were reduced in all patients with temporal lobe epilepsy when contrasted with autopsy controls; and measures of long term memory retrieval were correlated significantly with pyramidal cell densities in CA3 and the hilus for patients with left temporal seizure foci only. No significant correlations were found between measures of memory retrieval and the cell densities of CA1, CA2 or the granular layer. Left temporal seizure foci were associated with significantly greater preoperative verbal memory impairment than right temporal seizure foci. (Sass KJ et al. Verbal memory impairment correlates with hippocampal pyramidal cell density. *Neurology* Nov 1990; *40*:1694-1697).

COMMENT. This study demonstrates impaired verbal memory in patients with confirmed hippocampal damage. The verbal memory impairment was significantly correlated with hippocampal pyramidal cell density in patients with left temporal seizure foci. A history of febrile seizures in 77% of this group of patients with subsequent complex partial seizures is noteworthy. Lennox WG (*Pediatrics* 1953; *11*:341) found a significantly higher incidence of psychomotor seizures among patients with a history of febrile seizures compared to those with generalized tonic-clonic and absence patterns; psychomotor seizures were diagnosed in 17% of the febrile seizure group and in 5.9% of the grand mal and petit mal groups. - Editor. *Ped Neur Briefs* November 1990.

Autoscopic Phenomena

Ten patients with seizures and autoscopic phenomena, such as seeing one's double, are reported and 33 additional cases in the literature are reviewed from the Medical Neurology Branch, Division of Intramural Research, National Institute of Neurological Disorders and Stroke, Bethesda, MD; and the Department of Neurology, New York Hospital, New York, NY. The ictal autoscopy began at a median age of 25 years (range, 8 to 62 years), and the mean age at the time of case reporting was 34 years (range, 13 to 73 years). Autoscopic phenomena occurred as symptoms of simple partial, complex partial, or generalized tonic-clonic seizures. Out-of-body experiences occurred in five patients who gave vivid descriptions of the seizures and a feeling of leaving one's body and viewing it from another vantage point, usually from above. One patient stated "I watched the whole episode as if I were at the movies". She felt herself "slip back into my body". The temporal lobe was involved in 18 (86%) of the 21 patients in whom the seizure focus could be identified. There was no clear lateralization of lesions. The response of autoscopic episodes to treatment usually paralleled that of the underlying seizure disorder. (Devinsky O et al. Autoscopic phenomena with seizures. *Arch Neurol* October 1989; *46*:1080-1088).

COMMENT. The authors comment that autoscopic phenomena are likely to be discovered only on specific questioning of patients with epilepsy and may be an important and distressing feature of a chronic seizure disorder. Fear is a common symptom of complex partial seizures in children and may be explained by autoscopic phenomena. Autoscopy, the hallucination or psychic experience of seeing oneself, may also occur in healthy persons in association with anxiety and fatigue. It is reported frequently in near death encounters such as drowning and automobile accidents. - Editor. *Ped Neur Briefs* Nov 1989.

Prognosis Of Partial Epilepsy

Children with onset of partial seizures from 10 mos to 13 yrs (average 4.9 yrs) were followed for an average period of 7.4 yrs at the Instituto di Neuropsichiatria, Rome, Italy. Of a total of 261 consecutive patients (136 male and 125 female) 89 had simple partial seizures, 109 had complex symptomatology, and 63 were partial with secondary generalization. Acquired etiological factors in 112 (43%) patients included cerebral birth injury in 62, head trauma in 31, and CNS infection in 19. Seizure outcome at 5 yr follow-up was favorable in 214 (82%); 153 patients had been seizure-free for 2 years and 61 showed improved seizure frequency. Factors predictive of seizure control and a good prognosis were as follows: 1) a positive family history for epilepsy, 2) absence of acquired etiologies, 3) no antecedent generalized seizures, 4) normal EEG background activity, and 5) absence of mental retardation, neurological abnormalities or behavior disorders. An unfavorable seizure outcome correlated with 1) early onset of partial seizures, and 2) generalized seizures predating partial seizure onset. Factors of no prognostic value were 1) febrile convulsions preceding partial seizure onset, 2) normal initial EEG, and 3) cognitive and behavioral disorders. (Porro G et al. *Arch Dis Child* Oct 1988; 63:1192-97).

COMMENT. Position emission tomography (PET) had been employed to determine metabolic patterns in 48 patients with complex partial seizures. Patients with frontal hypometabolism had shorter and milder seizures and those with multilobar hypometabolism had prolonged seizures. An aura correlated with temporal hypometabolism (Holmes MD et al. *Arch Neurol* Nov 1988; *45*:1191). SPECT (single photon emission computed tomography) in 14 children with seizure disorders was useful in localization and prognosis. In patients with radiological lesions, SPECT showed more extensive localizations and those with normal CTs often had areas of hypo- or hyperperfusion. The pattern seen on SPECT was related to the clinical course and prognosis: extensive metabolic impairment on SPECT correlated with frequent seizure recurrence and mental retardation whereas all children with a normal SPECT had less than 2 seizures per year and normal neurological and intellectual development. (Denays R et al. *Arch Dis Child* Oct 1988; *63*:1184). - Editor. *Ped Neur Briefs* October 1988.

PSEUDOSEIZURES

Pseudoseizure Diagnosis

A protocol for the presentation of a diagnosis of pseudoseizure to the patient is outlined from the Indiana University Medical Center, Indianapolis, IN. After the diagnosis of pseudoseizure arrived at by simultaneous video EEG recording, the authors had frequently noted a disintegration of the patient's medical care in their center, attributed in part to the presentation of the diagnosis. To address this problem, they developed a protocol which stressed the nonepileptic nature of the spells, defused tension resulting from the nature of the diagnosis, promoted compliance with medical and psychiatric follow-up, and provided hints to the patient for the voluntary control of attacks. The results of the video EEG monitoring were presented only if the patient agreed to long-term follow-up in the clinic. Of 8 patients followed by one of the authors, a history of sexual abuse was eventually discovered in six. A majority experienced an immediate reduction in the pseudoseizures after the diagnosis was conveyed and abortive maneuvers were encouraged. Psychosocial issues continue to handicap many patients on long-term follow-up. (Shen W et al. Presenting the diagnosis of pseudoseizure. *Neurology* May 1990; *40*:756-759).

COMMENT The term pseudoseizure may be pejorative and psychogenic seizure is preferred by some. "Nonepileptic attack disorder" (NEAD) is suggested as a better and nonaccusatory term by Betts T (*Lancet* July 21, 1990; *336*:163-164). Reporting from the Department of Psychiatry, University of Birmingham, UK, Betts classifies nonepileptic attack disorders into three groups: 1) organic attack disorders (neurological, cardiovascular), 2) psychiatric disorders mistaken for epilepsy (hyperventilation, panic, anxiety), and 3) emotionally based attacks (swoon, tantrum, abreaction or symbolic attack). The symbolic attack, described as "macabre pastiche of intercourse", is seen in patients who have been sexually abused. The author avoids blunt confrontation of the patient with the truth regarding the nature of the attack, a policy with which I personally concur particularly in adolescents and young adults. "The patient should be led gently into recognizing the nonepileptic nature of the attack and the diagnosis put in positive terms". "Above all do not reject the patient, but allow her to save face". Intensive anxiety management and counseling may be necessary, and the family or close relatives should be involved. Patients may learn to voluntarily control their "seizures", but relapses at times of stress are not uncommon. - Editor. *Ped Neur Briefs* August 1990.

EPIDEMIOLOGY OF SEIZURES

Risk Of Seizure Recurrence After First Seizure

The frequency of seizure recurrence in 283 children presenting with a first unprovoked seizure was studied in the Montefiore/Einstein Epilepsy Management Center, Bronx, NY; Yale University School of Medicine, New Haven, CN; and Columbia College of Physicians and Surgeons, New York, NY. Seizures recurred in 101 children (36%). The mean time interval of recurrence was 9.2 months (median 6 months). Risk of recurrence was greatest in the first few months after the first seizure; 51% within six months. The cumulative risk of seizure recurrence for the entire group was 26% at 12 months, 36% at 24 months, 40% at 36 months, and 42% at 48 months. The risk of recurrence in children with an idiopathic first seizure was significantly lower than those with symptomatic seizures. An abnormal electroencephalogram was the most important predictor of recurrence in children with an idiopathic first seizure. A history of epilepsy in a first degree relative was a significant risk factor only in idiopathic cases with abnormal electroencephalograms. A history of prior febrile seizures or a partial seizure were significant predictors of recurrence in children with a remote symptomatic first seizure. The age at the first seizure and duration of seizure were not predictive in either the idiopathic or remote symptomatic group. The majority (84%) were not treated with antiepileptic drugs or were treated for less than two weeks. The risk of recurrence was not affected by treatment. In the opinion of the authors even children with risk factors for recurrence should not be routinely treated following a first unprovoked seizure. In the two major high risk groups, 1) remote symptomatic patients; and 2) idiopathic patients with abnormal EEG's, recurrence risk is estimated at 50% at two years following the initial seizure. (Shinnar S et al. Risk of seizure recurrence following a first unprovoked seizure in childhood: A prospective study. *Pediatrics* June 1990; *85*:1076-1085).

COMMENT. The growing concern and awareness of the potential adverse effects of long-term antiepileptic medications in children have led to an increasing reluctance to prescribe regular prophylactic therapy except in patients with multiple risk factors. To treat or not to treat is an individualized decision depending on many criteria: 1) Risk of seizure recurrence and associated brain injury; 2) Adverse effects of antiepileptic medications particularly on cognitive function and behavior; 3) Psychosocial consequences; 4) Geographic location and proximity of physician or hospital emergency services; and 5) Parental compliance and ability to provide CPR and first aid care at seizure recurrence. The more conservative the treatment approach the greater the time required in counseling parents regarding emergency medical care and treatment of the acute seizure. Further trials of efficacy and safety of rectal preparations of anticonvulsants are needed so that FDA approval may be extended to their use by parents in the home. Epilepsy in brain-injured children and the effects of seizures on brain damage and brain function are reviewed by Aicardi J (*Dev Med Child Neur* March 1990; *32*:191-202). - Editor. *Ped Neur Briefs* June 1990.

Recurrence Risk After A Single Seizure
The risk of recurrence after a single, unprovoked, generalized tonic-clonic seizure was assessed in 119 children aged 2 to 16 years, resident in Normandy and examined at the Hopital General, Le Havre and the Hopital Charles Nicolle, Rouen, France. All children in the study had a normal neurological examination and intellectual development, and the EEG showed no focal abnormality. The risk of recurrence at six months was 22%, at one year 28.5%, at three years 32.6% and at eight years 37.7%. Fifty-eight percent of recurrences occurred within the first six months and 87% within the first two years. The risk of recurrence after two years in patients with EEGs showing spikes or spike-and-wave was 40% and this risk was not significantly different from that for 51 patients with normal EEGs (29%).

However, 73% of patients with abnormal EEGs were receiving treatment compared to 52% of those with normal EEGs. Phenobarbital was prescribed for 46 patients, sodium valproate 19, carbamazepine 4, phenytoin 1, trimethadione 1, and phenobarbital and clonazepam 2. Drug compliance was not evaluated. When the seizure lasted less than five minutes, the risk of recurrence at two years was 25% compared with 42% for those whose seizures lasted longer than five minutes. Age at onset of the initial seizure did not affect the risk of recurrence. Seizure duration and history of epilepsy in the family were not significant risk factors. In summary, single, short duration, convulsive seizures of the grand mal type should not be systematically treated, especially when clinical examination and EEG findings are normal. A diagnosis of epilepsy will be confirmed or disproved within two years of follow-up: if seizures do recur they usually do so within that period. A history of febrile seizures does not increase the risk of recurrence of a single unprovoked grand mal seizure. (Boulloche J et al. Risk of recurrence after a single, unprovoked, generalized tonic-clonic seizure. *Dev Med Child Neurol* October 1989; *31*:626-663).

> COMMENT. Seizures that are focal or associated with mental retardation or brain damage have a higher risk of recurrence and warrant prophylactic treatment with anticonvulsant drugs. A single unprovoked generalized tonic-clonic seizure does not require treatment but medication should be commenced if these seizures recur. In the present study, the cumulative risk of recurrence for treated patients was lower than that of untreated patients but the difference was not significant. One might speculate that the difference may have been significant if compliance with therapy had been monitored and adequate therapeutic drug levels maintained. - Editor. *Ped Neur Briefs* January 1990.

Epidemiology Of Epilepsy In Japan

All children 3 years of age on January 1, 1975 in Fuchu City, Tokyo, a total of 17,044 of a population of 182,000, were examined neurologically at the Health Center and the Dept of Genetics, Tokyo Metropolitan Institute for Neurosciences, Tokyo, Japan. Those with a history of seizures were compared with a randomly selected group of healthy children from the same population. The incidence of epilepsy (recurrent non-febrile seizures) up to age 3 yrs was .43% and that of a single nonfebrile seizure was .47%. Febrile convulsions had occurred in 8.2%. Epilepsy developed in 50% of children with single non-febrile seizures, in 2% of those with febrile convulsions, .2% of healthy 3-yr-old children, and in 2% of potential seizure patients with spike EEG abnormalities observed at 3 years of age. The author stresses identification and treatment of patients with potential seizure disorders. (Tsuboi T. Prevalence and incidence of epilepsy in Tokyo. *Epilepsia* March/April 1988; *29*:103-110).

COMMENT. This study provides detailed statistics of the incidence of febrile convulsions, nonfebrile seizures and epilepsy in Japan. Of particular interest are the relatively high frequency of febrile convulsions in Japan c.f. US and Europe (8.2 v 3%), and the low incidence of epilepsy among potential healthy carriers with EEG seizure activity in the general population (2%). Methods for the preven-tion of clinical seizures in potentially epileptic subjects were not addressed although this goal was proposed. Most authorities would not advocate the use of long-term pro-phylactic anticonvulsant medication in healthy children with abnormal EEGs or in those with a history of one febrile convulsion uncomplicated by nonfebrile seizures.

Two epidemiological studies of epilepsy in India reported in the same issue of Epilepsia showed prevalence rates of .3-.4% for children and adolescent age groups. Males predominated and mental retardation and cerebral palsy were the most frequently associated conditions. - Editor. *Ped Neur Briefs* April 1988.

Maternal Epilepsy And Child's IQ

The intelligence of 116 children of epileptic mothers enrolled in a prospective study during pregnancy was compared with that of 104 control children at the Univ of Helsinki and Children's Castle Hospital, Helsinki, Finland. The prevalence of mental deficiency was 1.4% in the study group and zero in controls. Mean IQ's at 5-1/2 yr examinations were significantly lower in the study group compared to controls but showed no relation to exposure to antiepileptic drugs or to brief maternal convulsions. Among phenytoin-exposed children, 1 of 103 (1%) was mentally retarded and 1 had borderline IQ, short stature, microcephaly, and 8 minor anomalies. Multiple minor anomalies were associated with a lower mean IQ in both study and control groups. Hypertelorism and digital hypoplasia, typical of the fetal hydantoin syndrome, did not predict a poor intellect. (Gaily E et al. Intelligence of children of epileptic mothers. *J Pediat* Oct 1988; *113*:677-684).

COMMENT. This study shows a slight increase in prevalence of mental deficiency among children of epileptic mothers compared with the general population. Exposure to nontoxic levels of phenytoin as monotherapy or in combination with one other antiepileptic drug did not impair IQ. These results are contrary to those of Hanson et al (*J Pediat* 1976; *89*:662) who found that intrauterine exposure to phenytoin was a major risk factor for mental subnormality in affected children. - Editor. *Ped Neur Briefs* October 1988.

Seizures In Offspring Of Epileptic Parents

The risks of unprovoked seizures in the offspring of parents with generalized versus partial epilepsies among 687 patients born in Rochester, MN between 1922 and 1985 and followed for the occurrence of seizures through 1986 are reported from the Division of Epidemiology and Department of Neurology, Columbia University, New York, the University of Texas Health Sciences Center, Houston, and the Section of Clinical

Epidemiology, Mayo Clinic, Rochester, MN. The incidence of recurrent unprovoked seizures in the total group was 3.3% and three times that expected. The incidence was approximately the same in the offspring of parents with either generalized or partial seizures. For parents with absence generalized seizures the incidence of epilepsy among offspring was substantially higher than that for offspring of parents with other types of generalized onset seizures and was three times as high as for partial cases. The early age of onset and idiopathic nature of the epilepsy explained only in part the higher incidence in offspring of absence cases. These offspring had a higher risk not only for absence seizures but for other seizures types as well, suggesting that absence epilepsy is not genetically distinct from other seizure types of epilepsy. For offspring of parents in the largest subset of generalized seizures (primary generalized tonic-clonic convulsions) there was no evidence of higher risk than for offspring of parents with partial seizures. (Ottman R et al. Seizure risk in offspring of parents with generalized versus partial epilepsy. *Epilepsia* March-April 1989; *30*:157-161).

COMMENT. These findings contrast with the widely held assumption that partial epilepsies are less likely than generalized epilepsies to be genetic. The dramatically elevated risks in offspring of probands with absence seizures agreed with the findings of Metrakos and Metrakos (1961). However, in the present study, the increased risk in offspring of absence cases was not restricted to absence seizures, but was observed in all seizure types. The authors suggest that the data are more consistent with a common genetic basis for all seizure types, with absence cases having a higher genetic liability than other cases, leading to a higher risk for all seizure types in their relatives. This study did not take into account the etiology of seizures and febrile convulsions were not included. - Editor. *Ped Neur Briefs* March 1989.

Cognitive Dyfunction In
Children Of Epileptic Mothers

Specific cognitive abilities and motor function were investigated at 5-1/2 years in 104 children of epileptic mothers and in 105 control children with normal intelligence at the Child Neurology Department, Children's Castle Hospital, Lastenlinnantie, Helsinki, Finland. The children of the epileptic mothers had been exposed to antiepileptic drugs during pregnancy, most commonly phenytoin (69%), and maternal seizures had occurred during pregnancy in 52%. The WPPSI and ITPA test results showed that the children of epileptic mothers had impaired visuospatial and auditory phonemic skills whereas motor development was normal. Increased risk was associated with maternal partial seizures, with seizures occurring during pregnancy, and with low paternal education, but not with exposure to antiepileptic drugs. The mechanisms suggested include subtle brain damage secondary to fetal asphyxia during the mother's convulsions, genetically transmitted brain abnormalities, and psychosocial disadvantage. Most mothers in the study had relatively low anticonvulsant drug levels during pregnancy and polytherapy was extremely rare. (Gaily E et al. Specific cognitive dysfunction in children with epileptic mothers. *Dev Med Child Neur* May 1990; *32*:403-414)

COMMENT. The mechanisms by which maternal epilepsy might affect a child's intellectual development may include a teratogenic effect of antiepileptic drugs, fetal brain damage or maldevelopment induced by maternal convulsions, or hereditary causes. In this study the prevalence of mental deficiency (1.4%) and borderline intelligence (1.7%) was not significantly higher than in the general population but specific cognitive dysfunctions were uncovered in children of epileptic mothers. - Editor. *Ped Neur Briefs* June 1990.

Movement Of X Chromosome In Epileptic Cortex

Chronic uncontrolled seizure activity was linked to specific positional changes of the X chromosome in neurons of cortical seizure foci from both male and female patients at Yale University School of Medicine, New Haven, CT. In normal female neurons, X homologs were typically either on the nucleolus or on the nuclear membrane, whereas one or both X chromosome signals were moved interiorly in seizure foci of 2 representative female patients. There was a gradient of X positional changes spreading from the seizure focus toward normal surrounding cortex. In seizure foci there was a decrease of 25% in membrane plus nucleolar signal neurons compared to more normal specimens, and a concomitant increase of 27% of cells with interior signals in seizure foci. These X chromosome movements were limited to epileptic foci and were not simply the consequence of generalized seizure activity. (Borden J, Manuelidis L. Movement of the X chromosome in epilepsy. *Science* Dec 23, 1988; *242*:1687-1691).

> COMMENT. Specifically altered nuclear patterns may become established and create the genetic memory for intractable seizures. These changes in chromosome arrangements may be caused by various lesions, including trauma, developmental abnormalities, and toxic factors. These studies provide a new approach to the mechanism of kindling, based on structural rearrangements of the X chromosome rather than functional alterations of the neuronal membrane and synapses. - Editor. *Ped Neur Briefs* January 1989.

EPILEPSY, BEHAVIOR AND LEARNING

Behavioral Complications Of Frontal Lobe Seizures

A 13-yr-old girl with marked behavioral and selective cognitive deficits associated with partial complex seizures of frontal lobe origin is reported from the Depts of Neurology, Psychiatry and Pediatrics, Harbor-UCLA Medical Center, 1000 W Carson St, Torrance, CA. Behavioral deterioration consisting of inattention, sexual disinhibition, loss of concern for personal hygiene, physical and verbal aggression and periodic incoherent and bizarre speech, was concurrent with a 6-week history of seizures manifested by turning to the right, staring, picking at her clothes, shaking and urinary incontinence. An EEG showed periodic bursts of 2-1/2 Hz spike and slow wave complexes originating in the left frontal lobe. CT and MRI of the brain were normal. Neuropsychological testing for frontal lobe dysfunction (finger tapping, digit span, trailmaking, WISC-R mazes, Stroop test) demonstrated deficits in attention, response inhibition, alteration between tasks, maze solving, word generation and motor functioning. Overall intelligence, basic language skills, visual perception, constructional ability and remote memory were spared. Seizures were controlled, the EEG became normal, and the cognitive and behavioral deficits disappeared within one month after treatment with carbamazepine. On re-examination, the patient was composed, quiet and well groomed, and the content of her speech was appropriate, including memory and expression of shame regarding her behavior during preceding months. (Boone KB et al. Neuropsychological and behavioral abnormalities in an adolescent with frontal lobe seizures. *Neurology* April 1988; *38*:583-586).

COMMENT. This case-report suggests that frontal lobe seizures and interictal dysfunction may be associated with acute psychiatric disturbance in children. Whereas this patient exhibited remarkable reversible behavioral and cognitive defects without an underlying structural cerebral lesion, in some adults with destructive and selective frontal lobe pathology neuropsychological testing has failed to demonstrate behavioral deficits. It is possible that the seizure activity in the present case may have spread to involve areas in addition to the frontal lobe. - Editor. *Ped Neur Briefs* April 1988.

Epilepsy In Autism

Epilepsy occurred in 27% (14/52) of children with autism under 10 years of age in a population-based study in the Dept of Child and Adolescent Psychiatry and Pediatrics, University of Goteborg, Sweden. Psychomotor seizure patterns in 71% of those with epilepsy were associate with temporal lobe EEG focal abnormalities. Infantile spasms and hypsarrhythmia occurred in 3 cases. Organic brain factors included perinatal asphyxia or hemorrhage, progressive encephalopathy, fragile X syndrome and tuberous sclerosis. The authors conclude that autistic behavior and epilepsy probably reflect underlying brain dysfunction and are not causally related. (Olsson I et al. Epilepsy in autism and autistic-like conditions. A population-based study. *Arch Neurol* June 1988; 45:666-668).

COMMENT. The association of autistic behavior with epilepsy and mental retardation in children is not uncommon. Some have a previous history of infantile spasms caused by tuberous sclerosis. In this group of cases the epilepsy is primary and the autism secondary. The authors of the above study correctly distinguish between these cases referred to as autistic-like conditions and those in whom infantile autism is primary and precedes the development of epilepsy.

Adults with left-sided epileptogenic temporal lobe lesions may be at a greater risk of developing schizophrenic-like psychoses than those with right-sided lesions (Sherwin I. *Acta Psychiatr Scand* 1984; *69* (Suppl 313):92). A review of the EEG findings in children with autism and epilepsy in the above study showed that of 10 with temporal lobe foci, 5 were left-sided, 4 right-sided and 1 bilateral. Of the 5 with left-sided foci, 3 had infantile autism and 2 were classified as autistic-like in behavior. - Editor. *Ped Neur Briefs* June 1988.

Suicide Attempts In Epileptics

Causative factors for the high epileptic suicide rate are reported from the Departments of Neurology, University Hospitals of Cleveland and the Johns Hopkins University, Baltimore, MD. Of 711 patients hospitalized for a suicide attempt by drug overdose, 22 patients had idiopathic epilepsy. Attempted suicide was coincident with increased seizure activity only in one epileptic patient. When matched by age, sex, and race with 44 nonepileptic controls, the patients with epilepsy had more borderline personality disorders with multiple impulsive suicide attempts, more psychotic disturbances, including hallucinations, fewer adjustment disorders, and a comparable frequency of depression. Suicide attempts in epileptics were primarily associated with interictal psychopathologic factors, such as borderline personality disorder and psychosis, rather than with specific psychosocial stressors, seizure variables, or anticonvulsant medications. (Mendez MF et al. Causative factors for suicide attempts by overdose in epileptics. *Arch Neurol* October 1989; *46*:1065-1068).

COMMENT. Epilepsy is associated with increased suicidal behavior and the risk of completed suicide among patients with epilepsy is four or five times greater than among nonepileptic patients. Patients with complex partial seizures have a particularly high risk. Of the 22 patients reported in this study with suicide attempts, five were under 20 years of age and the median age was 28 years. The ready access of anticonvulsant drugs facilitates impulsive suicide attempts in patients with epilepsy. - Editor. *Ped Neur Briefs* November 1989.

Effects Of Brief Seizures On Learning

The effects of frequent brief seizures on learning, memory, and behavior in the young animal were studied at the Department of Neurology, Children's Hospital, Harvard Medical School, Boston, MA; and Veterans Administration Medical Center and Medical College of Georgia, Augusta, GA.

Three groups of animals were used: Group 1 immature genetically epilepsy prone rats (GEPRs) subjected to 66 audiogenic stimulations; Group 2 GEPR littermates handled and placed in the sound chamber but not stimulated; Group 3 genetically epilepsy resistant rats (GERRs) who received audiogenic stimulations but had no seizures. Tests for learning, memory and behavior, using the T-maze, water maze, open field activity test, home cage intruder test and handling test, were investigated after three weeks of stimulations. Compared with GERRs and control GEPRs, experimental GEPRs performed less well in the T-maze and water maze tests of learning and memory. They also differed in behavior and activity level. The study demonstrated that frequent brief seizures in immature animals results in significant detrimental changes in learning, memory, activity level, and behavior. (Holmes GL et al. Effects of seizures on learning, memory, and behavior in the genetically epilepsy-prone rat. *Ann Neurol* Jan 1990; *27*:24-32).

COMMENT. Some children with poorly controlled epilepsy have a progressive decline of IQ on serial intelligence tests (Bourgeois BF et al. *Ann Neurol* 1983; *14*:438-444 and Rodin EA et al. *Dev Med Child Neurol* 1986; *28*:25-33). The cause of this epileptic dementia in children is not always clearly understood. The underlying disease process may be degenerative in nature and sometimes the adverse side effects of anticonvulsant medications have been implicated. In the present paper the potential cognitive depressant effects of repeated generalized seizures are emphasized and age of onset of the seizure disorder may be a critical factor in determining whether deficits in learning and behavior occur. - Editor. *Ped Neur Briefs* March 1990.

Prolonged Postictal Encephalopathy

Prolonged postictal confusion lasting from four to ten days is reported in 11 patients (ages 7-1/2 to 40 years) from the Epilepsy Research Center, Department of Neurology, University of Minnesota and MINCEP Epilepsy Care, P.A., Minneapolis. Age of seizure onset averaged 10.7 years. The remote etiology was meningitis in 5, trauma 2, genetic 1, and birth anoxia 1. Mild to borderline mental retardation was present in nine and nine had nonspecific structural abnormalities on MRI or CT, including mild cortical atrophy and mild ventricular enlargement. Previous episodes of status epilepticus had occurred in ten. The encephalopathy always occurred after a cluster of seizures which were generalized tonic-clonic in eight, complex partial in two, and atypical absence in one. The patient with absence seizures, a girl aged 7-1/2, would regress into what mother described as an "infantile stage" after each cluster of seizures lasting a period of a week. During this stage which persisted seven to ten days she would not be able to talk, sit, walk, feed herself, or even chew food placed in her mouth. She was awake and would respond very slowly. Repeated loads of diazepam, valproic acid, ethosuximide, and methsuximide did not result in any clinical or EEG improvement. Metabolic drug toxicity as well as ongoing nonconvulsive status was ruled out as the cause of the confusional state. (Biton V et al. Prolonged postictal encephalopathy. *Neurology* June 1990; *40*:963-966).

COMMENT. This study demonstrates the adverse effects of repetitive seizures on the state of consciousness and mentation, particularly in patients who have previously experienced status epilepticus. The lack of response of this confusional state to anticonvulsant drugs is documented but the details of treatment and serum levels of anticonvulsant medications are not provided. This report suggests that patients who have a tendency to clusters of seizures, mild cerebral atrophy, a history of status epilepticus, and mild to borderline intellectual retardation, are particularly vulnerable to develop transient encephalopathy and are candidates for vigorous and regularly monitored anticonvulsant treatment. - Editor. *Ped Neur Briefs* June 1990.

TREATMENT OF EPILEPSY

Phenacemide In Complex Partial Seizures

The anticonvulsant phenacemide (phenylacetylurea), discarded for 30 years because of serious toxicity, has been resurrected and used in the treatment of 13 children with refractory complex seizures at Loyola University, Maywood, and Christ Hospital, Oak Lawn, IL. Twelve responded, nine were seizure-free for 2-12 months, and one developed nausea and vomiting necessitating drug withdrawal. Other side-effects included aggressive behavior in 1, drowsiness (2), ataxia (2), headache (1), and elevated SGPT and GGT in one child aged 3 years with tuberous sclerosis. A liquid chromatography assay developed to determine plasma phenacemide concentrations showed a linear relationship between drug peak height and plasma concentration over a range of 0-150 mcg/ml. After a single oral dose the peak concentration in a 16 year old patient was at 1 to 2 hours and in a 40 year old volunteer, at 5 hours. Phenacemide half-life in the adult was 25 hours and was estimated at 25 and 22 hours in two children. A twice-daily dosage regimen seemed appropriate. Therapeutic levels ranged from 16-75 mcg/ml (median, 52 mcg/ml). (Coker SB, Holmes EW, Egel RT. Phenacemide therapy of complex partial epilepsy in children: Determination of plasma drug concentrations. *Neurology* 1987; *37*:1861-1866).

COMMENT. The authors rationalize their reevaluation of phenacemide as monotherapy, stating that the majority of phenacemide-related deaths from liver failure or aplastic anemia had occurred in adults receiving polytherapy. After 30 years of dormancy, it is surprising that the drug had not been withdrawn from the market, having regard to its well established toxicity. The efficacy of phenacemide in partial complex (temporal-lobe) seizures has been demonstrated repeatedly in earlier studies and reconfirmed in this reevaluation. Fortunately, none developed liver failure but one patient taking 4 gm daily had symptoms of nausea and vomiting suggestive of liver involvement and sufficient to warrant phenacemide withdrawal. Another showed a behavior or personality disorder, a common and troublesome side effect in previous trials. Is the reactivation of this drug necessary or advisable? - Editor. *Ped Neur Briefs* December 1987.

Rectal Anticonvulsant Therapy

The use of rectally administered antiepileptic drugs (AEDs) is reviewed by experts from the College of Pharmacy and Division of Pediatric Neurology, University of Minnesota, Minneapolis, MN. Paraldehyde, diazepam, secobarbital, and valproic acid (VPA) in solution are used when a rapid effect is desired for termination of prolonged or serious seizures. VPA, lorazepam, carbamazepine, and phenytoin in suspension or suppository can be used in maintenance therapy. The authors recommended the following rectal doses: *paraldehyde* 0.3 ml/kg diluted with an equal volume of mineral oil in glass, not plastic, syringe and rubber tube; *diazepam* 0.5 mg/kg as parenteral solution or commercially available rectal preparation in Europe; *valproic acid* 6-15 mg/kg as oral solution diluted with equal volume of water; *clorazepam* 0.05-0.1 mg/kg as parenteral solution; *clonazepam* 0.02-0.1 mg/kg as suspension; *secobarbital* 5 mg/kg as parenteral solution or suppository; and *carbamazepine* 5 mg/kg as oral suspension diluted with equal volume of water as maintenance therapy only. Experience with rectal phenobarbital and phenytoin is limited. (Graves NM, Kriel RL. Rectal administration of antiepileptic drugs in children. *Pediatr Neurol* 1987; 3:321-326).

COMMENT. This practical and informative article emphasizes the usefulness of the rectal route of administration of antiepileptic drugs in children. The method is particularly applicable for use in the home by parents of children with acute recurrences of refractory epilepsies and as prophylaxis for febrile seizures at times of fever. Diazepam is the agent most commonly employed, and a commercial rectal preparation similar to those available in Europe would be welcome in the US. - Editor. *Ped Neur Briefs* January 1988.

Flunarizine In Alternating Hemiplegia

The effects of flunarizine, a calcium-entry blocker, in alternating hemiplegia are reported in the first 12 children included in an international study coordinated from the Dept Pediatrics, University Hospital Gasthuisberg, B-3000 Leuven, Belgium. Cases from France, Italy, Portugal, Spain and Scotland meeting the following diagnostic criteria were included: onset before 18 months, repeated attacks at least 2 per month involving both sides of the body, associated oculomotor abnormalities and autonomic disturbances, and mental and neurological abnormalities. A family history of migraine was present in half the patients. Various anticonvulsants used in 10 patients were without benefit. The dose of flunarizine was 5 mg daily for 4 months. During the open study period, all but one patient had a reduction in frequency and/or duration and severity of attacks, and mental development improved in several. In a subsequent double-blind placebo-controlled withdrawal study lasting another 4 months, 6 patients received placebo, 3 continued flunarizine therapy, and 3 declined inclusion in the controlled trial. Deterioration occurred in 5 of the 6 placebo patients and 2 of the 3 flunarizine treated patients. Relapses were thought to be precipitated by parental anxiety occasioned by the double-blind protocol. Flunarizine was well tolerated except for somnolence and weight gain. The author is soliciting further investigators and patients for a larger, more definitive study. (Casaer P et al. Flunarizine in alternating hemiplegia in childhood. An international study in 12 children. *Neuropediatrics* 1987; *18*:191-195).

COMMENT. The failure of conventional anticonvulsant drugs in the treatment of alternating hemiplegia (AH) is well known. Propranolol (Inderal), of reputed benefit in childhood migraine, was without effect in 2 patients with AH followed personally, and flunarizine treatment observed in a 3-year-old boy had only an equivocal and partial effect.

The pathogenesis of alternating hemiplegia is unknown although a vascular mechanism related to migraine is probable. Calcium channel antagonists such as flunarizine, effective in the treatment of migraine, are vasodilators and prevent the influx of extracellular calcium into vascular smooth muscle (Peroutka SJ. *Headache* 1983; 23:278). The response of AH to flunarizine is certainly not proven but the results of these preliminary studies are promising. - Editor. *Ped Neur Briefs* January 1988.

Vigabatrin In Drug-Resistant Epilepsy

A double-blind, placebo-controlled, crossover study of oral Vigabatrin (2-3 g/d) as add-on therapy for 31 patients with drug-resistant seizures is reported from the Neurological Clinic, Univ of Bologna School of Med, Italy. Both children and adults were included. Those with complex partial seizures and temporal spikes responded whereas patients with mixed seizure types and multifocal EEG abnormalities were not benefitted. Drowsiness was the most frequent side-effect and concomitant phenytoin serum concentrations fell during Vigabatrin treatment. (Tassinari CA et al. Double-blind study of Vigabatrin in the treatment of drug-resistant epilepsy. *Arch Neurol* 1987; 44:907-910).

COMMENT. Vigabatrin (y-vinyl GABA) is an inhibitor of y-aminobutyric acid (GABA)-transaminase. Increases in CNS-GABA concentrations in laboratory animals and CSF-GABA in patients treated with Vigabatrin have been associated with anticonvulsant activity. Several laboratory and clinical reports of this drug have appeared in the literature in the past decade, mostly with favorable results in patients with complex partial seizures (see Browne TR et al. *Neurology* 1987; 37:184. Rimmer EM, Richens A. *Lancet* 1984; 1:189).

The finding of microvacuoles in the white matter of the CNS of laboratory animals has not been duplicated in autopsy reports on patients who have died from causes independent of Vigabatrin therapy or in CT scans but has prompted the FDA to put a hold on clinical trials in the USA since 1983. At present, 31 adult patients with complex partial seizures are in the ongoing collaborative study but no patient may be added (R. Miketta, M.D., Merrell Dow Pharmaceuticals, personal communication). Phase III trials are continuing in other countries and registration of the drug is expected in France in 1988. Side effects in adults treated with Vigabatrin for complex partial seizures have included drowsiness, ataxia, dizziness, headache and skin rash. Levels of SGPT have shown decreases, as might be expected, but no liver or blood disorders have been reported.

Every anticonvulsant drug, both old and new, has its problems, and clinical trials are fraught with potential hazards (e.g. liver fatalities with valproate, leukopenia with carbamazepine, erytheme multiforme and lymphoma with phenytoin, and learning disorders with barbiturates). Hopefully, the Vigabatrin-induced CNS vacuoles in animals will prove to be a species specific effect but close monitoring in man is required. - Editor. *Ped Neur Briefs* October 1987.

Diazepam Sensitivity And Intractable Seizures

The benzodiazepine sensitivity test, an intravenous bolus of diazepam (0.2 mg/kg) under EEG control, was used in 40 children with intractable seizure disorders treated in the Paediatric Neurology Service and the Dept Neurology and Clinical Neurophysiology, Royal Hospital for Sick Children, Edinburgh. The etiology and clinical patterns of seizures were heterogeneous, 50% symptomatic of various causes and 63% with a mixed seizure disorder, atypical absences, myoclonic and drop or atonic seizures predominating. EEG abnormalities were severe and persistent. Many different drugs had been used but 29 (73%) patients had not received benzodiazepines.

A positive effect, defined as abolition of abnormal EEG activity often with appearance of fast activity, was obtained in 53% of the total group. The response was negative in 6 of 7 patients in non-convulsive status and in 7 of 9 patients with Lennox Gastaut syndrome, 2 showing exacerbations of EEG paroxysms and clinical seizures. All 5 with focal spikes responded whereas only 3 of 6 with hypsarrhythmia showed improvement in the EEG.

Of 32 patients treated subsequently with long-term oral benzodiazepines, 21 (66%) showed improvement in seizure control. Among those benefitted, the diazepam sensitivity test had been positive in 76%. Of 11 patients unresponsive to oral benzodiazepines, only 36% had shown a positive sensitivity test. The authors conclude that the test is of value in long-term management of intractable childhood seizures but emphasize the variability and unpredictability of the response to oral benzodiazepines. (Livingston JH et al. Benzodiazepine sensitivity testing in the management of intractable seizure disorders in childhood. *Electroencephalography and Clin Neurophysiol* 1987; *67*:197-203).

COMMENT. This practical study confirms the value of the EEG and intravenous drug sensitivity in the management of childhood epilepsy but with some limitations. It contradicts the recommended choice of benzodiazepines in the treatment of non-convulsive status (Gastaut H. *Adv Neurol* 1983; *34*:15-36). Editorial, *Lancet* 1987; 1:958). Development of tolerance is the greatest limitation to the long-term use of benzodiazepines in myoclonic and other epilepsies, occurring in 80% of 36 children treated with nitrazepam at Children's Memorial Hosp, Chicago (Millichap JG, Ortiz W. *Amer J Dis Child* 1966; *112*:242). - Editor. *Ped Neur Briefs* October 1987.

Causes Of Antiepileptic Treatment Failure

The Veterans Administration Epilepsy Cooperative Study Group (Regional Epilepsy Center, VA Med Cntr, 4500 S Lancaster Rd, Dallas, TX) have evaluated monotherapy with carbamazepine, phenobarbital, phenytoin, and primidone in a total of 622 patients with previously untreated partial seizures, with particular attention to seizure frequency, neurotoxicity, and systemic toxicity. These 3 factors contributed equally to failure in the first 6 months but systemic toxicity, primarily skin rash, played a relatively minor role in drug failure after that time interval, with the same pattern seen for all drugs studied. After 6 months, failure is determined by seizure frequency and neurotoxicity and is relatively low. A failure rate of 25.3 patients/month during the first 6 months was approximately 6.5 times that during the following 18 months (3.9 patients/month). The first 24 months were critical for successful control since after that time the failure rate falls rapidly to 0.83 patients/month during a 12 month period follow-up. (Homan RW, Miller MS. Causes of treatment failure with antiepileptic drugs vary over time. *Neurology* 1987; *37*:1620-1623).

COMMENT. Such studies would be difficult to duplicate in children although similar results might be expected. That dermatologic, hypersensitivity reactions should occur primarily during the first few months of a new antiepileptic drug (AED) treatment is not surprising. It is likely that the majority would have developed within the first 2 weeks. The incidence of skin rash in the first 6 months of this study involving only adults was 6% and similar to that encountered in children taking phenytoin but higher than that usually reported for carbamazepine (3 to 5%), phenobarbital (1 to 2%), and primidone (rare). AED hypersensitivity reactions are generally more prominent in young children than in adults (e.g. phenytoin, valproate). - Editor. *Ped Neur Briefs* October 1987.

Corn Oil Ketogenic Diet

The successful substitution of corn oil for MCT oil in 6 children treated with the ketogenic diet for intractable seizures is reported from the Depts of Pediatrics, Neurology and Psychiatry, University of Arkansas for Medical Sciences and Arkansas Children's Hospital, 804 Wolfe St., Little Rock, AR. Seizure types were mixed in all 6 patients, absence in 5, minor motor in 4, myoclonic in 3, and complex partial and generalized tonic-clonic in 1. All had been controlled with MCT oil diets but corn oil has the major advantages of being less expensive, more readily available without prescription, and better tolerated. Anticonvulsants were reduced in 5 patients and eliminated in 3, without deterioration in seizure control. (Woody RC et al. Corn oil ketogenic diet for children with intractable seizures. *J Child Neurol* Jan 1988; *3*:21-24).

> COMMENT. The medium chain triglyceride (MCT) oil was advocated by Huttenlocher et al (*Neurology* 1971; *21*:1097) as a substitute for dietary fats in the ketogenic diet. MCT's are more ketogenic and less restrictive of carbohydrates, they are more rapidly absorbed than dietary fat and may induce ketosis more quickly. A disadvantage of the MCT diet is the frequency of gastrointestinal side-effects, many patients suffering from bulky, loose stools, diarrhea, vomiting, and abdominal pain. Perhaps the superiority and availability of corn oil will encourage a renewed interest in the ketogenic diet for the treatment of refractory seizures in children. - Editor. *Ped Neur Briefs* April 1988.

Ketogenic Diets In Epilepsy

The classical ketogenic diet, the medium chain triglyceride (MCT) diet, and a modified MCT diet were used in the treatment of 55 children and 4 adults with intractable epilepsy at the University and Clinical Departments of Paediatrics, John Radcliffe Hospital, Oxford, England. The main types of seizures were drop attacks (24), infantile spasms (7), tonic-clonic (6), partial complex (5), primary absence (2), myoclonic absence (2), complex absence (4), and partial simple (4). Forty-five of the patients were under ten years of age. Cooperation and compliance were good and 57 patients completed at least six weeks dietary management and some continued for periods up to four years. Fifty-six had significantly elevated blood ketones bodies and all were reported to have ketonuria. Eighty-one percent showed greater than 50% reduction in seizure frequency. The response was independent of the type of diet used; all three diets appeared to be equally effective in children under the age of 15 years. The high fat diet was found to be palatable by all of the children but the adults found the restrictions unacceptable. Large quantities of MCT oil were also found to be unpalatable by all age groups. No patient found the cream and butter content of the classical diet to be unacceptable. Analysis of variance failed to show any significant difference between the type of seizure and the success of treatment. The EEG showed improvement in 14 cases, 9 while the children were on the MCT diet and 5 while on the classical diet. Nausea, vomiting or abdominal discomfort occurred in approximately one-half the patients taking the MCT diet; drowsiness occurred in 25% at the introduction of the diet. Loss of ketosis occurred during the prodromal phase of an intercurrent illness and was often accompanied by an increase in the frequency of seizures. Two children under one year of age showed no increase in weight, length or head circumference during a six month period on the diet. (Schwartz R H et al. Ketogenic diets in the treatment of epilepsy: Short term clinical effects. *Dev Med Child Neurol* April 1989; *31*:145-151).

Metabolic Effects Of Ketogenic Diets

The results of 24 metabolic profiles performed on 55 epileptic children receiving the classical ketogenic diet, the MCT diet, a modified MCT diet, and normal diets are reported from the University Department of Paediatrics, John Radcliffe Hospital, Oxford, England. The clinical effects of the diets are reported in the previous paper. All three therapeutic diets improved the control of epilepsy and induced a significant increase in the concentrations of blood aceto-acetate and 3-hydroxybutyrate, the greatest elevation being seen in patients on the classical diet (4:1). The pre- and post-prandial blood ketone levels with the classical diet reached a mean of 2.6 mmol/L before breakfast and 4 mmol/L before supper. The three ketogenic diets led to a buildup of ketone body concentrations during the day, reaching maximum levels in the afternoon. This was in contrast to the normal diet which led to slightly higher levels in the morning fasting samples. The Ketostix reagent strip test for urinary ketone bodies reflected these changes and showed higher levels in the afternoon and lower levels in morning samples. Children between 5 and 10 years of age showed the highest blood ketone levels. Levels of blood glycerol were highest while fasting and lowest after meals. Despite the high fat content of the diets none of the concentrations of plasma cholesterol, high density lipoproteins, low density and very low density lipoproteins was significantly raised in any of the therapeutic diet groups. Hypoglycemia was not documented in any patient at any time but blood concentrations of pyruvate were significantly lower. Lower blood levels of alanine occurred on all three diets, the most marked difference being in children receiving the classical diet. The remaining plasma amino acid concentrations tended to be lowest on the classical diet but other than alanine values, the mean concentrations of individual amino acids on the three diets failed to show any significant change. Plasma insulin concentrations corresponded to the blood glucose profiles, showing elevations after each meal, the highest levels occurring with the normal and modified MCT diet and the lowest responses occurring with the classical ketogenic diet. The mean plasma concentrations of sodium, potassium, chloride and bicarbonate did not differ significantly between the four diets, and plasma urea, creatinine, calcium, phosphate, total protein, albumin and bilirubin levels were also similar. Plasma uric acid levels were higher on all three ketogenic diets with the highest increase on the MCT diet. The mechanism of action of the ketogenic diet was not determined. (Schwartz R M et al. Metabolic effects of three ketogenic diets in the treatment of severe epilepsy. *Dev Med Child Neurol* April 1989; *31*:152-160).

COMMENT. The above two studies performed at the John Radcliffe Hospital in Oxford and including patients from the pediatric practice of Dr. B.D. Bower have reconfirmed the efficacy of the ketogenic diet in the management of intractable epilepsy in children under 15 years. The classical diet was more acceptable than the MCT diet, being equally effective and better tolerated by most patients. The authors were unable to document any significant changes in blood lipid profiles in the short term study, and the theoretical risks of inducing ischemic heart disease appeared to be outweighed by the benefit of the diets in controlling disabling seizures. With the increasing concern and attention to cholesterol and heart disease, however, this aspect of treatment must be followed carefully and patients with a family history of hypercholesterolemia or ischemic heart disease should probably be excluded from the ketogenic treatment program.

Balance studies are needed to determine the effect of the ketogenic diet on body water and electrolytes. In a balance study performed at the Mayo Clinic (Millichap JG, Jones JD. Acid-base, electrolyte, and amino-acid metabolism in children with petit mal. Etiologic significance and modification by anticonvulsant drugs and the ketogenic diet. *Epilepsia* 1964; 5:239-255) we found a decrease in the blood pH, CO_2, and standard bicarbonate during short ketogenic periods. . The urinary excretion of electrolytes was increased and particularly that of calcium, magnesium and sodium, and the balance of sodium, potassium, calcium, magnesium, phosphorus and nitrogen was negative. The excretion of alphaaminonitrogen was reduced, the excretion of free amino acids was variable, and the level of leucine in the serum was elevated. Fluid intake and urine output were reduced and the fall in body weight was rapid and marked in the initial week of treatment. The total lipids, fatty acid and cholesterol in the serum were increased but not significantly during the ketogenic diet period; they became elevated significantly when carbohy-drates and the antiketogenic diet were reintroduced. The anticonvulsant action of the ketogenic diet was unrelated to diuresis, independent of acidosis and was correlated with an increased urinary excretion and a negative balance of sodi-um and potassium. Calcium supplements are usually advised with the ketogenic diet and in addition magnesium supplements should probably be included. The ketogenic dietary therapy of childhood epilepsies deserves further attention from pediatric neurologists. Assurance of parental and patient cooperation is essential as well as skilled dietetic advice and follow-up. The classical diet is probably more acceptable and has less gastrointestinal side-effects than the MCT diet; a lower and more palatable ratio (3:1) than that used in the Oxford study is usually sufficient and effective. If the diet is continued for long periods, consultation with a specialist in lipid metabolism should be obtained and ultrasound of the liver ordered to exclude fatty infiltration of the liver. (See *Ped Neur Briefs*, April 1988; 2:28). - Editor. *Ped Neur Briefs* April 1989.

Oligoantigenic Diet For Epilepsy And Migraine

A diet low in antigenic items was used to treat 63 children with epilepsy refractory to medication at the Depts of Neurology, Immunology, and Dietetics, The Hospital for Sick Children, Great Ormond Street, and the Institute of Child Health, London, England. The authors had previously reported beneficial effects of the "oligoantigenic" diet in the treatment of migraine (*Lancet* 1983; 2:865) and the hyperkinetic syndrome (*Lancet* 1985; 1:940). The diet consisted of 2 meats (lamb and chicken), 2 carbohydrates (potatoes and rice), 2 fruits (banana and apple), vegetables (cabbage, sprouts, cauliflower, broccoli, cucumber, celery, carrots, parsnips), water, salt, pepper, pure herbs, and calcium and vitamins for 4 weeks. Patients who responded (no seizures or migraine for the last 2 weeks) were reintroduced to essential foods (e.g. milk, cheese, wheat) at the rate of one a week. If symptoms were provoked, soy-based or goat milk products, rye or oats were substituted. Setbacks were avoided by first giving foods least likely to be antigenic (e.g. beef, oats, peaches, or grapes). Of 45 children who had epilepsy with recurrent headaches, abdominal symptoms, or hyperkinetic behavior, 25 had no seizures and 11 had fewer seizures during diet therapy. Foods most likely to provoke seizures when reintroduced were cow milk and cheese, citrus fruits, wheat, tartrazine and benzoic acid food additives, eggs, tomato, pork, and chocolate. In double-blind, placebo-controlled provocation studies introducing cow milk, orange juice, wheat, pork, egg, and benzoate, symptoms recurred in 15 of 16 children, including seizures in 8; none recurred with placebo. The oligoantigenic diet was unsuccessful in the treatment of 18 children who had epilepsy uncomplicated by migraine or hyperkinetic behavior. (Egger J et al. Oligoantigenic diet treatment of children with epilepsy and migraine. *J Pediatr* Jan 1989; *114*:51-58).

> COMMENT. If reproducible and sustained, these results are impressive and deserve further investigation in children with frequently recurrent seizures and headache resistant to anticonvulsant medication. The authors point out that the diets are socially disruptive and may cause malnutrition. In the US, pediatric allergists are not generally impressed with the theory of food hypersensitivity as a cause of neurological disease and their enthusiastic collaboration in studies of this type is not readily available. -Editor. Ped Neur Briefs December 1988.

Vitamin E And Epilepsy

The value of D-alpha-tocopheryl acetate (Vitamin E 400 IU/day) as an adjunct therapy for drug resistant epilepsy is reported from The Hospital for Sick Children and the University of Toronto Faculty of Medicine, Canada. In a randomized, double-blind, placebo-controlled trial, 10 of 12 children aged 6-17 years showed a greater than 60% reduction in seizure frequency whereas none in the control group showed a significant change. One-half of the responders had concomitant

EEG improvements. The study period was 9 months: 3 mo pre-trial, 3 mo double-blind, and 3 mo open-label trial in which patients receiving placebo initially changed to Vitamin E as their own controls. The majority had generalized tonic-clonic seizures and anticonvulsant drug levels showed no significant change during treatment with Vitamin E. Plasma Vitamin E levels increased from 5 to 37 mcM during the treatment phase, the variability dependent on body size. Improvement in seizure control was similar in the open-label phase and no clinically significant alterations of blood counts, SGOT, alkaline phosphatase, and amylase were noted. (Ogunmekan AO, Hwang PA. A randomized, double-blind, placebo-controlled, clinical trial of D-a-tocopheryl acetate (Vitamin E), as add-on therapy, for epilepsy in children. *Epilepsia* Jan/Feb 1989; *30*:84-89).

COMMENT. These authors and others have reported reduced plasma levels of Vitamin E in children taking antiepileptic drugs. Hyperbaric oxygen-induced seizures in rats are prevented by prior administration of Vitamin E. (Jerrett SA et al. *Aerospace Med* 1971; *44*:40-4). The clinical trial reported here and a previous uncontrolled study support the experimental findings in animals that Vitamin E may inhibit the effects of oxidation in brain tissue and act as a membrane stabilizer in epileptic cerebral cortex. Further trials of this adjunctive treatment for refractory epilepsies are certainly warranted. - Editor. *Ped Neur Briefs* December 1988.

Acetazolamide For Partial Seizures

Acetazolamide (Diamox) (AZM) was tried as an adjunct to carbamazepine (CBZ) in 48 refractory partial seizure patients, the majority being adults and only 5 under 12 years of age. The seizures were complex partial in 80%, and idiopathic in 67%. A response measured by a 50% reduction in seizure frequency was obtained in 44% of patients, and side effects - lethargy, paresthesias, anorexia - were generally mild or transient. The duration of response ranged from 3 to 30 months and tolerance was not a major problem. Initial effective doses ranged from 3.8 to 16.5 mg/kg/day (mean, 8.2), and the maximum effective dose used was 22 mg/kg/day. The study was retrospective and uncontrolled, but the authors considered their results impressive and recommend AZM in preference to clonazepam as adjunctive therapy for partial seizures. (Oles KS, Penry JK, et al. Use of acetazolamide as an adjunctive to carbamazepine in refractory partial seizures. *Epilepsia* Jan/Feb 1989; *30*:74-78).

COMMENT. Having been an advocate of acetazolamide for the treatment of refractory childhood seizures for several years (Millichap, JG et al. *J Pharmacol & Exptl Therap* 1955; *115*:251; *Neurology* 1956; 6:552; *Lancet* July 18, 1987; *2*:163), I am happy to see that Dr. Penry and his associates now support its use in adults with partial seizures. AZM had previously been proposed as an alternative agent in the management of petit mal (absence) seizures in children, in menstrual-related seizures, and as an adjunct treatment in other refractory generalized and partial seizures of childhood. Despite the tendency for development of tolerance, which is also shared by the benzodiazepine agents, a review of published work in 1967 showed that AZM was equal in efficacy to ethosuximide and had a lower incidence of side effects (Millichap JG, Aymat F. Treatment and prognosis of petit mal epilepsy. *Pediatr Clin N Am* 1967; *14*:905). At least as an adjunct therapy, the drug deserves wider recognition and confirmation of efficacy by controlled studies. - Editor. *Ped Neur Briefs* January 1989.

Acetazolamide Monotherapy For Myoclonic Epilepsy

Chronic acetazolamide monotherapy controlled generalized tonic-clonic seizures in 14 of 31 patients with juvenile myoclonic epilepsy treated in the Department of Neurology, Columbia University College of Physicians and Surgeons, New York, NY, and the Department of Neurology, Stamford Hospital, Stamford, CT. The daily dose varied from 500 mg in six patients to 1750 mg in one (average 893 mg). Acetazolamide was less effective in controlling myoclonus than in the control of generalized tonic-clonic seizures. Six (43%) of 14 adults with generalized seizures responding to acetazolamide developed renal calculi. (Resor SR, Resor LD. Chronic acetazolamide monotherapy in the treatment of juvenile myoclonic epilepsy. *Neurology* Nov 1990; *40*:1677-1681).

> COMMENT. The frequency of renal calculus as a side effect of chronic acetazolamide therapy in the adults in this study is alarming and sufficient to contraindicate its use. In children, however, renal calculus is a rare side effect of acetazolamide, and this report in adults should not negate the efficacy and clinical use of acetazolamide in the treatment of childhood epilepsy.

In a double blind, placebo controlled trial of acetazolamide in 14 children, ages 6 months to 11 years, an anticonvulsant effect was demonstrated in all patients. Both generalized tonic-clonic and myoclonic seizures were reduced in frequency and in eight patients the maximal reduction in seizures was more than 75%. The control of generalized tonic-clonic seizures was superior to that of the myoclonic type. Acetazolamide monotherapy was used in two patients and additional antiepileptic drugs were continued in the remainder. Tolerance to the effect of acetazolamide shown in eight patients was a greater limiting factor than toxicity in this study. Polyuria and nocturnal enuresis were the only renal side effects and renal calculus did not occur. (Millichap JG. Anticonvulsant action of acetazolamide (Diamox) in children. *Neurology* 1956; *6*:552-559). Acetazolamide treatment of absence seizures reviewed in 620 children and young adults provided complete control in 50% and a 3/4 or greater reduction in an additional 26%. Side effects were reported in 60 (10%) patients and renal calculus occurred in one, a 20 year old adult. (Millichap JG, Aymat F. Treatment and prognosis of petit mal epilepsy. *Ped Clin N Amer* 1967; *14*:905-920). - Editor. *Ped Neur Briefs* November 1990.

Carbamazepine Therapy And Long-Term Prognosis Of Epileptic Children

The long-term prognosis in 90 children with partial or generalized tonic-clonic seizures treated with CBZ has been evaluated in the Department of Pediatrics, Myoto University, Myoto, Japan. Sixty-seven (74%) treated with CBZ monotherapy were seizure free for more than three years. Fifty (56%) had no epileptiform discharge on the follow-up EEG. Patients with mental retardation and a genetic predisposition were more likely to have an abnormal EEG. The incidence of mental retardation was significantly higher in those treated with polytherapy. The prognosis of patients with partial seizures secondarily generalized was less favorable than that of the other patients. Patients without mental retardation more often received CBZ monotherapy and patients with seizures of undetermined etiology more often received polytherapy. The lowest blood level of CBZ for maintenance was 4 mcg/ml and maximum blood levels ranged from 6-12 mcg/ml. Side effects were observed in 20 patients who had drowsiness, 4 ataxia, 2 a rash and 1 had anorexia. The SGOT, SGPT, or both were elevated in 16 patients. Leukopenia between 2,000 and 4,000 occurred in 32 patients. (Okuno T et al. Carbamazepine therapy and long-term prognosis in epilepsy of childhood. *Epilepsia* Jan/Feb 1989; *30*:57-61).

COMMENT. There was no correlation between the type of seizure and the prognosis of the patients in this study. All patients with simple partial seizures and benign epilepsy of children with centrotemporal foci were seizure free for more than one year and the majority were seizure free for more than three years. There was no correlation between a history of febrile convulsions and the prognosis of children with partial or generalized tonic-clonic seizures. Patients with partial seizures secondarily generalized had a less

favorable prognosis than that of other patients. - Editor.
Ped Neur Briefs March 1989.

Mechanisms Of Antiepileptic Drug Action

The mechanisms of antiepileptic drug action are reviewed from the University Pediatric Epilepsy Program and Division of Pediatric Neurology, University of Minnesota Hospital, Minneapolis, MN. Phenytoin, carbamazepine, and valproic acid decrease sustained repetitive firing of action potentials at therapeutic concentrations. Unlike phenytoin and carbamazepine which block the sodium channel, valproic acid blocks sustained repetitive firing by activation of calcium-dependent, potassium conductance. Phenytoin and carbamazepine also have the ability to block post-tetanic potentiation, an effect mediated by blocking the sodium channel. Benzodiazepines and barbiturates enhance GABA-mediated inhibition. Other mechanisms of antiepileptic drug action include inhibition of calcium influx, inhibition of excitatory receptors, or excitation of inhibitory receptors. Glutamate and aspartate are the major excitatory neurotransmitters in the central nervous system and glutamate binds to excitatory receptors, including N-Methyl D-aspartate (NMDA). NMDA receptors which regulate channels permeable to sodium and calcium and are blocked by magnesium play a role in the pathogenesis of some forms of epilepsy. Lamotrigine is an NMDA antagonist with antiepileptic potential. (Talwar D. Mechanisms of antiepileptic drug action. *Pediatr Neurol* Sept/Oct 1990; 6:289-295).

COMMENT. This excellent review of antiepileptic drug action might also include acetazolamide, a carbonic anhydrase inhibitor with an anticonvulsant mechanism that is unique and not shared by the drugs noted in the review. Acetazolamide is a sulfonamide containing a free-SO2NH2 group which is essential for inhibition of carbonic anhydrase. The anticonvulsant effect of acetazolamide is not abolished by nephrectomy and is independent of the action of the drug on the kidney and the resultant metabolic acidosis. The anticonvulsant effect is correlated directly with the inhibition of brain carbonic anhydrase. (Millichap JG et al. Mechanism of the anticonvulsant action of acetazolamide, a carbonic anhydrase inhibitor. *J Pharm Exp Ther* 1955; *115*:251-258). The inhibition of carbonic anhydrase located in glial cells results in CO_2 accumulation and changes in acid-base and electrolyte balance that reduce neuronal excitability. - Editor. *Ped Neur Briefs* November 1990.

Generic Substitutions For Antiepileptic Drugs

The hazards and problems of generic substitutions for antiepileptic drugs are reviewed in a Report of the Therapeutics and Technology Assessment Subcommittee of the American Academy of Neurology (*Neurology* Nov 1990; *40*:1641-1643) and are discussed by Nuwer MR et al (*Neurology* Nov 1990; *40*:1647-1651). According to the present Federal guidelines for manufacturers a generic product may be approved as equivalent to a brand name product even if it produces widely varying bioavailability in some individuals. Implicit in the FDA guidelines is the assumption that a ± 20% change in mean steady-state serum concentration of antiepileptic drugs can be tolerated safely. However, there is no scientific evidence to support this assertion. When substitution of different formulations of an antiepileptic drug occurs, the patient is put at risk of drug intoxication or breakthrough seizures. Generic substitution of drugs such as phenytoin and carbamazepine which have a narrow therapeutic range is especially problematic.

COMMENT. Economic benefits because of lower cost of generic substitutions may be outweighed by the need for more frequent serum concentration determinations and costs of follow-up visits. - Editor. *Ped Neur Briefs* November 1990.

Psychological Treatment Of Epilepsy

Three children, ages 12-15, with frequent refractory seizures were treated by behavioral intervention techniques in the Depts of Medical Rehabilitation and Clinical Neurophysiology, Orebro Medical Center Hospital, Orebro, and Dept of Clinical Psychology, University of Uppsala, Sweden. Seizure types described as myoclonic in pt 1, Jacksonian (pt 2), and minor motor (pt 3) were associated with mental deterioration. Behavioral countermeasures, consisting of tensing of muscle groups and screaming "stop"! (pt 1), massaging the affected limb (pt 2), and fixing eye movements on an object (pt 3), resulted in an immediate reduction in both the seizures and paroxysmal EEG activity in all three cases. Other behavioral strategies, including biofeedback training in awareness of early seizure signals, applied relaxation, and positive reinforcement, were without beneficial effect. The authors propose that countermeasures in the level and speed of arousal may be the mechanism of the treatment intervention. (Dahl J, Melin L, Leissner P. Effects of behavioral intervention on epileptic seizure behavior and paroxysmal activity: a systematic replication of three cases of children with intractable epilepsy. *Epilepsia* March/April 1988; *29*:172-183).

COMMENT. Countermeasures involving sensory stimulation for the treatment of Jacksonian seizures have been advocated for centuries, dating back to the time of Galen and Aretaeus. Brown-Sequard (1872) proposed an encircling blister and Gowers (1901) found that forcing the closed fingers to open or preventing a leg from flexing would break up a motor march (quoted in Lennox WG. *Epilepsy and Related Disorders Vol 1*, 1960, Little, Brown & Co, Boston). The value of these methods in the treatment of other seizure types should be explored further. - Editor. *Ped Neur Briefs* April 1988.

STATUS EPILEPTICUS

Status Epilepticus Prognosis

The mortality and incidence of sequelae of status epilepticus of varying causes were studied in 193 children, age 1 month to 18 years (mean, 5 years), followed for a mean period of 13.2 months in the Division of Pediatric Neurology, Montefiore Medical Center, 111 E. 210th St, Bronx, NY. The cause of the status epilepticus was idiopathic in 46 cases, symptomatic of a previous CNS insult (stroke, head trauma, meningitis, or static encephalopathy) in 45 cases, febrile in 46, acute symptomatic with neurologic insult or systemic metabolic dysfunction in 45, and progressive neurologic with neurodegenerative, malignant, and neurocutaneous syndromes in 11. The mortality and incidence of sequelae following status epilepticus was low and primarily a function of etiology. Seven children (3.6%) died within three months of the episode of status epilepticus. All seven deaths occurred among the 56 children with status epilepticus associated with an acute CNS insult or progressive encephalopathy. The mortality in this group was 12.5%. Only two of the 137 children with unprovoked (idiopathic), remote symptomatic, or febrile status epilepticus sustained neurologic deficit attributable to the status epilepticus. None of the 67 children in the unprovoked or febrile groups studied prospectively had any residual motor or cognitive disability. The difference in the rate of neurologic sequelae between different causes was highly significant (P<.001). A total of 17 (9.1%) children sustained new motor or cognitive deficits following status epilepticus. The incidence of significant sequelae was a function of age; it declined from 29% among infants less than 1 year of age to 11% in children between 1-3 years of age and 6% for children older than 3 years of age (P<.001). The majority of the patients with sequelae were in the acute symptomatic or progressive encephalopathy groups and these consisted of extremely young patients. Within each etiologic group, age did not significantly affect the outcome. The incidence of severe sequelae in the younger age group was related to the more frequent occurrence of acute symptomatic status epilepticus and progressive encephalopathy in that age group. The risk of unprovoked seizures following status epilepticus in 125 surviving children with no history of prior seizures was 30%. The authors concluded that the morbidity of aggressively treated status epilepticus in children in the absence of an acute neurologic insult or progressive neurologic disorder was low. (Maytal J et al. Low morbidity and mortality of status epilepticus in children. *Pediatrics* March 1989; *83*:323-331).

COMMENT. Dr. John M. Freeman of Johns Hopkins Hospital, Baltimore, commented that status epilepticus is "not what we've thought or taught." He asks the question: "Does the morbidity of the treatment of seizures in the emergency room to prevent status epilepticus now exceed the morbidity of the status epilepticus itself? He states that "just as it is not necessary to administer long term anticonvulsant medication to a child after a first seizure, it seems also not necessary to initiate long term therapy when a child's first seizure is status epilepticus."

Many will not agree with this advice, however. An incidence of 30% of unprovoked seizures in children surviving status epilepticus is sufficiently high to warrant long term preventive anticonvulsant therapy. Furthermore, status epilepticus if not treated aggressively is a serious and potentially fatal complication of convulsive disorders. The conclusion to this study and commentary should not permit a diminished respect for the hazards of status epilepticus nor change the accepted methods of treatment with maximally tolerated intravenously administered anticonvulsant therapy. The use of rectal anticonvulsant therapy (see *Ped Neur Briefs* Jan 1988; *2*:7) by parents in selected patients may prevent prolongation of seizure recurrences and avoid the necessity for toxic levels of anticonvulsant drugs for refractory cases. - Editor. *Ped Neur Briefs* March 1989.

Treatment Of Status Epilepticus

Very-high-dose phenobarbital was used for refractory status epilepticus in 50 children treated in the Neurology Division, Children's Hospital, University of Southern California School of Medicine, Los Angeles, CA. Intravenous boluses of 5-20 mg/kg, in increments of 10 mg/kg at 30-60 min intervals, produced a linear increase in drug level of 9.7 mcg/ml over a 24- to 48-hour time span. All patients were intubated prior to treatment. Side-effects, principally depression of respiratory drive and cardiac suppression with hypotension, were influenced more by the severity of the underlying disease and the seizures than by the use of the drug. Phenobarbital controlled seizures in all cases where limits were not imposed on the maximum dose by uncontrollable hypotension. Seven patients died, none during a period of rising drug level. Maximum serum levels ranged from 70-344 mcg/ml. (Crawford TO et al. Very-high-dose phenobarbital for refractory status epilepticus in children. *Neurology* July 1988; *38*:1035-1040).

COMMENT. Phenobarbital in adequate amounts given intravenously is a relatively safe and effective treatment for status epilepticus, but in those cases not responding to initial doses of 10-20 mg/kg, further amounts should be used only after the patient has been intubated. Pressor agent may be required to treat hypotension and assisted ventilation for respiratory depression. When the intravenous administration of drugs is not possible or practical, rectal therapy with paraldehyde, diazepam, or valproic acid has been recommended (see *Ped Neur Briefs* Jan 1988; *2*:7) for termination of prolonged or serial seizures. The treatment of status epilepticus in children with rectal sodium valproate was reported from the Children's Hospital, Birmingham, Alabama (Snead OC, Miles MV. *J Pediat* 1985; *106*:323). A loading dose of 20 mg/kg was effective but a marked rise in serum glumatic oxaloacetic transaminase activity occurred in 3 of 7 patients treated, requiring cessation of valproate therapy. - Editor. *Ped Neur Briefs* July 1988.

ANTICONVULSANT WITHDRAWAL

Seizure Recurrence After Medication Withdrawal

The relapse rate after withdrawal of antiepileptic medication was investigated in 146 children with epilepsy seen at the Dept of Child Neurology, University Hospital, Rotterdam, and Research Unit for Clinical Neurophysiology, Westeinde Hospital, The Hague, The Netherlands. The cumulative probability of remaining seizure-free after a 2 year period of control and normalization of the EEG was 75%. Three-quarters of relapses occurred during the withdrawal period and in the following 2 years. A significantly higher relapse rate was present in girls and with seizures of known etiology. In patients with partial epilepsy, recurrence may be predicted by the presence of focal neurological signs and/or mental retardation, female sex, a positive family history for epilepsy, and polytherapy. In those with primary generalized epilepsy, no predictive factor was uncovered. The recurrence rate did not change between groups of children who were treated for 2, 3, 4, or 5 years before withdrawal was attempted and EEG epileptiform abnormalities had disappeared. (Arts WFM et al. Follow-up of 146 children with epilepsy after withdrawal of antiepileptic therapy. *Epilepsia* May/June 1988; *29*:244-250).

COMMENT. A relapse rate of 25% in this study is similar to that reported previously, and the relatively short treatment period did not appear to increase the risk of recurrence compared to studies requiring a minimum 4 year seizure-free period before discontinuing medicines. However, the absence of EEG epileptiform discharges at the time of drug withdrawal did not improve the outcome by reducing relapse rate compared to studies in which the EEG was not used in decision to withdraw. The results of this investigation emphasize the dangers of antiepileptic drug withdrawal in mentally retarded female patients with neurological deficits. - Editor. *Ped Neur Briefs* July 1988.

Withdrawal Of Antiepileptic Treatment

Investigators at the Division of Neurology and Clinical Neurophysiology, Hospital General de Catalunya, Barcelona, Spain, evaluated the withdrawal of antiepileptic treatment over a one year period in 608 epileptics who had been seizure-free for 5 years. Relapses occurred in 144 (23.7%) of the total group. Among 474 patients in whom details of seizure types were available, relapses occurred in 119 (25.1%) of the total. Idiopathic generalized epilepsies showed a 19.6% relapse rate whereas symptomatic generalized epilepsies relapsed in 37.9% of patients. The lowest relapse rate occurred in patients with absence seizures (9.9%) and the highest rates in those with West (50%) and Lennox-Gastaut (43.7%) syndromes. Grand mal and complex partial seizures recurred in 27.8% and 23.3% of patients, respectively. The majority of relapses were single isolated seizures and occurred in the first year after drug withdrawal.

Risk factors for seizure relapse included 1) delay in initiating anticonvulsant therapy, 2) a symptomatic etiology, 3) mixed seizure types, 4) status epilepticus occurrence, and 5) signs of permanent neurologic damage. (Oller-Daurella L, Oller, F-V L. Suppression of antiepileptic treatment. *Eur Neurol* 1987; *27*:106-113).

COMMENT. The 5 year seizure-free period before drug withdrawal in this study is longer and approximately twice that employed by other investigators. Shinnar S et al (*N Engl J Med* 1985; *313*:976) reported the same 25% relapse rate among 89 children who had been seizure free for only 2 years.

The withdrawal of antiepileptic medication should not be determined by a set seizure-free time-period for all types of epilepsy. Each patient should be evaluated individually, having regard to several factors, including psychological, predictive of potential relapse. Withdrawal is probably contraindicated or likely to be unsuccessful in patients with the following: 1) symptomatic epilepsies with radiological or neurological evidence of structural cerebral defect, 2) mixed seizure types, Lennox-Gastaut syndrome, focal seizures, complex partial with secondary generalized tonic-clonic patterns, 3) history of status epilepticus, and 4) psychological stress, especially in adolescents and young adults.

The prognostic value of the EEG is controversial; these authors and Thurston JH et al (*N Engl J Med* 1982; *306*:831) found a negative correlation whereas others regard the EEG as an important factor, predictive of a good outcome when normal (Shinnar S et al 1985). An abnormal EEG was one of the most significant predictors of relapse after drug withdrawal in the study by Emerson R et al (*N Engl J Med* 1981; *305*:1125). - Editor. *Ped Neur Briefs* August 1987.

Relapse After Antiepileptic Drug Withdrawal

The recurrence risks and predictive factors of relapse after antiepileptic drug (AED) discontinuation in a prospective analysis of 425 children with epilepsy are reported from the Instituto di Neuropsichiatria Infantile, Universita La Sapienza, Via dei Sabelli, Rome, Italy. AEDs were discontinued in children who had not had seizures for at least two years and the follow-up after withdrawal was 1.6 to 12 years, mean 8 years. The relapse rate after drug withdrawal was 12% and the risk was greatest in the first year. Factors related by multivariate analysis to relapse were neurologic abnormalities and organic etiology, mental retardation, seizure type (infantile spasms, absence seizures), and appearance or persistence of EEG abnormalities during the course of the illness and before discontinuation of the drugs. (Matricardi M et al. Outcome after discontinuation of antiepileptic drug therapy in children with epilepsy. *Epilepsia* October 1989; *30*:582-589).

COMMENT. The authors believe that drug withdrawal can be attempted in patients with well controlled idiopathic epilepsy, without signs of brain damage and without persistent EEG abnormalities. They stress that predictive factors must be considered to individualize the risk of relapse for each patient. - Editor. *Ped Neur Briefs* November 1989.

Drug Withdrawal And Relapse Rate For Grand Mal Seizures

The relapse rate when monotherapy was discontinued in 187 children who were seizure-free for three consecutive years was studied at the Leeds General Infirmary and St. James University Hospital, Leeds, England. Of a total group of 640 children with grand mal seizures 30% had become seizure-free on monotherapy. Children were assigned to one of three groups: 1) Normal neurologically and EEG; 2) normal neurologically, abnormal EEG; and 3) abnormal neurologically, including mental retardation with or without abnormal EEG. Relapse occurred in 22 of the total (12%). The relapse rate was the same in groups 1 and 2 and lower in the group 3 patients with abnormal neurologic exams (7.7%). Relapse was related to the age of onset of the seizure disorder; the younger the age of onset the greater the risk of relapse. Of the 22 children who relapsed 67% had a seizure while drug therapy was being withdrawn or within one year of withdrawal, and 86% relapsed within two years. Of 49 children who had EEGs before drug withdrawal the incidence of relapse was 19% in the normal EEG group (37) and 25% in the abnormal group (12) and the difference was not significant. The authors concluded that prewithdrawal EEG for a neurologically normal child is not of prognostic benefit. Since some relapses occurred as late as eight years after withdrawal the authors recommended that follow-up should continue for ten years. (Ehrhardt P, Forsythe WI. Prognosis after grand mal seizures: A study of 187 children with three-year remissions. *Dev Med Child Neurol* October 1989; *31*:633-639).

COMMENT. Recommendations for the withdrawal of anticonvulsant treatment vary, some employing a two year remission, others a three year remission, and some four, five, and even ten year remission before withdrawing treatment. The present paper was more specific than some regarding the relationship of the clinical characteristics of the patients in relation to prognosis. The group of children with neurological dysfunction and mental retardation was small comprising only 13 of the total group and the actual risks of drug withdrawal could not be assessed in this investigation. Of those patients who had EEGs before drug treatment was discontinued, the relapse rate was almost double the relapse rate in the total group. In those with abnormal EEGs the relapse rate was 25%. It would be interesting to know the factors involved in deciding which of these patients required EEGs. This group may deserve further study.

A paper reviewed in the last issue of *Ped Neur Briefs* (1989; *3*:83) showed that the relapse rate after drug withdrawal in 425 children with epilepsy was 12% (the same rate of relapse as in the present study) and the risk was greatest in the first year. Factors related to relapse were neurologic abnormalities and organic etiology, mental retardation, seizure type (infantile spasms, absence seizures), and the appearance or persistence of EEG abnormalities during the course of the illness and before discontinuation of the drugs. The value of the EEG before drug withdrawal as a predictive factor for relapse cannot be discounted. - Editor. *Ped Neur Briefs* January 1990.

ANTICONVULSANT TOXICITY

Side Effects Of Anticonvulsant Monotherapy

The severity and nature of side effects and doses and plasma levels of phenobarbital (PB), primidone (PRM), phenytoin (PHT), carbamazepine (CBZ), and valproate (VPA) were examined in 392 pediatric outpatients at the Division of Paediatric

Neurology, National Hospital "Marques de Valdecilla", University of Cantabria, Santander, Spain. Side effects occurred in 50%, necessitating changes in medication in 18% and withdrawal of drug in 7%. The incidence of side effects was highest with PHT (71%) and lowest with PRM (29%). Serious side effects requiring drug withdrawal occurred with PHT (10%), VPA (8%), and PRM (8%), and less frequently with PB (4%) and CBZ (3%). The best tolerated drug was CBZ, and the least tolerated was PHT. Behavioral side effects were noted most commonly with PB (60%), neurological abnormalities such as ataxia and nystagmus with PHT (22%), digestive tract disorders with VPA (28%), and gingival hyperplasia and hirsutism with PHT (58%). The side effects that most often necessitated changes in treatment were behavioral disorders, especially excitement and hyperactivity, with PB and PRM, hirsutism and gingival hyperplasia with PHT, restless sleep and vomiting with CBZ, and digestive disorders with VPA. Behavioral disorders produced by PB and PRM disappeared in half of the patients if the dosage of the drug was increased. (Herranz JL et al. Clinical side effects of phenobarbital, primidone, phenytoin, carbamazepine, and valproate during monotherapy in children. *Epilepsia* Nov/Dec 1988; *29:*794-804).

COMMENT. A collaborative group for epidemiology of epilepsy reports a 42% incidence of adverse reactions to antiepileptic drugs in 355 patients followed for an average of 11 months in 15 university and hospital centers in Italy (Beghi E et al. Institute for Pharmacological Research (Mario Negri," Milan. *Epilepsia* Nov/Dec 1988; *29:*787). Clinical judgment provided the most valid basis for the evaluation of drug toxicity, and "toxic" plasma drug levels were not correlated with adverse reactions. Of 31 patients with "abnormal" plasma levels, only 1 had an adverse drug reaction. The authors stress the importance of reporting adverse drug reactions as a means of improving the quality of care for the epileptic in routine clinical practice. Physicians are sometimes reluctant to get involved, fearing legal repercussions or lengthy and tedious questionnaires from drug companies. Perhaps a system permitting anonymity might encourage more active physician participation. Addition, more sensitive, methods of monitoring drug treatment should expand the concept of "intolerable" side effects to include subtle psychological and behavioral effects. (Vining EPG et al. *Pediatrics* 1987; *80*:165). - Editor. *Ped Neur Briefs* January 1989.

Fetal Hydantoin Syndrome

In a prospective study of 19 pregnancies monitored by amniocentesis at the Center for Human Genetics and the Meyer Rehabilitation Institute, University of Nebraska, Omaha, an adverse outcome was predicted for four fetuses on the basis of low epoxide hydrolase activity (<30% of standard). The mothers were receiving phenytoin monotherapy and the infants had clinical characteristics of the fetal hydantoin syndrome. Fifteen fetuses with enzyme activity above 30% of the standard had no features of the syndrome. The authors suggest that this enzymatic biomarker may be useful in the prediction of infants at increased risk for congenital malformations induced by anticonvulsant drugs. (Buehler BA et al. Prenatal prediction of risk of the fetal hydantoin syndrome. *N Engl J Med* May 31, 1990; *322*:1567-72).

COMMENT. Anticonvulsant drugs that are metabolized to form oxidative intermediates (epoxides) pose the greatest teratogenic risk to the fetus. The measurement of the enzyme involved with the biotransformation of the epoxide to a less toxic metabolite may serve as a biomarker of the fetus at high risk for the fetal hydantoin syndrome.

The clinical characteristics of the fetal hydantoin syndrome include upturned nose, midfacial hypoplasia, long upper lip, absent cupid's bow, hirsutism of face, back, arms, and legs, nail hypoplasia, hypotonia with delayed motor development, and poor weight gain. - Editor. *Ped Neur Briefs* May 1990.

Fetal Anticonvulsant Syndrome With Neocerebellar Hypoplasia

An infant with dysmorphic features and hypoplasia of the cerebral hemispheres and cerebellum is reported from the John Radcliffe Hospital, Oxford, England as an extreme example of anticonvulsant teratogenicity. The mother was epileptic and she had taken phenytoin and sodium valproate throughout pregnancy. The infant was cyanosed and hypotonic at birth with Apgar scores of 4 at one minute and 6 at five minutes. She had abnormalities of the toes, fingers, nails, elbows, hips, ears, and an anti-mongoloid slant to the eyes with hypertelorism. Intractable seizures began ten minutes after delivery and she died at 66 hours of age. Postmortem neuropathological examination showed a thickened skull, reduced size of the pons and neocerebellum and widespread neuronal loss and gliosis. (Squier W et al. Neocerebellar hypoplasia in a neonate following intra-uterine exposure to anticonvulsants. *Dev Med Child Neurol* August 1990; *32*:725-742).

COMMENT. The authors felt that this clinical picture may represent the most severe end of the spectrum of fetal abnormalities attributable to phenytoin and/or sodium valproate. The anticonvulsant drug dosages taken by the mother were phenytoin 175 mg and sodium valproate 1 gram daily but the serum levels were not reported. - Editor. *Ped Neur Briefs* September 1990.

Phenobarbital-Induced Depression

Twenty-eight epileptic children aged six to 16 years were assessed for psychopathology in relation to anticonvulsant monotherapy at the Western Psychiatric Institute and Clinic, Children's Hospital of Pittsburgh and Mercy Hospital, Pittsburgh, PA. Eight patients were treated with phenobarbital, 17 carbamazepine, and three had been withdrawn from their anticonvulsant regimen. The phenobarbital treated group showed a higher rate of major depression than did those treated with carbamazepine or no anticonvulsant (38% vs 0%). The frequency of suicide attempts was similar between groups (13% vs 12%). The phenobarbital treated group had higher scores on the Children's Depression Inventory than did the carbamazepine treated patients. The patients who discontinued phenobarbital therapy recovered from major depressive disorder whereas those who continued the treatment remained depressed. (Brent DA et al. Phenobarbital treatment and major depressive disorder in children with epilepsy: A naturalistic follow-up. *Pediatrics* June 1990; *85*:1086-1091).

> COMMENT. Despite the relative safety of phenobarbital compared to other anticonvulsants, the increasing number of reports regarding adverse effects on behavior and cognition preclude its use in children whenever possible. Patients should be monitored closely for symptoms of an affective disorder and intellectual deterioration, and if signs of depression or regression are detected, a change to an alternative anti-convulsant should be considered. (See *PNB* January 1990; 4:2). - Editor. *Ped Neur Briefs* May 1990.

Carbamazepine-Exacerbated Epilepsy

Reporting from Denver, Colorado, the authors studied 49 children and adolescents whose seizures reportedly worsened during carbamazepine (CBZ) therapy. In 26 well documented cases, the drug at therapeutic dose levels induced exacerbation of absence, atonic myoclonic and generalized tonic-clonic seizure patterns. The effect was dose-related in 10 patients. Three of 11 patients who had their first absence seizure when CBZ was introduced developed absence status. In addition to childhood absence, the epileptic syndromes worsened by CBZ included focal symptomatic (frontal lobe), Lennox-Gastaut, and severe myoclonic epilepsy of childhood. (Horn CS, Ater SB, Hurst DL. *Pediatric Neurology* 1986; *2*:340-345).

> COMMENT. This is the sixth report concerning seizures induced or exacerbated by carbamazepine. Partial complex

seizures are frequently responsive but absence, generalized tonic-clonic, focal, or myoclonic epilepsies may be worsened by CBZ. A slow withdrawal of the CBZ results in improved seizure control. - Editor. *Ped Neur Briefs* June 1987.

Carbamazepine And Cognitive Impairment

Members of the Departments of Pediatrics, Neurology, and Clinical Pharmacology and Toxicology at the Children's Hospital and Ohio State University, Columbus, OH 43205, assessed neuropsychological function before and after carbamazepine monotherapy at low (<7.5, ug/ml) and moderate (>8.0, ug/ml) plasma levels in 11 children (4 boys 7 girls, mean age 9.8 yrs) with controlled complex partial epilepsy. Carbamazepine caused significant impairments (P<.03) of efficiency in learning of new information (Paired Associates Test) and short-term memory scanning (Sternberg Memory and Reaction Time Paradigm) that were associated with moderate plasma concentrations within the therapeutic range. The decline in performance was not accompanied by a greater abnormality on the EEG or carbamazepine-induced seizure exacerbation (see *Ped Neur Briefs* 1987; *1*:2). A mild beneficial effect on speeded eye-hand coordination was suggested at moderate plasma levels but only in the nonpreferred hand. Except for a trend toward more rapid memory scanning, there was no change in performance from the baseline to low drug level assessment. (O'Dougherty M, Wright FS et al. Carbamazepine plasma concentration. Relationship to cognitive impairment. *Arch Neurol* 1987; *44*:863-867).

COMMENT. These results are in agreement with previous studies in adults that have shown impairments in concentration and memory-processing with higher but therapeutic serum concentrations of carbamazepine (Thompson PJ, Trimble MR. *J Neurol Neurosurg Psychiatry* 1983; *46*:227-233). It has been suggested that the so-called "psychotropic" effect of carbamazepine reported in crossover antiepileptic drug studies may have been related to the discontinuance of previous drugs rather than a positive carbamazepine effect and that crossover studies are potentially open to error by practice effects (Schain RJ et al. *Neurology* 1977; *27*:476-480). The present study confirms the importance of comprehensive neuropsychological assessments to evaluate possible adverse cognitive side effects of antiepileptic drugs in children particularly at higher dose levels. The theoretical advantages of monotherapy, notwithstanding, the tendency to rigid persistence of large and potentially toxic doses and delay in change to alternative therapy may result in subtle deficits in learning that might be avoided by selective combination therapies at lower dose levels. - Editor. *Ped Neur Briefs* August 1987.

Behavioral Effects Of Antiepileptic Drugs

Parental responses to a Child Behavior Checklist were compared before and after changing antiepileptic therapy in an open, parallel design study in the School of Pharmacy and Department of Neurology and Pediatrics, School of Medicine, University of North Carolina, Chapel Hill, North Carolina. Patients were evaluated just before and again three to four months after starting or stopping phenytoin (PHT), carbamazepine (CBZ), phenobarbital (PB), or primidone (PMD). Patients 4-16 years of age whose antiepileptic regimens were being altered by either adding or discontinuing one of the four drugs were included. Behavioral types were in two groups: 1) Externalizing (aggressive and hyperactive), and 2) Iternalizing (depressed, withdrawn, schizoid, somatic complaints). Individual T scores were calculated and compared with and without treatment using the two tailed t test for paired data. In the CBZ group (n=6), there were significant improvements in aggression, in the externalizing broad band group and in the T behavior score. Significant changes did not occur in the PHT (n=6) or in the PB/PMD (n=7) groups: externalizing behavior was worse in certain individuals receiving PB or PMD. The Child Behavior Checklist was a sensitive instrument for assessing the behavioral effects of antiepileptic agents in epileptic children. Carbamazepine appeared to have a more consistent beneficial effect on child behavior than phenytoin, phenobarbital, and primidone. (Miles MV et al. Assessment of antiepileptic drug effects on child behavior using the Child Behavior Checklist. *J Epilepsy* Dec 1988; *1*:209-213).

COMMENT. The Child Behavior Checklist (CBCL) consists of 112 behavior problem items to which a parent responds: very (or often) true, somewhat (or sometimes) true, or not true, as a description of their child. The CBCL has been standardized for both sex and age. The CBCL can be completed by the parents in 15-20 minutes and may be computer scored allowing for rapid individual and group evaluation. This study confirms the value of the CBCL in detecting behavioral changes secondary to antiepileptic therapy in children. All antiepileptic drugs may adversely affect child behavior and cognition but carbamazepine seems to be least likely to increase behavioral problems. - Editor. *Ped Neur Briefs* February 1989.

Cognitive Effects Of Anticonvulsants

The neuropsychological effects of carbamazepine, phenobarbital, and phenytoin in 15 patients with partial complex epilepsy were investigated at the Department of Neurology, Medical College of Georgia, Augusta, GA. Patients were treated with each drug for three months, using a randomized double-blind, triple crossover design. Neuropsychological tests included digit span, selective reminding test, digit symbol, finger tapping, grooved pegboard, choice reaction time, P3 evoked potential, and profile of mood states. Anticonvulsant blood levels were converted to a percentage of the standard therapeutic ranges. Separate analyses of covariance using percentage blood levels and seizure frequency were performed for each of the cognitive variables. Digit symbol performance with phenobarbital was significantly worse than with the other two anticonvulsants but otherwise the neuropsychological performance was comparable during treatment with each of the drugs. (Meador KJ et al. Comparative cognitive effects of anticonvulsants. *Neurology* March 1990; *40*:391-394).

> COMMENT. All major anticonvulsant drugs may produce cognitive deficits. The effects are dose dependent and may occur even when anticonvulsant blood levels are well within the established therapeutic ranges. Cognitive deficits are particularly prominent with polypharmacy (Trimble MR. *Epilepsia* 1987;*28* (suppl 3):S37-S45). The present study conducted in adults has shown that any differential cognitive effects of anticonvulsants must be subtle. Neuro-psychological deficits commonly associated with anticonvulsant drugs include impairments in attention and concentration, memory, information processing and motor speed. A double-blind crossover study of phenobarbital and valproic acid treatment in 21 epileptic children has shown that neuropsychological functioning was significantly worse during phenobarbital treatment (Vining et al. *Pediatrics* 1987; *80*:165). - Editor. *Ped Neur Briefs* March 1990.

Carbamazepine Induced Malformations

A study of the pattern of malformations in children of women treated with carbamazepine during pregnancy is reported from the Division of Dysmorphology, Department of Pediatrics, University of California - San Diego, La Jolla, CA. The authors evaluated eight infants identified retrospectively as having had prenatal exposure to carbamazepine, alone or in combination with other drugs except phenytoin. In addition, in a prospective study they documented the outcome of the pregnancies of 72 women who were concerned early in their pregnancies about the potential teratogenicity of carbamazepine. The pattern of malformation including minor craniofacial defects, fingernail hypoplasia and developmental delay identified in the eight children in the retrospective study was confirmed through the evaluation of 48 children born alive to the women in the prospective study. The incidence of craniofacial defects was 11%, fingernail hypoplasia 26%, and developmental delay 20%. The pattern of malformation with carbamazepine was similar to that of fetal hydantoin syndrome, suggesting that the epoxide intermediate metabolite is the teratogenic agent rather than the drug itself. (Jones KL et al. Pattern of malformation in the children of women treated with carbamazepine during pregnancy. *N Engl J Med* June 22, 1989; *320*:1661-6).

> COMMENT. We can now add carbamazepine (Tegretol) to the list of anticonvulsants with teratogenic effects. A new use for carbamazepine is described from the Department of Pediatrics, 1011 Lausanne, Switzerland (Roulet E Deona T. *Pediatrics* June 1989; *83*:1077). Hereditary dominant chorea in an 11-1/2 year old girl and in her mother was treated successfully with carbamazepine, confirming the experience of some other authors that this drug may have an effect on various choreas in a lower dose than that required for an antiepileptic effect. - Editor. *Ped Neur Briefs* June 1988.

Carbamazepine-Induced Hepatotoxicity

Three children who developed acute liver failure while taking carbamazepine are reported from the Department of Child Health, King's College Hospital, Denmark Hill, London, England. A girl aged 11 developed a severe maculopapular rash, intermittent fever, arthralgia, anemia, and vomiting four weeks after starting carbamazepine. The blood concentration was 32 mcmol/l (therapeutic range 16-50). She developed jaundice two weeks later and on admission six days later she had a generalized exfoliative rash, periorbital edema, generalized lymphadenopathy, and hepatomegaly. Her platelets and differential white count were normal. Concentrations of IgG, IgM, and IgE were increased. Liver biopsy showed acute hepatitis. Steroid treatment with prednisolone (0.7 mg/kg/24 hours) caused a dramatic symptomatic and biochemical improvement. She was discharged one week later after complete recovery and prednisolone was stopped after 18 days. The second child, aged 7, again presented with fever, generalized maculopapular rash, arthralgia, and lymphadenopathy four weeks after starting carbamazepine. She developed jaundice, ascites, and generalized edema 17 days later. Total bilirubin concentration was 236 mcmol/1. Hepatic encephalopathy developed four days after admission and the child died of infectious complications three months after a liver transplantation. The third patient, a 3 year old child, had a fulminant hepatic failure due to carbamazepine toxicity which was treated successfully by transplantation. (Hadzic N et al. Acute liver failure induced by carbamazepine. *Arch Dis Child* March 1990; *65*:315-317).

> COMMENT. The authors identified three previous cases of fatal acute liver failure directly attributable to carbamazepine, one in a child. Four other children with fatal hepatitis while on carbamazepine were also taking several drugs, some being potentially hepatotoxic such as phenytoin. Clinical and laboratory findings in the authors cases suggested an immunoallergic reaction although only one patient improved with steroids. It was suggested that determination of liver function during the first few weeks of treatment and early detection of signs of idiosyncrasy may help detect patients at risk of developing acute liver failure. Two of the three patients had rash preceding the development of jaundice. A warning to the parents to discontinue medication at the first sign of skin rash might be more important than reliance only on serial liver function tests. Two cases of carbamazepine-induced liver failure were reported at the 1989 meeting of the Child Neurology Society (Murphy JV et al). At the recent 42nd annual meeting of the AAN there were two reports of systemic lupus erythromatosis induced by carbamazepine and the manufacturer (Ciba-Geigy) had knowledge of 18 unpublished cases. (*Neurology* April 1990; *40*:Suppl I:137). - Editor. *Ped Neur Briefs* April 1990.

Valproate Hepatotoxicity In Children With Epilepsy

Authors from the University Children's Hospital in Heidelberg estimate the incidence of fatal valproate (VPA) hepatotoxicity in West Germany at around 1 in 5000 and find it hard to justify the use of VPA as a drug of first choice for children with generalized epilepsies. Analyses of data on 16 cases (15 between 1980 and 1986) and 75 additional published cases (a total of 91 cases) showed that no single high-risk age group could be defined; only 2 of the 16 German cases (12%) and 26% of the 91 cases reviewed were under 3 years of age. Fatalities were more frequent in young children on polytherapy, but 14 (15%) followed monotherapy with VPA and 10 (71%) of these were in patients older than 3 years. (Scheffner D. *Lancet* 1986; *ii*:511. Scheffner D, Konig St. *Lancet* 1987; *i*:389-390).

COMMENT. I agree with the authors that valproate, a drug with known hepatotoxicity and potentially fatal side-effects, should not be used as a first-line therapy in children with epilepsy. Also, its use in the treatment of febrile convulsions seems unacceptable. Despite the less worrisome estimates of fatalities from the US (1 in 10,000; 1 in 7,000 for polytherapy and 1 in 37,000 for monotherapy)[1] and from England (1 in 20,000)[2], careful monitoring of valproate therapy should be mandatory. Fatalities for VPA polytherapy in children <3 yr was 1/500. ([1]Dreifuss FE, Santilli N. *Neurology* 1986; *36* (Suppl 1):175. Dreifuss FE et al. *Neurology* 1987; *37*:379. [2]Jeavons PM. *Epilepsia* 1984; *35* (Suppl 1):50-55). - Editor. *Ped Neur Briefs* June 1987.

Valproate-Induced Malformations

Two children born with birth defects after intrauterine exposure to valproic acid are reported from the Dept Pediatrics Hopital Sainte-Justine, University of Montreal, Quebec, Canada. The drug was taken by the mothers throughout pregnancy as monotherapy for primary generalized epilepsy. One baby had facial dysmorphism, hypertelorism, anti-mongoloid palpebral fissures, a naevus flammeus on the forehead, portwine palpebral and nasal angiomas, arachnodactyly, triphalangeal thumbs, syndactyly, and a septum pellucidum cyst and dilated ventricles on CT scan. The second baby had facial dysmorphism, laryngeal hypoplasia, tracheomalacia, aberrant innominate artery and hydronephrosis. The authors concluded that valproic acid has probable teratogenic potential in humans but the spectrum of anomalies is broad and a definite fetal valproate syndrome is difficult to delineate. (Huot C et al. Congenital malformations associated with maternal use of valproic acid. *Can J Neurol Sci* 1987; *14*:290-293).

COMMENT. Approximately 50 malformed babies born to epileptic mothers taking valproate monotherapy have been reported. Contrary to the above opinion, Diliberti et al (*Amer J Med Genetics* 1984; *19*:473-481) have recognized a "fetal valproate syndrome", and the frequency of reports of valproate-induced congenital malformations together with other side-effects (liver failure, pancreatitis, endocrine abnormalities, weight gain) tend to contraindicate its use in pregnancy.

Portwine angioma noted in the first baby in this study of valproic acid toxicity may also be induced by thalidomide and alcohol ingestion during pregnancy (Jones et al. *Lancet* 1974; *1*:1076. Colver GB, Savin JA. Editorial. J *Roy Soc Med* 1987; *80*:603). Dilated ventricles, defined by CT in the first baby, are reported as a reversible cerebral pseudoatrophy for the first time as a side-effect of valproic acid monotherapy in a 17-year-old with epilepsy (McLachlan RS. *Can J Neurol Sci* 1987; *14*:294).

For an update of antiepileptic drugs and teratogenicity, refer to Weber M. *Rev Neurol (Paris)* 1987; *143*:413. According to this report, the frequency of congenital malformations among children of epileptic mothers is twice that in the general population, genetic factors play a major role, and generally the teratogenic potential of antiepileptic drugs is low and does not contraindicate pregnancy in epileptic women. Many neurologists and certainly geneticists would advise stricter selectivity and caution in the choice of anticonvulsant for epileptic women contemplating pregnancy. Drugs with especially high or relatively frequent teratogenic potential (e.g. trimethadione, phenytoin) are usually contraindicated, those with moderate or unknown degrees of propensity (primidone, valproic acid, carbamazepine, clonazepam) are avoided when possible, and the drug of choice, least likely to induce malformations and most often recommended, is probably phenobarbital. - Editor. *Ped Neur Briefs* November 1987.

Valproate-Induced Gastritis

Gastritis and erosion of the gastric mucosa is reported in 10 children who presented with feeding difficulties after long-term treatment with divalproex sodium (Depakote) and valproic acid (Depakene) at the Departments of Neurology, Pediatrics, and Pediatric Surgery, University of Oklahoma Health Sciences Center, Oklahoma City. Anorexia and refusal to eat were complicated by vomiting in 8 patients, abdominal pain in 5, weight loss in 3, and diarrhea in 2. Endoscopy confirmed erosive gastritis. Treatment with oral antacids (Maalox) and cimetidine resulted in clinical improvement. (Marks WA et al. Gastritis with valproate therapy. *Arch Neurol* August 1988; *45*:903-905).

COMMENT. Gastrointestinal disturbances are common at the initiation of valproate therapy but have not previously been reported following its long term use. The diagnosis of gastritis in mentally retarded patients with epilepsy may be difficult, and delay may lead to gastric erosion, resulting in malnutrition, weight loss, and dehydration. If liver and pancreas disease has been excluded as a side-effect, the treatment of valproate-induced gastritis includes antacids and an alteration of anticonvulsant regimen in some cases. - Editor. *Ped Neur Briefs* August 1988.

Valproate-Induced Edema

Facial and limb edema in seven patients during long-term valproate therapy are reported from the Montefiore/Einstein Epilepsy Center, Albert Einstein College of Medicine, Bronx, NY. Ages ranged from 6 to 43 years; four were 6 to 17 years. All received dosages greater than 1500 mg/day for a prolonged time and trough levels ranged from 36 to 107 mcg/ml. Four patients were receiving other medications. All had normal liver and renal function tests. Reduction in the edema occurred in four following a reduction in valproate dosage, and one resolved spontaneously. (Ettinger A, Moshe S, Shinnar S. Edema associated with long-term valproate therapy. *Epilepsia* March/April 1990; *31*:211-213).

COMMENT. In a recent case report of a three year old boy from Japan a fulminant hepatic failure induced by valproate was associated with a marked increase in *w*-oxidation of the drug. The patient died on the seventh hospital day and autopsy findings showed acute liver necrosis with congestion and cholestasis. (Kuhara T et al. *Epilepsia* March/April 1990; 31:214-217). Valproate-induced thrombocytopenia was reported in a total of 35 patients at the 42nd annual meeting of the AAN. (Delgado et al: Sherbany AA et al. *Neurology* April 1990; *40 (Suppl I)*:136-137). Close monitoring of platelet counts is recommended particularly when high doses of valproate are necessary in treatment of children with epilepsy. Thrombocytopenia may develop after several years of therapy and seems to be dose related. - Editor. *Ped Neur Briefs* April 1990.

Valproate, Carnitine, And Lipid Metabolism

The effects of valproate (VPA) on carnitine and lipid metabolism and on liver function were assessed in 213 outpatients from five centers and reported from the Instituto di Ricerche Farmacologiche "Mario Negri," Milan, Italy. The mean total and free carnitine levels were significantly lower in patients on polytherapy. A significant correlation was found between serum ammonia levels and VPA dosage. VPA monotherapy and polytherapy were associated with significantly elevated cholesterol levels, especially "HDL". The authors concluded that impairment of carnitine metabolism and liver function by VPA does not appear to be a clinically important phenomenon especially when VPA is administered as monotherapy to well nourished patients. There was no correlation between carnitine deficiency and reports of anticonvulsant clinical toxicity, e.g. somnolence, behavioral disturbance, headache, increased appetite, weight gain, anorexia, ataxia, and tremor. (Beghi E et al and the Collaborative Group for the Study of Epilepsy. Valproate, carnitine metabolism, and biochemical indicators of liver function. *Epilepsia* May/June 1990; *31*:346-352).

COMMENT. These data confirm previous findings that VPA impairs carnitine metabolism. In contrast to other reports, this study showed a significant correlation between serum ammonia and VPA dosage. The observed change in lipid metabolism with increased cholesterol levels during treatment with VPA and other anticonvulsants is important in the evaluation of children receiving the ketogenic diet as a supplement to anticonvulsant drugs. Carnitine deficiency has been found in hyperlipemic patients and carnitine replacement therapy may correct the hyperlipemia. Children, especially females and younger males, should be tested for carnitine deficiency during treatment with anticonvulsant drugs and particularly with VPA polytherapy. - Editor. *Ped Neur Briefs* June 1990.

Valproate-Induced Cytopenias

A 16 year old white boy with trisomy 21 and valproic-acid induced erythrocyte aplasia is reported from the Divisions of Hematology and Oncology, University of Alabama, Birmingham, AL. Suppression of hematopoiesis was demonstrated by in vitro studies of colony-forming-unit granulocyte/macrophage (CFU-GM) assays using bone marrow from healthy adult volunteers cultured in the presence of increasing doses of valproic acid (60, 120, and 240 mcg/ml). At a VPA concentration of 120 mcg/ml, similar to that observed in the patient with erythrocyte aplasia, macrocytosis and neutropenia, there was a 67% CFU-GM growth inhibition, and at VPA levels of 240 mcg/ml, 84% of the colony growth was inhibited. The inhibition was specific to VPA and was not related to a change in pH. The addition of the patient's serum to the assays had no significant effect. The results suggested a direct dose dependent suppression of bone marrow neutrophilic progenitors by valproic acid. (Watts RG et al. Valproic acid-induced cytopenias: Evidence for a dose-related suppression of hematopoiesis. *J Pediatr* Sept 1990; *117*:495-499).

COMMENT. This patient had no family history or medical history of anemia, congenital or acquired bone marrow failure, or malignancies. The only recent drug exposure was valproic acid. The authors recommend close hematologic monitoring of patients receiving valproic acid therapy and especially when larger doses are employed.

Of practical importance in the management of a severe overdose of valproic acid, studies of the elimination half life and clearance of valproic acid in a patient with dialysis-induced encephalopathy who was taking divalproic sodium for a seizure disorder showed that hemodialysis and hemoperfusion had little effect on the removal of valproic acid from the body. The equilibrium shifted so that valproic acid redistributed back into the blood from the tissues. (Kandrotas RJ et al. *Neurology* Sept 1990; *40*:1456-1458). Hemodialysis is unlikely to benefit patients with toxic overdose of valproic acid. - Editor. *Ped Neur Briefs* October 1990.

Toxicity Of Nitrazepam (Mogadon)

A pediatric neurologist and his associates at the Children's Mercy Hospital, Kansas City, report 6 deaths among 80 patients with intractable epilepsy treated with nitrazepam. The patients who died were 13-39 mos of age (mean 28 mos) and had received nitrazepam for 2 to 19 months (mean 8 mos) in a dosage of 0.9-2.7 mg/kg/d (mean 1.4). Up to 2 additional but unnamed antiepileptic drugs were used concurrently but no patient received other benzodiazepines. The dosage of nitrazepam in the 6 fatal cases was significantly higher and approximately double that in 22 survivors of the same age range (mean 0.7 mg/kg/d). Patients in both groups had multiple seizures, including generalized tonic-clonic, myoclonic and focal types but none had infantile spasms or absence attacks. Perinatal asphyxia, Prader-Willi syndrome, pertussis vaccine-related encephalopathy, and nonketotic hyperglycinemia were the etiological diagnoses in 4 of the 6 fatal cases. Three of the 6 had known factors contributing to death: congestive heart failure, aspiration of gastric contents, and unexplained hyperthermia, shock, and respiratory failure. Three patients died unexpectedly and autopsies in 2 were unrevealing. The cause of death was undetermined but a nitrazepam-induced swallowing disturbance and aspiration was suspected. The authors recommend that the use of nitrazepam in young children should be restricted to those resistant to other antiepileptic drugs, the dose should not exceed 0.8 mg/kg/d, and children with prior swallowing difficulties should be observed closely. (Murphy JV et al. Deaths in young children receiving nitrazepam. *J Pediat* 1987; *111*:145-147).

COMMENT. Nitrazepam (Mogadon) is considered the most effective benzodiazepine for control of infantile spasms ad other myoclonic seizures. It is not usually recommended for the treatment of generalized tonic-clonic seizures, as employed in this study, which might explain the necessity for the larger doses in the affected infants.

In a study at Children's Memorial Hospital, Chicago (Millichap JG, Ortiz WR. *Am J Dis Child* 1966; *112*:242), the side effects of nitrazepam in a trial involving 36 infants and children with myoclonic seizures included drowsiness (50%), ataxia (20%), hypotonia (20%), and muscular weakness (9%). Anorexia and vomiting developed in 2% and skin rash in 2%. The most serious adverse effects of nitrazepam in our study were symptoms suggesting autonomic dysfunction, previously unreported. Excessive drooling of saliva occurred in 9 (25%) infants and pulmonary congestion with wheezing developed in 4 (11%) debilitated infants with diplegia and severe retardation. Miosis of the pupils was also noted. The pulmonary symptoms required withdrawal of the drug or reduction of the dose to less effective levels and possible fatalities were avoided. The nitrazepam-induced drooling and aspiration in some cases have recently been explained by a delay of cricopharyngeal relaxation (Wyllie E et al. *N Engl J Med* 1986; *314*:35-38). The tolerance that develops to nitrazepam and the autonomic and sedative side-effects of larger doses seriously detract from the usefulness of this agent in long-term therapy of infantile spasms. In debilitated infants, perhaps nitrazepam should be contraindicated. - Editor. *Ped Neur Briefs* August 1987.

Teratogenic Effects Of Diazepam

Eight children exposed in utero to benzodiazepines, diazepam or oxazepam, and having dysmorphic characteristics resembling the fetal alcohol syndrome (FAS) are reported from the Department of Pediatrics, Gothenburg University, Sweden. The most common craniofacial abnormalities were slanted eyes, epicanthic folds, short, uptilted nose, flat upper lip, and hypoplastic mandible. All were hypotonic from birth and had neonatal drug withdrawal symptoms of opisthotonos and convulsions. Low Apgar scores were recorded in 6, mainly because of apnea, and 5 were resuscitated. Rooting and sucking reflexes were absent and feeding difficulties prominent. Gross motor disability in all children, 2 having spastic hemiparesis, was seen during early life, and fine motor incoordination and tremor were common in older children. One infant who died had neuronal migration defects and heterotopias. (Laegreid L et al. Teratogenic effects of benzodiazepine use during pregnancy. *J Pediatr* Jan 1989; *114*:126-31).

COMMENT. Alcohol ingestion in these mothers was excluded. The fetal diazepam syndrome (FDS) differed from the FAS in a greater focal involvement of cranial nerves, a sullen and expressionless facies, and more frequent occurrence of low Apgar scores, apneic spells, delayed motor development, and neonatal hypotonia. There have been numerous previous reports of the "floppy infant syndrome" in babies born to women treated with long-term diazepam during pregnancy. Bilateral opercular polymicrogyria and grey matter heterotopias found at autopsy of 2 cases of Foix-Chavany-Marie syndrome (facio-pharyngealglossomasticatory diplegia) (Becker PS et al. *Ann Neurol* Jan 1989; *25*:90) might sometimes be explained by diazepam teratogenicity. This syndrome is rare and usually follows stroke and vascular infarction in adults. There are very few reports of the pathology in developmental varieties of the syndrome. - Editor. *Ped Neur Briefs* January 1989.

Benzodiazepine-Induced Congenital Malformations

The potential teratogenic properties of benzodiazepine (BZD) intake during early pregnancy were investigated at the Departments of Pediatrics, Pathology and Genetics at Goteborg University, Sweden. Four neonatal diagnoses of congenital malformations known to be characteristic of infants born to mothers with excessive intake of BZD in early pregnancy were present in 25 of 10,646 live born infants (2.3/1,000) delivered by mothers living in the city of Gothenburg in 1985 and 1986. The maternal plasma was analyzed in 18 of these cases 1.2 to 1.5 years after the birth of the probands; eight samples (44%) were BZD positive. Of 60 controls, two maternal blood samples (3%) were positive for BZD. The difference was highly significant and suggests an association between the congenital malformation and BZD consumed during early gestation. (Laegried L et al. Congenital malformations and maternal consumption of benzodiazepines: A case-control study. *Dev Med Child Neur* May 1990; *32*:432-441).

COMMENT. The diagnoses considered to be specific for BZD-induced congenital malformations were embryopathy and fetopathy, nervous system malformations, cleft lip and cleft palate, congenital malformations of the urinary tract. The authors considered that their findings strengthened the hypothesis that BZD intake during early pregnancy is associated with teratogenicity in man but there is as yet no firm proof of association. Diazepam in early pregnancy should be avoided on the basis of this and other studies which strongly suggest a teratogenic effect of BZD - Editor. *Ped Neur Briefs* May 1990.

Lorazepam-Induced Memory Deficits

The effects of low doses of lorazepam (Ativan) 0.03 mg/kg IV, on episodic versus long-term memory, attention, and somatic and affective symptoms were investigated in a group of 16 children aged 2.8 to 14.2 years at St. Jude Children's Research Hospital, Memphis, and the Center for Pediatric Pharmacokinetics and Therapeutics, Departments of Clinical Pharmacy and Pediatrics, University of Tennessee, Memphis. Psychological assessments were performed twice before drug administration and 1-1/2 hours and 24 hours after intravenous lorazepam. A selective anterograde amnestic effect was observed in 5 of 16 children as measured by a picture recognition test. There were no significant changes in long term memory, attention or somatic symptoms but affective symptoms were significantly decreased at 1-1/2 hours and a trend toward decreased anxiety was seen at 1-1/2 and 24 hours after lorazepam injection. The half life of lorazepam was 10.5 ±2.9 hours. (Relling MV et al. Lorazepam pharmacodynamics and pharmacokinetics in children. *J Pediatr* April 1989; *114*:641-646).

COMMENT. Lorazepam is a short acting benzodiazepine that is used in children most commonly as a preoperative sedative and as an anticonvulsant. In adults it is used as an antiemetic agent during chemotherapy for cancer, an effect largely due to its amnestic properties. This study shows that it is possible to produce a selective amnestic effect on episodic memory in children without significantly impairing long-term memory or attention.

Lorazepam has become increasingly popular for the treatment of status epilepticus in children; the usual median dose is 0.1 mg/kg. Midazolam, a benzodiazepine used primarily for induction of anesthesia, in contrast to lorazepam and diazepam, is water soluble and its injection is neither painful nor irritating by the intramuscular route. Midazolam 15 mg *IM* was as effective in abolishing spikes as 20 mg of diazepam *IV* five minutes after administration in a study in adults with epilepsy. (Jawad S et al. *J Neurol Neurosurg Psychiat* 1986; *49*:1050). The half life of lorazepam is longer than that of diazepam or midazolam, however, and its duration of action is more prolonged. - Editor. *Ped Neur Briefs* March 1989.

HORMONES AND EPILEPSY

Post-Ictal ACTH And Prolactin Plasma Levels

Significant elevations in ACTH and prolactin plasma levels were found within one hour after generalized tonic-clonic seizures in 10 epileptic patients but not in patients with syncopal attacks investigated at the Service de Neurologie, Hopital General 3, rue Faubourg Raines, Dijon, France. The mean ACTH and prolactin levels were 72.6±37.7 pg/ml and 13.9±1.9 ng/ml at one hour compared to 17.1±2.1 pg/ml and 4.1±1.2 ng/ml, respectively, at three to five days after seizures; the differences were significant (p<0.01) and independent of anticonvulsant effects. Levels of FSH, LH, and TSH were unchanged. The postictal rise of ACTH and prolactin levels may be used in the differentiation of epileptic seizures and syncope. (Giroud M et al. Les troubles neuro-endocriniens observes en phase post-critique chez les epileptiques. *Rev Neurol* (Paris) 1987; *143*:620-623).

COMMENT. In the last 10 years, numerous studies have demonstrated the hormonal effects not only of generalized convulsive seizures but also of complex partial seizures and of interictal epileptiform discharges (Molaie M, Culebras A, Miller M. *Epilepsia* 1986; *27*:724). Plasma prolactin elevations are used to differentiate epileptic from pseudoseizures (Collins WCJ et al. *J Neurol Neurosurg Psychiatry* 1983; *46*:505). It is postulated that persistent elevations of prolactin may contribute to endocrine dysfunctions in epileptic patients.

In the same issue of *Rev Neurol (Paris)* (1987; *143*:559), Landrieu P of the Hospital de Bicetre reviews the recent progress and perspectives in pediatric neurology in France. - Editor. *Ped Neur Briefs* December 1987.

Serum Hormones And Anticonvulsants

Circulating sex and thyroid hormones were assessed in 63 male young adults with epilepsy in the Departments of Neurology and Clinical Chemistry, University of Oulu, Finland. All therapeutic regimens that included carbamazepine and/or phenytoin were associated with low levels of circulating thyroxine (T4), free thyroxine (FT4), and dehydroepiandrosterone sulfate, and low values for the free androgen index. Phenytoin, alone or combined with carbamazepine, was associated with high serum concentrations of sex hormone - binding globulin. Hormone values were unaffected by valproate monotherapy, but the combination of carbamazepine plus valproate had the most marked effect on serum thyroid hormone levels and the free androgen index. Serum T3 concentrations were unaffected by any of the medications or combinations. Serum thyrotropin concentrations were not elevated despite low serum thyroid hormone levels. (Isojarvi JIT et al. Serum hormones in male epileptic patients receiving anticonvulsant medication. *Arch Neurol* June 1990, *47*:670-676).

COMMENT. This study supports the hypothesis that an increased metabolism of thyroid hormones in the liver is the main reason for decreased T4 and FT4 serum levels in epileptic patients receiving carbamazepine and/or phenytoin treatment. The combination of valproate and carbamazepine has the most marked effect on thyroid hormone balance and both drugs are highly bound to serum proteins. Valproate displaces T4 from its binding sites on plasma proteins thereby leading to a larger amount of T4 subject to the liver enzyme inducing properties of carbamazepine. Thyroid supplements are usually not required in patients with a low serum T4 associated with anticonvulsant drug therapy. If the free T3 and T4 are normal thyroid supplements should be withheld.

To avoid criticism of a gender bias, a reference is included to "Serum steroid hormones and pituitary function in female epileptic patients during carbamazepine therapy" (Iojarvi JIT. *Epilepsia* Aug 1990; *31*:438-445). In 13 female epilepsy patients receiving long-term carbamazepine (CBZ) monotherapy, serum sex hormone binding globulin levels increased and dehydroepiandrosterone sulfate levels decreased during CBZ treatment. Increased metabolism of steroid hormones caused by liver enzyme inducing properties of CBZ and a direct inhibitory effect of CBZ on hormone synthesis and hypothalamic function are possible explanations. Despite the many changes in the serum sex hormone balance, the patients appeared to maintain ovulatory cycles during the first year of CBZ treatment. -Editor. *Ped Neur Briefs* August 1990.

ELECTROENCEPHALOGRAPHY

Cassette EEG Monitoring

The importance of interictal epileptiform abnormalities discovered with cassette electroencephalographic (EEG) monitoring has been assessed in a group of 184 nonepileptic patients referred because of headache and reported from the Department of Neurology, Yale University School of Medicine, New Haven, CT; and the Neurology Service, Veterans Administration Medical Center, West Haven, CT. Only one (0.5%) of these patients had epileptiform abnormalities on cassette EEG and the incidence was no higher than on routine EEG. In contrast, the authors have found more than 50% of episodes characterized as seizures to be accompanied by cassette EEG seizure activity. Consequently, the detection of such abnormalities seems a worthwhile aspect of cassette EEG interpretation when the goal of monitoring is the detection of evidence to support diagnosis of epilepsy. (Bridgers SL et al. Estimating the importance of epileptiform abnormalities discovered on cassette electroencephalographic monitoring. *Arch Neurol* October 1989; 46:1077-1079).

COMMENT. The mean age of patients reporting headache in this study was 30 years, and only five patients were age 10 years or less. The incidence of epileptiform activity may well be higher in a group of children with headache. (Millichap JG. Recurrent headaches in 100 children, electroencephalographic abnormalities and response to Phenytoin (Dilantin). *Child's Brain* 1978; 4:95-105). - Editor. *Ped Neur Briefs* November 1989.

Biomagnetometry In Seizure Localization

Biomeganetometry was discussed at the 75th Annual Meeting of the Radiological Society of North America. Unlike ultrasound, CT, and MRI (which provide anatomic information) and PET (metabolic information), biomagnetic imaging provides spatial and temporal data on the electrical activity of the brain. It may help locate the foci of epileptic seizures and show locations for language, auditory and visual processing. Unlike the EEG which is crude and looks at ripples in the water, biomagnetometry shows the stone and the source of the ripples (Dr. Harwood-Nash, Toronto). EEG signals travel through many types of tissue with varying degrees of electrical resistance and consequent distortion. The magnetic flux generated by neurons are not distorted by bone or other biologic tissues, they are picked up and converted to electrical signals by detection coils, amplified, filtered and processed for display on a computer screen to show spatial distribution and time evolution of the electrical activity being scanned. The information is presented graphically superimposed over a single plane MRI image so that correlations with the anatomical structures can be made. In 15 of 40 patients with epilepsy who received biomagnetic scans and underwent surgery for the removal of epileptic foci, there was good correlation between EEG and biomagnetometry mapping of the epileptic foci. (Sato S. Bethesda, MD). (Skolnick A. Biomagnetometry provides a new compass for exploring the brain and heart. *JAMA* Feb 2, 1990; *263*:623-627).

COMMENT. Biomagnetic Technologies (BTi), a San Diego company, has installed more than 50 seven channel machines and announced the availability of a 37 channel biomagnetometer at the RSNA November 1989 meeting. Siemen's expects to install its first 37 channel system (Krenikon) in West Germany and three at research centers in the U.S. A large area, 7-channel, magnetometer (SQUID) was used to preoperatively determine the sites of epileptic foci in two patients with intractable temporal lobe seizures and results are reported from the Department of Neurosurgery, Kuopio University Hospital, Finland. Preop localization agreed with electrocorticogram and depth electrode operative recordings. (Tiihonen J et al. *Ann Neurol* March 1990; *27*:283-290). - Editor. *Ped Neur Briefs* March 1990.

DRIVING AND EPILEPSY

Auto Accidents And Epilepsy

Of 400 drivers with epilepsy questioned, 133 admitted having one or more seizures at the wheel, and 17% had resulting accidents. The authors from the Institut de Reserches Neurologiques, Marseille, France, and Dept Neurology, SUNY Health Sciences Center at Brooklyn, NY, attempting to relate the risk of accidents to the type of seizure, were able to characterize 109 attacks in 82 subjects of which 55% led to an accident. Young drivers accounted for one half those with seizures at the wheel and a complex partial seizure usually without aura was the most common pattern, being responsible for 88% of the accidents. Those with auras were significantly less likely to lead to accidents. Many of the patients were driving illegally, 46% having seizures at least monthly and 74%, at least yearly. Males, 19 to 30 years, in higher socioeconomic classes, formed the majority continuing to drive without adequate seizure control. Based on the recommendations of the Ad Hoc Committee of Epilepsy International, the authors proposed that: 1) a driving license may be granted only to an epileptic who has been seizure-free for at least 1 year; 2) temporary permits may be granted in exceptional circumstances to certain individuals on the advice of a certified neurologist having special interest and competence in epilepsy. (Gastaut H, Zifkin BG. The risk of automobile accidents with seizures occurring while driving: relation to seizure type. *Neurology* 1987; *37*:1613-1616).

COMMENT. In the State of Illinois, patients with epilepsy may obtain a license to drive at the discretion and on the advice of the neurologist in charge of treatment. Temporary permits are not issued. Although questioned concerning the duration of care, the occurrence of attacks in the past 6 months, of a type without warning and with loss of consciousness, and the patient's compliance in taking medication, a neurologist's certificate to the effect that the patient is medically fit to operate a motor vehicle is usually sufficient, irrespective of the frequency or pattern of seizures. A more restrictive policy toward epileptics and driving, including a one year period of control, was counterproductive, forcing patients to deny the recurrence of seizures and thereby preventing the prescription of optimal therapy. The present study appears to support the discretionary policy based on individualized applications for driving licenses of epileptics, but the monitoring of young male drivers with complex partial seizures should be close and frequent and should include serum drug levels and when appropriate, repeated EEG's to check drug compliance and seizure susceptibility. - Editor. *Ped Neur Briefs* October 1987.

SURGERY AND EPILEPSY

Surgical Treatment Of Intractable Epilepsy

Seventy-five children, ages 5 months to 15 years, were treated for intractable seizures in the Neurosurgical Dept. of Washington University School of Medicine, St. Louis, MO, USA. The use of implantable arrays of epidural electrodes facilitated extraoperative electrocorticography (ECOG) and simultaneous video monitoring provided localizing information prior to cortical excision in 53 patients. The pathological lesions were chronic encephalitis of Rasmussen (9), cortical sclerosis with infantile hemiplegia (7), mesial temporal sclerosis (6), extratemporal sclerosis (6), cortical dysplasia (4), tuberous sclerosis (3), porencephalic cyst (3), Sturge-Weber (3), polymicrogyria (2), heterotopia (2), occult vascular malformation (1), misc (7). Results were good in 32 (65%): 16 seizure-free and 16 improved control after follow-up of 1-14 years. Gliomas were found in an additional 17 cases and were the most common single cause of intractable seizures; 82% were seizure-free for more than 1 year (mean follow-up of 4.5 years) since surgery. (Goldring S. Pediatric epilepsy surgery. *Epilepsia* 1987; *28* (Suppl *1*):S82-102).

COMMENT. With an increasing awareness of the adverse effects of antiepileptic drugs on learning and behavior in children (see *Ped Neur Briefs* 1987; 1:20; Vining EPG et al. *Pediatrics* 1987 ; *80*:165; Freeman JM. *Epilepsia* 1987; *28S*:103) the need for alternative therapies becomes more apparent. The ketogenic and MCT diets could be used more frequently, metabolic causes requiring specific therapy (e.g. biotin, pyridoxine), though rare, should not be overlook; and psychological factors especially important in the adolescent and young adult should be investigated and remedied. Dr. Goldring offers another alternative in surgical intervention which he believes to be a much under utilized therapeutic approach to intractable epilepsy in children. Although the emphasis and reliance on drugs in the management of seizures cannot be discounted, their promotion must not permit the neglect of preventive and alternative approaches to the child with seizures. - Editor. *Ped Neur Briefs* September 1987.

Hemispherectomy For Childhood Epilepsy

Seventeen patients treated for hemiplegic epilepsy by hemispherectomy between 1950 and the present day have been followed up at the National Centre for Children with Epilepsy, The Park Hospital for Children, Oxford. The causes of the seizures were associated with perinatal complications in 8 and early febrile status epilepticus, prolonged and unilateral, in 9. Two of the 17 had congenital abnormalities: Sturge-Weber disease in one and a heterotopia found at operation in the other. Habitual seizures began at age 1 to 10 yrs after an interval of relative freedom varying from 8 mos to 10 yrs. Gross behavior disorder was a major handicap, schooling was interrupted, and intelligence deteriorated in the years before operation. EEG was of limited value, both hemispheres often being involved. High-voltage discharges occurred in the preserved hemisphere. The median age at operation was 11-1/2 years (7-17 yrs). Follow-up ranged from 1-36 yrs.

Post-operatively, 1) habitual epilepsy was interrupted with complete freedom in 11 (65%); 2) behavior improved, sometimes dramatically; 3) drop in IQ was halted; 4) the residual homonymous hemianopia was not a major handicap; and 5) one patient developed hemosiderosis of the postoperative cavity and died 11 years after operation.

The authors make the following recommendations: 1) establish that the lesion is unilateral and medication has been tried fully, 2) weigh dangers of status epilepticus, escalating behavior disorder, and deterioration of IQ when operation is delayed compared to benefits and low risks of early surgery; 3) use improved operative techniques with dissection of cortex in single piece (Falconer and Rushworth) and reconstruction and closure of cavity (Adams), and 4) regular follow-up with CT scans. (Lindsay J, Ounsted C, Richards P. Hemispherectomy for childhood epilepsy: A 36-year study. *Dev Med Child Neurol* 1987; *29:*592-600).

COMMENT. These authors have found hemispherectomy to be of considerable benefit to children with hemiplegic epilepsy and its concomitant social, psychological, and medical disabilities. The surgical treatment of intractable epilepsy offers an alternative to chronic anticonvulsant drugs with their attendant adverse effects. With improved techniques now available the surgical approach should be considered more frequently in preference to a dogged persistence and reliance on medicines alone. (*Ped Neur Briefs* 1987; *1*:24). - Editor. *Ped Neur Briefs* November 1987.

Surgery For Partial Epilepsy In Infancy

Focal resection of epileptic tissue was performed in five infants under one year of age with malignant partial seizures and deteriorating developmental status at Miami Children's Hospital and the Comprehensive Epilepsy Center, Miami, FL. Surgery was performed between two and 11 months of age. Pathology of resected specimens was as follows: Dysplastic gangliocytoma, hamartoma with tuberous sclerosis, gliosis and neuronal degeneration, and localized cortical gliosis. Remission of seizures was obtained in three of five infants and surgery did not result in significant neurologic deficit. (Duchowny MS et al. Focal resection for malignant partial seizures in infancy. *Neurology* June 1990; *40:*980-984).

COMMENT. The authors conclude that excisional surgery can be performed safely in selected infants with medically uncontrolled malignant partial seizures and may improve long-term seizure outcome. They emphasize referral to a center specializing in early childhood epilepsy surgery. The same authors report at the 42nd Annual Meeting of the AAN that intractable focal seizures in childhood have a histopathological spectrum distinct from that of adults. Malformations, particularly neuronal migration disorders are most frequent in infants whereas hippocampal sclerosis, a common pathology in adult epileptics, did not occur in the infants or the children in this report. (*Neurology* April 1990; *40 (Suppl I)*:187). - Editor. *Ped Neur Briefs* June 1990.

Anterior Temporal Lobectomy
In Refractory Complex Partial Seizures

The outcome of 22 patients with onset of complex partial seizures (CPS) in early childhood and treated by anterior temporal lobectomy after intervals varying from three to 28 years, is reported from the Epilepsy Research Center, Baylor College of Medicine, Houston, TX. All patients showed improved seizure control, the majority having a greater than 95% reduction in seizure frequency. Psychosocial, behavioral, and educational problems occurred more frequently in patients whose surgery was delayed until adult life. Neuropathologic abnormalities were found in both the mesial and lateral portions of the temporal lobe. Mesial abnormalities included the classical Ammon's horn sclerosis and ganglioglioma. All the brain specimens showed congenital malformations or "microdysgenesis". The authors considered surgery, performed soon after medical intractibility has been determined, may limit the problems associated with prolonged uncontrolled seizures. (Mizrahi EM et al. Anterior temporal lobectomy and medically refractory temporal lobe epilepsy of childhood. *Epilepsia* May/June 1990; *31*:301-312).

COMMENT. In these patients with seizure onset between two and ten years of age Ammon's horn sclerosis occurred in 16 of the 22 patients. This finding contrasted with the absence of hippocampal sclerosis in patients with seizures beginning in infancy. (See Duchowny et al. *Neurology* 1990; *40*:980). - Editor. *Ped Neur Briefs* June 1990.

Surgery For Neonatal-Onset Seizures

Four children with intractable neonatal-onset seizures treated successfully by hemispherectomy at 1 -5 years of age are reported from UCLA School of Medicine, Los Angeles, CA. Positron emission tomography (PET) with fluoro-D-glucose provided accurate localization of seizure foci whereas CT and MRI were either normal or showed mild generalized cerebral atrophy. The report illustrates the important role of PET in the evaluation of children with intractable epilepsy of neonatal onset. (Chugani HT et al. Surgical treatment of intractable neonatal-onset seizures: The role of positron emission tomography. *Neurology* Aug 1988; *38*:1178-88).

COMMENT. The criteria for hemispherectomy were as follows: 1) Intractable unilateral seizures with diffuse epileptic activity in the affected hemisphere. 2) Persistent neurologic deficit on the contralateral side. 3) Malfunction of the affected hemisphere and intact function of the opposite hemisphere as tested by interictal EEGs, evoked potentials, thiopental test, and PET. At UCLA the results of surgery are impressive: the patients were seizure-free for periods up to 1-1/2 years and 3 patients were off all anticonvulsants. The surgical approach to treatment of refractory seizures appears superior to the conservative method with potentially toxic anticonvulsant drugs. The authors are to be complemented for their aggressive approach and search for alternate forms of early treatment. - Editor. *Ped Neur Briefs* August 1988.

Seizures And Ventricular Shunts

The role of ventricular shunts as a cause of seizures in children with hydrocephalus was studied in 190 patients treated for myelomeningocele in the Dept of Neurosurgery, Arkansas Children's Hospital, Little Rock, AR. The period of follow-up was 1-26 yrs, with an average of 9 yrs. The frequency of seizures in 144 shunted compared to 46 nonshunted patients was 22% and 2%, respectively. If modification of the shunt was unnecessary, only 9% had seizures, whereas in those requiring modification the incidence was 22%. A shunt infection raised the risk of seizures to 47%. Seizure frequency was approximately the same in those with frontal or parietal location catheters, 20 and 26%, respectively. Of 7 patients with unorthodox locations of shunt placements, near the motor cortex, 4 (57%) developed seizures. (Chadduck W, Adametz J. Incidence of seizures in patients with myelomeningocele: a multifactorial analysis. *Surg Neurol* Oct 1988; *30*:281-5).

COMMENT. One in four infants with myelomeningocele who are shunted for hydrocephalus develop seizures. Cortical injury at the time of shunt placement is a likely factor in etiology, and a complicating bacterial infection, even low-grade in type, will lead to diffuse cerebral injury and will double the risk of seizures. Candida meningitis has been reported in patients with CSF shunts (Surgarman B. *Arch Neurol* 1980; *37*:180), and a single colony of yeast should not be considered a contaminant especially in infants with hydrocephalus, ventricular shunts and cranial nerve palsies (Coker SB, Beltran RS. Candida meningitis; Clinical and radiographic diagnosis. *Pediatr Neurol* 1988; *4*:317). McLone et al (*Pediatrics* 1982; *70*:338) have alluded to the effect of CNS infections on the intelligence of children with myelomeningocele, and the occurrence of seizures is a further complication of surgery. Delay in operative closure of the spina bifida may reduce the severity of hydrocephalus and lessen the need for shunting with its attendant risks (see *Ped Neur Briefs* 1988; 2:52). - Editor. *Ped Neur Briefs* October 1988.

Surgery For Intractable Epilepsy Reviewed

The outcome and implications of early surgery for epilepsy are reviewed from the literature by the Comprehensive Epilepsy Center, Miami Children's Hospital, Miami, FA. Focal resection, corpus callostomy, and hemispherectomy are the three major neurosurgical procedures for epilepsy. In 40 children less than 15 years of age treated by removal of the anterior temporal lobe 23 were completely free of seizures postoperatively, eight almost seizure free and five improved significantly. (Davidson, Falconer. *Lancet* 1975; *1*:1260). Subsequent studies have confirmed these early results and freedom or near freedom from seizures is usually achieved in 50-90% of selected cases. The indications for *focal resection* are 1) intractable partial seizures, 2) localized structural lesion, 3) behavioral and academic deterioration, and 4) localized seizure focus. The contraindications are 1) medication noncompliance, 2) neurodegenerative disorder, and 3) multifocal seizure origin. Complication risks include quadrantanopic visual field deficit, transient dysphasia, third nerve palsy, cerebrovascular accident, and infection. *Corpus callostomy* is indicated for primary generalized seizures - atonic, tonic, clonic; partial seizures with secondary generalization; Lennox Gastaut syndrome; bilateral synchronous seizure discharges; multifocal seizure foci. Atonic seizures are particularly benefitted by corpus callostomy with 80% relief or reduction; tonic, clonic and partial seizures are improved in only 25-75% of cases. *Hemispherectomy* is indicated for partial seizures with hemiparesis, hemianopic visual field deficit, behavioral and cognitive disorder, and lateralized electroencephalographic focus. The lateralized (partial) seizures may be reduced by 80-90% and behavioral and cognitive status improved. The risks of hemispherectomy include hemosiderosis, hydrocephalus, and greater cognitive deficit. (Duchowny MS. Surgery for intractable epilepsy: Issues and outcome. *Pediatrics* November 1989; *84*:886-894).

COMMENT. The author comments that the psychosocial benefits constitute the most important argument in favor of early surgical intervention for intractable epilepsy in children. Relatively little is known about neural reorganization after early focal resection of hemispheric disconnection. The benefits of hemispherectomy for childhood epilepsy were described in a 36 year study (Lindsay J et al. See *Ped Neur Briefs* 1987; *1*:24 and 45). It has been used successfully in some children with intractable neonatal onset seizures with hemispherectomy performed as early as 1 to five years of age. (See *Ped Neur Briefs* 1988; *2*:62). - Editor. *Ped Neur Briefs* November 1989.

NARCOLEPSY

Symptomatic Narcolepsy With Diencephalic Lesions

Three patients with symptomatic narcolepsy are reported from the Departments of Neurology and Psychiatry, University of Michigan Medical Center, Ann Arbor, MI. One was a girl who developed polyphagia, weight gain, decreased growth, headaches with visual blurring, and excessive daytime sleepiness with frequent, irresistible brief naps at age 7 years. At age nine, she developed hyperprolactinemia and galactorrhea. At age 11 she had diabetic ketoacidosis, temperature dysregulation, hypothalamic hypothyroidism, partial diabetes insipidus, and hepatitis. The CT was normal. MRI showed mild diffuse brain substance loss. Following treatment with methylphenidate, sleepiness and irresistible sleep attacks improved. Tissue typing was positive for HLA-DR2 and HLA-DQw1. The authors refer to ten additional cases of symptomatic narcolepsy with documented brain lesions reported in the literature. (Aldrich, MS, Naylor, MW. Narcolepsy associated with lesions of the diencephalon. *Neurology* November 1989; *39*:1505-1508).

COMMENT. In these cases the REM sleep abnormalities and excessive daytime sleepiness were documented by polysomnography and Multiple Sleep latency Tests. Two of the three patients were HLA-DR2 positive while the third was negative. In an addendum, the authors note an additional report of symptomatic narcolepsy in a nine year old HLA-DR2-positive boy following removal of a craniopharyngioma (Kowatch RA, et al. *Sleep Res* 1989; *18*:250). Other brain lesions associated with narcolepsy have included midbrain glioblastoma, cerebral sarcoidosis, pontine infarcts, 3rd ventricle glioma, pituitary adenoma, 3rd ventricle colloid cyst, multiple sclerosis, encephalitis, ischemia, head trauma, as well as craniopharyngioma. - Editor. *Ped Neur Briefs* November 1989.

NON-EPILEPTIC EYE DEVIATION

Tonic Upgaze In Infancy

Tonic upward ocular deviation without seizure activity or neurologic disease is reported in 3 infants from the Pediatric and Neuroophthalmology Units, School of Medicine, University of California, San Francisco. The frequency and duration of the tonic upgaze episodes decreased with time but were exacerbated by fatigue or illness. Downward eye movements were normal. (Ahn JC et al. Tonic upgaze in infancy. A report of three cases. *Arch Ophthalmol* Jan 1989; *107*:57-58).

COMMENT. Transient tonic downward gaze in newborns is a fairly common phenomenon whereas tonic upgaze deviation is rarely reported, except with seizure activity, visual loss, or brain-stem disease. The pathophysiology of this transient variety of tonic upgaze is unknown but appears to differ from that of the downgaze type, being more persistent and exacerbated by fatigue or illness. - Editor. *Ped Neur Briefs* January 1989.

CHAPTER **2**

MIGRAINE AND OTHER HEADACHES

ETIOLOGIC FACTORS

Migraine As A Neurovascular Metabolic Disorder

Brain oxidative metabolism has been studied in nine patients with classical migraine at the Neurological Institute, University of Bologna, Italy. An increase in plasma lactate was found after standardized muscular effort and deficits of various mitochondrial respiratory chain enzymes in muscle biopsies occurred in 7. Two patients had 72% and 60% depression of cytochrome C oxidase activity, 1 also showed ragged red fibers and subsarcolemmal clusters of giant mitochondria with paracrystalline inclusions. The findings indicated a dysfunction of mitochondrial energy metabolism and suggested that migraine is the result of a defect of brain oxidative metabolism. The authors conclude that neural energetic lability, especially if coupled with vascular metabolic dysfunction, could result - particularly under stressful conditions - in the neurological deficits of classical migraine. It was their hypothesis that a metabolic oxidative defect involving brain cells and possibly brain vessels represents the critical factor predisposing migraineurs to transient or persistent neurological deficits. (Mantagna P et al. Migraine as a defect of brain oxidative metabolism: A hypothesis. *J Neurol* Feb 1989; *236*:124-125).

> COMMENT. The neurological deficits of migraine have been attributed to brain ischemia or a primary derangement of brain metabolism. The progression of the aura and the prodromal symptoms are difficult to reconcile with a purely vascular problem and changes in platelet function suggest a diffuse extracerebral metabolic disturbance. Migraine attacks sometimes occur as complications of mitochondrial encephalomyopathies which reinforces the suggestion that migraine is the result of a defect of brain oxidative metabolism. - Editor. *Ped Neur Briefs* March 1989.

Psychological Factors In Adolescent Headache

Seventy high school students between 16 and 18 years of age reporting a headache frequency of once a week or more were compared with a headache-free control group and were studied by questionnaires for psychosocial, health-behavior, and medical problems at the Dept of Child and Youth Psychiatry, University Hospital of Uppsala, Sweden. Adolescents with recurrent tension and migraine headaches reported significantly more somatic symptoms and psychological distress than controls, they were more often absent from school, and used the school health service more than controls. Their parents were more often divorced and suffered more frequently from headache and abdominal pain. Nervous problems, anxiety, depression, homework time, somatic symptoms and absence from school were psychosocial predictors of headache susceptibility. (Larsson B. The role of psychological, health-behavior and medical factors in adolescent headache. *Dev Med Child Neurol* Oct 1988; *30*:616-625).

COMMENT. These results differ from a previous study of anxiety in childhood migraine. Patients with migraine and their parents who completed standardized anxiety, personality, and life-event scales showed no significant difference from controls. All patients had anxiety scores within normal. Patient selection and the omission of tension headache suffers could explain the difference in findings. - Editor. *Ped Neur Briefs* December 1988.

Environmental Factors In Headache

The environmental conditions related to headache in 38 children are reviewed from the Illinois Institute of Technology and the Franciscan Children's Hospital and Rehabilitation Center, Boston, MA. Parents filled out the Children's Headache Assessment Scale (CHAS) at an evaluation for behavioral medicine treatment and the parent rating questionnaire was completed again after therapy. The frequency of specific CHAS categories (stress antecedents, physical antecedents, attention consequences, escape consequences, coping responses, and medication use) varied widely and were changed by behavioral medicine treatment. There was less interference of headache with school attendance and improved coping responses after treatment. (Budd KS, Kedesdy JH. Investigation of environmental factors in pediatric headache. *Headache* October 1989; *29*:569-573.

COMMENT. The Children's Headache Assessment Scale focuses on situations and events surrounding the headaches rather than questioning parents about the symptoms. This study shows that the parent rating questionnaire is of value in behavioral assessment of pediatric headache and in following responses to behavioral treatment. - Editor. *Ped Neur Briefs* November 1989.

METHODS OF MANAGEMENT

Self-Hypnosis Control Of Migraine

In a prospective study at the Minneapolis Children's Medical Center 28 children with classic migraine were treated with propranolol (3 mg/kg/d) or placebo for 3 months, using a cross over design, followed by an equal period of self-hypnosis. The mean number of headaches per child during placebo and propranolol periods were similar (13.3 and 14.9, respectively) and was significantly reduced (5.8) with self-hypnosis (P=.045), a standard progressive relaxation exercise. (Olness K, Macdonald JT, Uden DL. *Pediatrics* 1987; *79*:593-597.

COMMENT. Non-pharmacological methods (biofeedback, self-hypnosis, dietary) of treatment of juvenile migraine are displacing the previously popular pharmacologic options e.g. propranolol and phenytoin. Phenytoin prophylactic treatment is attended by potential adverse toxicity and propranolol in controlled studies has been found ineffective (Forsythe WI et al. *Develop Med Child Neurol* 1984; *26*:737-741). - Editor. *Ped Neur Briefs* June 1987.

Relaxation Treatment For Migraine

Relaxation training was compared to two control placebo psychological methods of treatment in 99 children and adolescents with frequent migraine at the Children's Hospital of Eastern Ontario, University of Ottawa, Canada. Relaxation methods consisted of 6, one-hour, weekly sessions in which children were taught sequential tensing and relaxation of large muscle groups and the use of deep breathing. Placebo treatment consisted of therapy sessions to teach recognition of emotions, relating them to life situations, and to urge discussion of feelings daily with a friend or parent. A second control method labeled "own best efforts" consisted of a single session to discuss the use of the headache diary to determine triggering factors. The value of the treatments were determined by questionnaires concerning headache frequency and severity and confidence in the method and therapist. Patients in all three treatment groups showed a significant reduction in headaches following treatment for 4 weeks and at 3 and 12 month follow-up. Relaxation training was no more effective than brief reassurance and self-control suggestion techniques in treating pediatric migraine. (McGrath PJ et al. Relaxation prophylaxis for childhood migraines: a randomized placebo-controlled trial. *Dev Med Child Neurol* Oct 1988; *30*:626-631.

COMMENT. The incidence of migraine in children and adolescents has been estimated at 5-7%. Pharmacological intervention has been the usual approach to treatment but self-regulation methods may be helpful and may reduce reliance on drugs of doubtful efficacy. In one well-controlled trial, propranolol was ineffective when compared to placebo (Forsythe WI et al. *Dev Med Child Neurol* Dec 1984; *26*:737). The average duration of headache was greater during the propranolol period (40 mg two or three times daily) and the frequency was not reduced. Food allergy has been emphasized as a causative factor, and dietary therapy eliminating such foods as cow's milk, egg, chocolate, orange, and wheat, or other allergenic items has been proposed as an alternative to drugs in childhood migraine (Egger J et al. *Lancet* 1983; *2*:865; and *J Pediatr* Jan 1989; *114*:51). - Editor. *Ped Neur Briefs* December 1988.

Aspirin Prophylaxis In Chronic Paroxysmal Hemicrania

A nine year old child with chronic paroxysmal hemicrania (CPH) was treated successfully using small dose aspirin prophylaxis at the California Medical Clinic for Headache, Encino, and the Harbor-UCLA Medical Center, Torrance, CA. Attacks occurred every 1-1/2 hours throughout the day and awakened him from a sleep at night. They lasted a minimum of ten minutes and a maximum of 20 minutes and were localized to the left retroorbital and supraorbital areas. Pain was excruciating and nonthrobbing and was associated with ipsilateral lacrimation, nasal stuffiness, ptosis, and conjunctival injection. No relief was obtained with acetaminophen or phenobarbital. Baby aspirin, (243 mg b.i.d., prevented the headaches and the dosage was decreased to 162 mg b.i.d. without further attacks. The aspirin was discontinued after three months without recurrence of headaches. The authors consider that this case is the first report of chronic paroxysmal hemicrania observed in a child, the earliest onset of CPH, and the first case obtaining relief from low dose prophylactic aspirin therapy. The effective daily dose of aspirin used (14.7 mg/kg) was less than the lowest mean level at risk for Reye's syndrome (25.1 mg/kg). (Kudrow DB, Kudrow L. Successful aspirin prophylaxis in a child with chronic paroxysmal hemicrania. *Headache* March 1989; *29*:280-281).

COMMENT. Indomethacin prophylaxis is considered the treatment of choice in adults with chronic paroxysmal hemicrania whereas salicylates are usually ineffective. Aspirin prophylaxis for chronic headache in children would not be a popular therapy generally because of the concern about Reye's syndrome. - Editor. *Ped Neur Briefs* March 1989.

DIETARY TREATMENT

Diet And Migraine

A team of investigators at the Department of Paediatrics, Rotherham District General Hospital, and Sheffield Children's Hospital, have carried out a controlled study in 39 children to assess the effects of exclusion of dietary vasoactive amines in migraine. The children were allocated at random to either a high fibre diet low in these substances or a regular high fibre diet for an 8 week period. Foods excluded were chocolate, cheese, yogurt, citrus fruits, bananas, pineapple, raspberries, plums, peas, beans, yeast, shellfish, smoked pickled fish, game, tea, coffee, and cola drinks containing caffeine.

Both test and control groups showed a significant decrease in the number of headaches and there was no significant difference between the two groups. A placebo effect was considered a probable explanation for the improvement in many. (Salfield SAW et al. *Arch Dis Child* 1987; *62*:458-460).

COMMENT. The relation of tyramine and other amine-rich foods to the occurrence of headaches in certain migraineurs is a theory frequently proposed (Hanington E. In *Clinical Reaction to Food*. New York, Wiley, 1983). The authors of the present study admit that their group was small and an idiosyncrasy to amines in occasional patients with migraine could not be ruled out.

An allergic mechanism for dietary migraine is an alternative theory investigated by use of a so-called "oligoantigenic diet", a diet that eliminates all but a few sensitizing food antigens. Cow's milk, egg, and wheat cereals were the most frequent offenders (Egger J et al. *Lancet* 1983; *2*:865). To strictly avoid all foods listed as possible migraine precipitants is usually unnecessary and possibly hazardous to the child's health. If the possible benefits of an elimination diet are to be confirmed, however, the use of a control diet would be essential to exclude a placebo effect. - Editor. *Ped Neur Briefs* July 1987.

Oligoantigenic Diet For Migraine And Epilepsy

A diet low in antigenic items was used to treat 63 children with epilepsy refractory to medication at the Depts of Neurology, Immunology, and Dietetics, The Hospital for Sick Children, Great Ormond Street, and the Institute of Child Health, London, England. The authors had previously reported beneficial effects of the "oligoantigenic" diet in the treatment of migraine (*Lancet* 1983; *2*:865) and the hyperkinetic syndrome (*Lancet* 1985; *1*:940). The diet consisted of 2 meats (lamb and chicken), 2 carbohydrates (potatoes and rice), 2 fruits (banana and apple), vegetables (cabbage, sprouts, cauliflower, broccoli, cucumber, celery, carrots, parsnips), water, salt, pepper, pure herbs, and calcium and vitamins for 4 weeks. Patients who responded (no seizures or migraine for the last 2 weeks) were reintroduced to essential foods (e.g. milk, cheese, wheat) at the rate of one a week. If symptoms were provoked, soy-based or goat milk products, rye or oats were substituted. Setbacks were avoided by first giving foods least likely to be antigenic (e.g. beef, oats, peaches, or grapes). Of 45 children who had epilepsy with recurrent headaches, abdominal symptoms, or hyperkinetic behavior, 25 had no seizures and 11 had fewer seizures during diet therapy. Foods most likely to provoke seizures when reintroduced were cow milk and cheese, citrus fruits, wheat, tartrazine and benzoic acid food additives, eggs, tomato, pork, and chocolate. In double-blind, placebo-controlled provocation studies introducing cow milk, orange juice, wheat, pork, egg, and benzoate, symptoms recurred in 15 of 16 children, including seizures in 8; none recurred with placebo. The oligoantigenic diet was unsuccessful in the treatment of 18 children who had epilepsy uncomplicated by migraine or hyperkinetic behavior. (Egger J, Wilson J, et al. Oligoantigenic diet treatment of children with epilepsy and migraine. *J Pediatr* Jan 1989; *114*:51-58).

COMMENT. If reproducible and sustained, these results are impressive and deserve further investigation in children with frequently recurrent seizures and headache resistant to anticonvulsant medication. The authors point out that the diets are socially disruptive and may cause malnutrition. In the US, pediatric allergists are not generally impressed with the theory of food hypersensitivity as a cause of neurological disease and their enthusiastic collaboration in studies of this type is not readily available. - Editor. *Ped Neur Briefs* December 1988.

Aspartame And Headache

At a recent meeting of the American Academy of Neurology, neurologists at the Albert Einstein College of Medicine, Bronx, NY and the Montefiore Headache Unit reported that aspartame was a headache precipitating factor in 8.2% of 171 patients evaluated consecutively. Migraineurs were three times as likely to complain that aspartame triggered their headaches than those with muscle contraction or mixed headache types. The authors concluded that aspartame may be an important dietary trigger in a significant proportion of headache suffers, particularly in migraineurs. (Lipton RB et al. *Neurology* March 1988; *38*(Suppl 1):356); and *N Engl J Med* May 5, 1988; *318*:1200).

> COMMENT. Although the above study was conducted mainly in adults, the findings would probably apply equally to children with migraine. The role of aspartame in aggravating migraine and other vascular headaches is confirmed by investigators at the Cleveland Clinic and at Emory University School of Medicine and negated by those at Duke University (*N Engl J Med* May 5, 1988; *318*:1201-2). Diet drinks containing NutraSweet should be on the list of items to be avoided by migraineurs until further studies are completed. - Editor. *Ped Neur Briefs* May 1988.

Diet Related Migraine And The Electroencephalogram

Thirty-eight patients with a history of diet induced migraine were studied with recording of clinical responses and electroencephalography at the Departments of Neurology and Biometry, Kansas University Medical Center, Kansas City, Kansas. The subjects consisted of 30 females and 8 males aged from 17 to 38 years, all having a history of migraine attacks consistently provoked by either chocolate, cheese, or alcohol. With the exception of one patient with a febrile seizure at age 2, none had a seizure history. There was a family history of migraine in first degree relatives in 22 patients (58%). Tests were carried out on an initial baseline day and on a second day, after challenge with chocolate, red wine, cheese, and fasting. Migraine headache occurred in 16 (42%), four with scintillating scotomata. Electroencephalograms were abnormal in 12 subjects (32%); most abnormalities being nonspecific slow waves. In three cases there were paroxysmal features. Electroencephalographic response to hyperventilation was exaggerated in eight subjects

(21%) but was not related to the occurrence of a headache. Photic stimulation showed high frequency driving in all 16 patients who developed headache but in only 15 out of 22 (64%) who did not develop headache (Lai C et al. Clinical and electrophysiological responses to dietary challenge in migraineurs. *Headache* March 1989; *29*:180-186).

> COMMENT. Foods are commonly cited by patients as the cause of some migraine attacks. Tyramine is present in high concentrations in certain substances frequently producing migraine (various cheeses, beer and wine). Electro-encephalographic abnormalities are found during asymptomatic periods in patients with migraine, and focal and unilateral delta rhythms have been described in patients with migraine during symptomatic states. Paroxysmal epileptiform discharges are unusual in adults with migraine but not uncommon in children. Temporal relationships between headache and severe episodic EEG abnormality ("ictal headache") have been reported (Isler H et al in Andermann F, Lugaresi E (eds): *Migraine and Epilepsy*, Boston, Butterworths, 1987). - Editor. *Ped Neur Briefs* March 1989.

ASSOCIATED SYMPTOMS AND SYNDROMES

Somnambulism And Migraine

Neurologists in the EEG laboratory of the Hopital d'Enfants, Dijon, France, have continued their interests and research concerning the association of somnambulism and migraine in childhood. Among 25 children with migraine developing between 8 and 15 years of age, 7 (28%) had a history of somnambulism beginning at age 5 to 10 years (mean 7 years). In normal controls and in children with epilepsy, the incidence of somnambulism was only 5% and 6%, respectively. A history of somnambulism may be a useful aid in the diagnosis of migraine in a child with headaches. (Giroud M, Nivelon JL, Dumas R. *Arch Fr Pediatr* 1987; *44*:263-5).

COMMENT. The early differentiation of migraine from nonmigraine headaches is important (1) to expedite relief by appropriate treatment and (2) to spare the child unnecessary radiological and other extensive testing. This study confirms that of Barabas G et al (*Neurology* 1983; *33*:948) that showed an incidence of sleep walking of 30% in migraineurs compared to 5 to 6% with learning disabilities. Additional childhood precursors of migraine include cyclic vomiting, abdominal pain, motion sickness, and paroxysmal vertigo. - Editor. *Ped Neur Briefs* July 1987.

Tolosa-Hunt Syndrome

The authors report a case in a 10.5 year old girl admitted to the Centre hospitalier Guy-de-Chauliac, Montpellier, France, with a left painful ophthalmoplegia. She had a convulsion with fever and a left facial palsy at 6 years of age and since then complained of headaches. Four years later she had diplopia, left-sided ocular pain and ptosis. On admission, there was a complete III nerve and a VI nerve paralysis on the left. CT, EEG, evoked potentials, spinal tap, blood and immunologic tests were normal. Steroid therapy resulted in a rapid remission. The authors point out that the diagnosis is by exclusion of local and systemic disease and that the syndrome is difficult to differentiate from ophthalmoplegic migraine. (Rapin F, Echenne B. *Arch Fr Pediatr* 1987; *44*:299-301).

COMMENT. Tolosa, in 1954, described this syndrome as a periarteritic lesion of the carotid syphon with the clinical features of a carotid infraclinoidal aneurysm. Hunt et al, in 1961, involved an indolent inflammation of the cavernous sinus and described the beneficial response to steroids.

Ophthalmoplegic migraine, in the differential diagnosis, has been reported in infants (*Pediatrics* 1978; *61*:886) and usually presents early in childhood. The III nerve palsy develops 24 hours or more after the onset of the migraine headache and coincides with the stage of vasodilation; presumably it is due to a localized pressure effect of the carotid artery. - Editor. *Ped Neur Briefs* July 1987.

Amaurosis Fugax And Migraine

Amaurosis fugax, a sudden, transient monocular loss of vision resolving in 5 to 10 minutes, is reported in five teenagers from the British Columbia's Children's Hospital, Vancouver, BC, and The Hospital for Sick Children, Toronto, Canada. Four patients had a history of common migraine at other times or a family history of migraine. Unlike adults in whom amaurosis fugax is associated frequently with atherosclerosis of the internal carotid artery and a herald of stroke, these symptoms in children may represent a migraine variant, and cerebral angiography is usually unwarranted. (Appleton R et al. Amaurosis fugax in teenagers. A migraine variant. *AJDC* March 1988; *142*:331-3).

COMMENT. The causes of amaurosis fugax are diverse and include carotid atheromatous disease, Raynaud's disease, temporal arteritis, sickle cell anemia, optic nerve tumor, hysteria, as well as migraine. Patients who describe a characteristic mosaic or jigsaw pattern of transient monocular blindness are more likely to be suffering from migraine than carotid atheromatosis, especially in children and adolescents.

On the subject of migraine, Peroutka SJ of Stanford University Medical Center has demonstrated that a large number of migraine prophylactic agents, including propranolol, methysergide, cyproheptadine, and pizotifen, share an ability to interact with 5-hydroxytryptamine (serotonin) receptor subtypes in human brain. This property is offered as a method of selection of drugs for clinical trial in migraine. (*Ann Neurol* May 1988; *23*:500). - Editor. *Ped Neur Briefs* May 1988.

Posttraumatic Headache

The occurrence and persistence of headache after closed head injury was investigated in 129 children, 70 boys and 59 girls, during a follow-up period, average 5.9 yrs, in the Depts of Neuropsychology and Child Neurology, State University Hospital, P.O. Box 9600, 2300 RC Leiden, The Netherlands. During hospitalization, complaints of headache occurred in 34 children (29%), especially in girls and in those with serious EEG abnormalities. The incidence of headache at 6 mos, 1 year, and 6 yrs after the accident was 23%, 23%, and 25%, respectively. The patients with complaints were different in each group and could not be distinguished from headache-free patients with regard to age, sex, duration of coma, skull fracture, and the EEG. Complaints of headache after hospitalization for closed head injury did not appear to be accident related. (Lanser JBK, Jennekens-Schinkel A, Peters ACB. Headache after closed head injury in children. *Headache* April 1988; *28*:176-179).

COMMENT. The percentage of children (25%) suffering from headache at an extended period after closed head injury in this study is similar to that previously reported by others (Rothner AD, *Headache* 1978; *18*:169). Assumptions that the headaches are accident-related do not appear to be justified, and other possible causes should be investigated. - Editor. *Ped Neur Briefs* May 1988.

Migraine-Related Stroke

The diagnosis of migraine-related stroke is reviewed and case histories provided from the Center for Stroke Research, Department of Neurology, Henry Ford Hospital, Detroit, MI. The collaborative group for the study of stroke in young women defined the relative risk for thrombotic stroke as two-fold for women with migraine when compared with a neighbor but not with a hospital control. In 448 total stroke cases 4% were attributed to migraine. The classification of migraine-related stroke is in three categories: 1) Coexisting stroke and migraine, 2) stroke with clinical features of migraine, and 3) migraine-induced stroke. Several arteriovenous malformations frequently masquerade as migraine with aura, oral contraceptives increase stroke risk and may cause coexisting stroke and migraine, and ergot therapy for migraine is sometimes complicated by stroke. The pathogenesis of migraine-induced stroke includes coagulation, hemodynamic and neuronal factors. The initiation of a migraine attack is a primary neuronal phenomenon with metabolic and cerebral hemodynamic consequences. A low cerebral blood flow combined with factors which predispose to coagulopathy may lead rarely to intravascular thrombosis and migraine-induced cerebral infarction. (Welch KMA, Levine SR. Migraine-related stroke in the context of the international headache society classification of head pain. *Arch Neurol* April 1990, *47*:458-462).

> COMMENT. Stroke associated with migraine in children is rare and is an indication for exclusion of an underlying structural cerebral lesion, e.g. arteriovenous malformation, congenital cerebral arterial occlusion, and encephalomalacia. Classical migraine associated with intractable epilepsy and multiple strokes has been described with mitochondrial encephalopathies. (Dvorkin GS, Andermann F et al, 1987). - Editor. *Ped Neur Briefs* April 1990.

Migraine And Cerebellar Ataxia

A four year old boy with migraine associated with focal cerebral edema, CSF pleocytosis, and progressive cerebellar ataxia is reported from the Departments of Neurology and Radiology, Yale University School of Medicine, New Haven, CT. The onset was at one year of age with an episode of unresponsiveness which resolved within one day. At three years of age he suffered acute cortical blindness for 36 hours. At four years of age he presented with a pulsating left-sided headache and an acute right hemiparesis. An MRI showed increased signal in the left parietooccipital region, enhanced with Gadolinium. The next day he had a right focal seizure lasting five minutes and a seizure occurrence with persistent nonresponsiveness and right hemiparesis. On recovery over several days, the hemiparesis fluctuated, a left-sided headache resolved, but cerebellar ataxia developed and persisted. The CSF was clear with 60 WBC, protein 12 mg/dl, and glucose 75 mg/dl. A course of Propranolol has prevented recurrence of hemiparesis and headache but lower extremity spasticity and gait ataxia have persisted. (Goldstein JM, Shaywitz BA et al. Migraine associated with focal cerebral edema, cerebrospinal fluid pleocytosis, and progressive cerebellar ataxia: MRI documentation. *Neurology* August 1990; *40*:1284-1287).

COMMENT. A so-called meningitic migraine with cerebral edema and autosomal dominant cerebellar ataxia has been reported previously in an adult (Fitzsimons RB, Wolfenden WH. *Brain* 1985; *108*:555) but the present case is the first report in a child and with MRI documentation of a transient lesion. Severe prolonged migrainous symptoms and prolonged partial status epilepticus are characteristic features of the MELAS syndrome or mitochondrial encephalomyopathy which should be considered in the differential diagnosis of patients with headache and seizures. (Montagna P et al. *Neurology* 1988; *38*:751). - Editor. *Ped Neur Briefs* September 1990.

Visual Evoked Responses In Migraine

The visual evoked responses (VERs) to flash and pattern stimulation were examined in 44 children with migraine and 8 with periodic syndrome at the Birmingham and Midland Eye Hospital, Birmingham, England. Patients younger than 13 years had higher fast wave amplitude and lower fast wave frequency than controls in the same age groups. In older children the fast wave amplitude was higher in those with migraine than in controls but fast wave frequencies were not different. Children with periodic syndrome had similar fast wave amplitudes to the younger children with migraine. The high fast wave frequency with superimposed intermittent high amplitude sharp waves after flash stimulation seen in patients with periodic syndrome are similar to those seen in acephalgic migraine in adults. The finding of similar VERs in migraine and periodic syndrome supports the inclusion of periodic syndrome in the international classification of migraine. (Mortimer MJ et al. Visual evoked responses in children with migraine: a diagnostic test. *Lancet* January 13, 1990; *335*:75-77).

COMMENT. The VER is proposed as a useful test in the diagnosis of migraine in children. The test may be especially valuable in the differentiation and diagnosis of cases of periodic or cyclical vomiting when a migrainous etiology is unclear. (Millichap JG. *Arch Fr Pediatr* 1987; *44*:231; *Pediatrics* 1955; *15*:705). - Editor. *Ped Neur Briefs* April 1990.

CHAPTER **3**

ATTENTION DEFICIT, BEHAVIOR, AND LEARNING DISORDERS

Progress in the neurology of behavior has emphasized the neurobiological basis for learning disabilities, the use of drugs in treatment, and the controversial topic of diet in relation to attention and motor activity.

The neurologic examination, evoked potentials, the electroencephalogram, MRI, PET, SPECT, and neuropsychological tests have been used to define the types and localization of brain pathologies underlying certain learning and behavior disorders. With the development of more sophisticated neuroscientific methods, evidence for a structural or biochemical brain defect as the basis for learning disabilities has been uncovered with greater certainty.

Attention deficit hyperactivity disorder is a heterogeneous problem necessitating the collaboration of parent, teacher, social worker, pediatrician, psychologist, psychiatrist, and neurologist. Subtle signs of neurological dysfunction aid in the differentiation of the various causes of ADHD and the pediatric neurologist has an important role in the management of the child with learning and behavior problems.

NEUROLOGICAL BASIS FOR ADHD

Attention Deficit Disorder Pathophysiology

Progress over the past 50 years in our understanding of the neurobiology of attention deficit disorder with hyperactivity is reviewed by child psychiatrists at the National Institute of Mental Health, Bethesda, MD. Since Bradley first described the paradoxical calming effect of the stimulant benzedrine on hyperactive children (*Amer J Psychiat* 1937; *94*:577), more than 20 neuropharmacological agents have been used for the study and treatment of children with attention deficit disorder with hyperactivity (ADDH).

Biochemical, pharmacological, and anatomical hypotheses are analyzed and may be summarized as follows: 1) stimulants are the treatment of choice and all beneficial drugs have effects on catecholamine metabolism; 2) alteration in noradrenergic function appears necessary for clinical efficacy; 3) a role for norepinephrine but not serotonin metabolism in the pathophysiology is likely; 4) support for a frontal lobe anatomical location of CNS dysfunction for ADDH seems more conclusive than hypothalamic dysfunction; 5) different sites of dysfunction in the cortical-striatal "circuit" might account for the varying symptoms of the ADDH syndrome. (Zametkin AJ, Rapoport JL. Neurobiology of attention deficit disorder with hyperactivity: Where have we come in 50 years? *J Amer Acad Child and Adolesc Psychiat* 1987; *26*:676-686).

COMMENT. The possible importance of brain injury or other neuropathological lesions in the pathogenesis of hyperkinetic behavior is often discounted in favor of environmental factors, and the authors emphasis on the neuroanatomical hypothesis and especially frontal lobe dysfunction in ADDH is refreshing. Some of the earlier experimental neuroanatomical studies of hyperkinesia have been concerned with the effects of ablation or destruction of different cortical and subcortical structures on locomotor activity. Bilateral removal of the prefrontal and frontal areas in the monkey causes the greatest total increase in activity (Kennard MA et al. *J Neurophysiol* 1941; 4:512).

Millichap JG et al. (*Excerpta Medica* Ed. Conners, CK 1974; 130-139) found an increase in locomotor activity of mice with prefrontal cortical lesions and those animals with the highest level of postoperative activity responded to methylphenidate with a reduction in locomotor activity. We suggested that animals with prefrontal cortical lesions should make valuable experimental models for testing new drugs. The beneficial effect of methylphenidate on hyperactivity in our patients was related to the level of motor activity before treatment and the degree of neurological abnormality. ADDH patients with the greatest number of neurologic signs were most active and were most likely to benefit from stimulant therapy. (Millichap JG. *N.Y. Acad Sci* 1973; 205:321). A neuroanatomical basis for ADDH in some children might be substantiated by the MRI. - Editor. *Ped Neur Briefs* October 1987.

ADDH, Auditory Evoked
Responses, And Delinquncy Subgroups

Two subgroups of hyperactive children (25 non-delinquent and 9 delinquent) and one group of 34 non-delinquent normal children were evaluated from childhood to adolescence at the National Center for Hyperactive Children, Encino, CA, using auditory evoked response potential (AERP) measures and EEG recordings. Abnormalities of CNS maturation and function related by longitudinal AERP changes and abnormal EEGs characterized the non-delinquent hyperactive subjects, while delinquent hyperactive subjects showed normal maturational changes. ADDH boys with neurologic abnormalities had a better outcome than those with normal CNS functions who later became delinquent and whose behavior was presumed secondary to environmental social factors. Two distinct subgroups of ADDH, one with and one without delinquency, were lineated. (Satterfield JH et al. Longitudinal study of AERP's in hyperactive and normal children: relationship to antisocial behavior. *Electroenceph Clin Neurophysiol* 1987; *67*:531-536).

COMMENT. In addition to psychiatric diagnosis, the neurologic exam, EEG, and evoked potentials are important in the differentiation of subgroups of hyperactive children. - Editor. *Ped Neur Briefs* January 1988.

Hyperactive Boys In Adolescence

The rates of dysfunction among male adolescents with a history of hyperactive behavior in childhood were examined in a follow-up study at the New York State Psychiatric Institute and Long Island Jewish Med Cntr, New York, NY. In a previous report, the authors found that half (48%) of the 101 formerly hyperactive subjects compared with 20% of 100 controls had psychiatric disorders at follow-up, including ADDH, antisocial personality disorder, and substance use disorder (SUD).

A comparison of the 52 patients and 80 controls who had not developed psychiatric disorders showed that hyperactivity in childhood did not lead to behavioral and social problems in later life. Academic functioning and conduct problems in high school, alcohol-related problems and conduct outside of school, and temper outbursts were not significantly different in the two groups. Inattention and hyperactivity were more prevalent in the former patient group, as expected, but drug use and drug-related problems, especially marijuana, were more frequent among the controls than in formerly hyperactive children.

These results suggest that the eventual occupational and social adjustment of hyperactive children is not different from that of controls and any tendencies to drug abuse may be less of a problem. Hyperactive children with psychiatric disorders form a deviant subgroup that must be identified for the purpose of treatment and prognosis. (Mannuzza S, Gittelman Klein R et al. Hyperactive boys almost grown up. II Status of subjects without a mental disorder. *Arch Gen Psychiatry* Jan 1988; 45:13-18).

> COMMENT. How many of these patients had neurological signs indicative of brain dysfunction in early childhood? The hyperactive patients without psychiatric disorders evaluated in this study are those often referred to the pediatrician or pediatric neurologist for management. They frequently have signs of minimal brain dysfunction during childhood that become less obvious in adolescence, many have electroencephalographic abnormalities, and the behavior and inattention respond to methylphenidate or other central nervous system stimulant medication. - Editor. *Ped Neur Briefs* February 1988.

Psychiatric Disorders And ADD

The frequencies of various psychiatric and neuromaturational disorders were compared in 22 ADD children aged 5-16 years and in 20 normal control subjects studied by structured diagnostic interviews with mothers in the Pediatric Psychopharmacology Clinic and Child Psychiatry Service, Massachusetts General Hospital, Boston.

Compared with controls, ADD patients had significantly higher rates of conduct disorder, oppositional disorder, major affective disorder, tics, language disorder/stuttering, encopresis and learning disorders. Enuresis occurred in seven (32%) ADD children compared to three (15%) controls. The rate of affective disorders in ADD children was significantly higher in subgroups with conduct/oppositional disorders and anxiety and significantly lower in the subgroup with neuromaturational disorders (enuresis, encopresis, language disorders, tics) when compared to normal control subjects. The incidence of conduct disorders was increased in the ADD subgroup with anxiety disorders. The recognition of ADD subgroups and psychiatric co-morbidity may be clinically useful in prognosis and treatment. (Munir K, Biederman J, Knee D. Psychiatric comorbidity in patients with attention deficit disorder. *J Amer Acad Child Adol Psychiat* 1987; *26 (6)*:844-848).

COMMENT. Previous studies have emphasized the need to correctly classify children with ADD into groups with or without conduct and anxiety disorders and those with abnormal neurologic signs and MBD when evaluating drug effects. (See *Ped Neur Briefs* 1987; *1 (2)*:14). - Editor. *Ped Neur Briefs* February 1988.

Attention Deficit Disorder:
Measure Of Impulsivity And Inattention
The go-no-go paradigm was used in the evaluation of children with attention deficit disorder (ADD) at the Dept of Pediatrics, Division of Neurology and Evaluation Center for Learning, Northwestern Univ Medical School, Evanston Hospital, Evanston, IL. The paradigm consisted of the taped presentation of 2 trials of 10 stimuli; 5 go signals (1 tap) to which the children were expected to respond by raising and lowering their index finger, and 5 no-go signals to which they should not respond. Commissions errors suggest impulsivity and omission errors suggest inattention. Children with ADD (44 boys) made more total errors than did 32 control subjects (P .03). Nonhyperactive (ADDnoH) subjects made more commission errors than controls initially but improved with practice. Hyperactive ADD subjects (ADDH) made the same number of early commission errors as controls but failed to improve with practice. Omission errors were highest in the ADDH group. The paradigm provided an objective measure of inattention and impulsivity and a distinction between hyperactive and nonhyper-

active children with ADD. (Trommer BL et al. The go-no-go paradigm in attention deficit disorder. *Ann Neurol* Nov 1988; 24:610-614).

> COMMENT. Errors of commission are more common than errors of omission in children with ADD which suggests that impulsivity is more easily demonstrated than inattention. The DSM-III "impulsivity" criteria include inability to wait in turn at games, calling out in class, and shifting activity. The go-no-go paradigm offers a test for impulsivity at a cognitive level, the inability to give the most correct answer in a multiple choice setting, and supplements reports of behavioral manifestations of ADD. - Editor. *Ped Neur Briefs* October 1988.

Mental Status Examination

The child neurologists' approach to the mental status examination of children with learning problems was examined by questionnaires randomly submitted to 163 attendees at the 16th Annual Child Neurology Society Meeting in 1987 and the results are reported from the Division of Neurology, Department of Pediatrics, Newington Children's Hospital and Biostatistics Research Center, Farmington, CT. The child neurologists were asked to score on a five point scale (0=never, 5=always) the frequency with which they test for 30 mental status items when examining school age children who present with learning problems. The 30 items were divided into six categories of mental status function in ascending order of complexity: 1) fundamental processes including level of responsiveness, attention and/or vigilance; 2) Language including handedness, spontaneous speech, comprehension, reading, writing, spelling; 3) Memory including orientation, immediate recall, remote memory; 4) Constructional ability with reproduction drawings, drawings to command and block designs; 5) Higher cortical function for fund of information, proverb interpretation, similarities, calculations; 6) Related cortical function including ideomotor apraxia, ideational apraxia, right/left disorientation, finger agnosia, childhood Gerstmann, visual agnosia, and geographic orientation.

The responders' frequency of testing in the six major categories of mental status function was independent of their age, sex, board certified/eligible status, type of practice and years elapsed since completion of training. The results of the entire group and comparison among demographic subgroups demonstrated a progressive decline in testing frequency with increasing complexity of mental status function. Higher and related cortical functions were tested significantly less often in children with learning problems than were the more elementary categories of mental status function. The diagnosis ascribed to a child with learning problems appeared to be based on findings other than those provided by the mental status examination. (Brunquell PJ et al. Mental status examination of children with learning problems. *Pediatric Neurology* Jan-Feb 1989; 5:32-36).

COMMENT. Pediatric neurologists are often consulted for the assessment of children with learning disabilities since many childhood learning disorders appear to have a primary neurologic basis. Sensory impairment, epilepsy, or progressive neurologic disease may require exclusion. The use of stimulant medication may need to be justified or its safety determined. The neurologist will use the all important history, the physical and neurological examination, an EEG and sometimes a neuro-imaging test. He will also rely on teacher evaluations and psychological testing by the school or privately.

The results of this survey indicate that although the elementary aspects of mental status function (e.g. attention, vigilance, language) are almost always assessed in these children, higher and related cortical functions are relatively ignored or may not be practical in an office setting. However, it is relatively simple to test for Gerstmann syndrome and for defects in the fund of information and calculations. The Draw A

Man test and parts of the Stanford-Binet may also be included in a routine pediatric neurology examination. Clinical-neuroanatomic correlations in LD children are not uncommon, particularly when the neurological exam is supplemented with the EEG, evoked potentials, and magnetic resonance imaging. In the future perhaps the mental status examination will play a larger role in the diagnosis of children with learning problems in the child neurologist's office setting. - Editor. *Ped Neur Briefs* February 1989.

Rating Scales In Attention Deficit Disorder

A comparison of parent, teacher, and child performance rating scales in the diagnosis and follow-up of methylphenidate treated children with ADDH is reported from Developmental Pediatrics, San Antonio, TX; Department of Pediatrics, Madigan Army Medical Center, Tacoma, WA; and Department of Pediatrics, William Beaumont Army Medical Center, El Paso, TX. The three clinical tools provided varying degrees of supportive data during diagnosis and treatment of 21 children with ADDH. The ADDH *Comprehensive Teacher Rating* Scale classified 67% as having ADDH and 14% as borderline. The *Conners' Parent Rating* Scale-Revised identified 71% as having ADDH. The *Gordon Diagnostic System* showed 52% as having ADDH and 29% as borderline. During treatment with methylphenidate, the teacher rating scale showed an increase in attention span and a decrease in hyperactivity, the parent rating scale showed a significant decrease in hyperactive behavior and the Gordon child performance scale showed no significant change. (Cohen ML et al. Parent, Teacher, Child: A trilateral approach to attention deficit disorder. *AJDC* October 1989; *143*:1229-1233).

COMMENT. The teacher and parent rating scales were helpful in monitoring the effects of treatment with methylphenidate while the child performance-dependent test was insensitive to drug effects. - Editor. *Ped Neur Briefs* October 1989.

Transient Infantile Hypertonicity
And Learning Disabilities

The neuromotor and developmental progress of 33 children who had transient hypertonicity during early infancy was analyzed and reported from the Stanley S. Lamm Institute, Long Island College Hospital, Brooklyn, NY. Seventeen children were mildly affected while 16 were moderately affected. Hypertonia was present in all four limbs in 24%, the lower limbs were more involved in 48% and hypertonicity was asymmetric in 24%. CT scans in the immediate newborn period showed subarachnoid hemorrhage in 6 and leukomalacia in 1. Subsequent CT scans were normal. EEG's showed no significant abnormality in 12 infants at 3-17 months of age. Gross motor milestones were fairly satisfactory in all children, and independent walking was achieved between 8-20 months of age, 75% by 15 months. Hypertonicity disappeared at 9-18 months of age. Independent walking occurred after 14 months of age in 12 patients whereas resolution of hypertonicity had occurred in the majority of the patients before 14 months of age. At 2-3 years of age developmental abnormalities were identified in more than 2/3 of the children. Delays in speech and language development and also fine motor, adaptive and behavior difficulties were most frequently present. At five years of age or older learning disabilities were frequent and they were associated with persistent language and perceptual problems. None had epilepsy and mental retardation occurred in only two. Reading disability was diagnosed in 14 of 25 children older than 5 years of age (42%) compared to a figure of 4% in the general population. (PeBenito, R et al. Residual developmental disabilities in children with transient hypertonicity in infancy. *Pediatr Neurol* May/June 1989; 5:154-60).

COMMENT. The hypertonic infant, at risk for language and learning disabilities, should receive regular neurological and developmental follow-up evaluations through early childhood despite resolution of the increased tone and normal motor milestones. Early therapeutic intervention is advised. - Editor. *Ped Neur Briefs* July 1989.

Neurological Tests In Predicting Learning Disabilities And ADD

A battery of 12 simple neurological test items that differentiated normal from at-risk children at three and five years of age is described from the Departments of Pediatrics and Education, Wyler Children's Hospital, University of Chicago, IL. A follow-up of the five year olds at age seven showed a significant linear relation between scores on neurological tasks and the Wechsler Intelligence Test for Children. A poor neurological test score at age five correlated with a lower Full-scale IQ at age seven. The correlation for Verbal IQ was -0.42 and slightly lower than that for Performance IQ (-0.48). Both the school system's assessment and the neurological screening test accurately identified nearly all the children who needed special educational help at age seven. The neurological tests of predictive value for learning disabilities in preschool children included walking on toes and heels, tandem gait forward and backward, touch localization, restless movements, downward drift of outstretched hands, rapid alternating movements of forearms, hopping, alternate tapping of the fingers, and complex tapping. The percentages of at-risk children failing each neurological task were significantly higher than the normal group in almost all categories. (Huttenlocher PR et al. Discrimination of normal and at-risk preschool children on the basis of neurological tests. *Dev Med Child Neur* May 1990; *32*:394-402).

COMMENT. The emphasis of attention deficits in the evaluation of children with learning disabilities has overshadowed the recognition of subtle or soft neurological signs in the evaluation of children who may need psychological testing and early remedial education. As a pediatric neurologist it is gratifying to review a report that demonstrates the importance of the neurological examination in children with potential learning problems.

Abnormal neurologic signs almost identical to those included in the above test battery have previously been correlated with hyperactive behavior and response to stimulant medication. In a study of 28 hyperactive children with learning disabilities and ADDH, those with the highest incidence of abnormal neurologic signs had the greatest degree of overactivity and were most likely to benefit from methylphenidate. (Millichap JG. Methylphenidate in hyperkinetic behavior: Relation of response to degree of activity and brain damage. In "Clinical Use of Stimulant Drugs in Children". Ed. Conners, CK. Amsterdam, *Excerpta Medica* 1974; 130-140). - Editor. *Ped Neur* Briefs May 1990.

Corpus Callosum And Cognitive Function

Cognitive function communicated between the cerebral hemispheres by the corpus callosum was studied in two patients with commissurotomies at the Cognitive Neuroscience Laboratory, Department of Psychiatry, Dartmouth Medical School, Hanover, NH and the Department of Neurosciences, University of California at San Diego, CA. The patients were asked to judge whether pairs of words rhymed. One word in each pair was presented to the left visual field and the other to the right visual field. The two words in each pair either sounded and looked alike (R+ L+), sounded alike but looked different (R+ L-), sounded different but looked alike (R- L+), or both sounded and looked different (R- L-). The two commissurotomy patients differed in that one had sparing of some rostral and splenial fibers of the corpus callosum verified by MRI while the second patient had MRI-verified full callosal section.

The patient with some sparing of fibers was able to perform the rhyming judgment significantly better than chance when the words both looked and sounded alike (R+ L+) whereas her accuracy did not differ from chance in the other three conditions. The second patient with full callosal section performed at chance in all conditions, and normal control subjects were significantly better than chance in all conditions except R+ L-. Both patients had callosal section performed at age 26 to control intractable epileptic seizures. These results indicated to the authors that the first patient was capable of comparing both phonologic and orthographic information across her hemispheres and this ability reflected the functioning of the callosal remnant fibers. The splenium of the corpus callosum interconnects visual association cortex and this patient's ability to transfer orthographic information was commensurate with the splenial locus of her spared callosal fibers. The surviving rostral fibers may have contributed to the transfer of phonologic information. (Gazzaniga MS et al. Human callosal function: MRI-verified neuropsychological functions. *Neurology* July 1989; *39*:942-946).

> COMMENT. The MRI has proved of value in defining the extent of brain lesions with greater precision than was previously possible and has provided more accurate information regarding the areas of the callosum that are cut in the split brain patient. This study has helped to specify the functional zones of the human callosum in regard to cognition.
>
> A second paper regarding magnetic resonance imaging morphology of the corpus callosum in monozygotic twins is published from the same Program in Cognitive Neuroscience of Dartmouth Medical School (*Ann Neurol* July 1989; *26*:100-104). There are wide variations in the size and shape of the human corpus callosum and measurements of size and shape revealed greater similarity in twin pairs than in randomly paired controls. The results were consistent with the view that the anatomy of the corpus callosum is under genetic control as well as being influenced by nongenetic factors. - Editor. *Ped Neur Briefs* July 1989.

Utilization Behavior And Frontal Lobe Lesions

Utilization behavior was investigated in an adult with an acute behavioral disturbance, memory deficits, and a localized inferior medial bifrontal lesion at the Psychology Department,

National Hospital, Queen Square, London; the MRC Applied Psychology Unit, Cambridge; and Department of Neurology, Atkinson Morley's Hospital, Wimbledon; and St. Andrews Hospital, Northampton, UK. Incidental utilization behavior was observed and categorized: 1) Toying, an object manipulated but not in a purposeful way (e.g. picking up a pencil but not using it for any purpose), 2) complex toying, two objects used in a linked way but in an incomplete fashion (e.g. picking up a pencil and using it to move objects), 3) coherent activity, set of actions integrated in a typical fashion (e.g. picking up a pen and paper and writing; picking up a pack of cards and dealing). Utilization behavior occurred when the patient was in conversation with the examiner and also when performing both verbal and nonverbal neuropsychological tests. His WAIS Verbal IQ was 73 and Performance IQ 79. Performance on spatial, perceptual, language, and simple praxic tests was satisfactory in contrast to tasks involving a frontal or long term memory component which were uniformly and severely impaired. The utilization behavior was present in the absence of confusion or dementia. The utilization behavior occurred most frequently in the brief intervals between tasks, and more often when auditory verbal rather than visual motor tasks were being performed. A differentiation was made between two forms of utilization behavior: 1) an incidental form, as exhibited by the patient; and 2) an induced form, occurring with Lhermitte's procedure where the examiner stimulates the palm and fingers of the patient's hands with the object. (Shallice T et al. The origins of utilization behavior. *Brain* Dec 1989; *112*:1587-1598).

COMMENT. Utilization behavior investigated in this adult patient might also be evaluated in children with learning and memory disorders and may assist in the neuroanatomical localization of lesions in the frontal lobe. Lhermitte's neuroanatomical account of utilization behavior is based on the theories of Denny-Brown and a possible imbalance between the activities of frontal and parietal lobes. Visual stimuli activate parietal lobe systems which in turn initiate actions normally inhibited by frontal lobe systems. Damage to the frontal lobes leading to unmodulated effects of parietal systems may result in utilization behavior. Children with minimal brain dysfunction and hyperactivity have an increased tendency to touch and toy with articles within their reach. - Editor. *Ped Neur Briefs* March 1990.

Focal Cerebral Dysfunction And Learning Disabilities

Single photon emission tomography was used to study regional cerebral activity in 24 children with developmental learning disabilities and 15 age matched controls at the John F. Kennedy Institute, Glostrup, and Department of Neurology, Rigshospitalet, Copenhagen, Denmark. The distribution of regional cerebral activity was abnormal - low in striatal and posterior periventricular regions and high in occipital regions - in nine children with pure attention deficit and hyperactivity disorder, low in striatal and posterior ventricular areas in eight children with ADHD plus phonologic-syntactic dysphasia, and low in the left temporofrontal regions in seven children with dysphasia without hyperactive behavior. (Lou HC et al. Focal cerebral dysfunction in developmental learning disabilities. *Lancet* Jan 6, 1990; *335*:8-11).

COMMENT. The use of PET in children is restricted by the radiation dose and invasive procedure. The smaller dose of radiation associated with SPET was considered less invasive and hazardous. The MRI avoids the risk of radiation side effects and has illuminated structural cerebral defects underlying various learning disabilities, e.g. cortical heterotopias in dyslexic patients, and temporal lobe cysts in children with auditory perceptual problems. The regional cerebral blow flow abnormalities demonstrated by SPET may reveal focal cerebral dysfunction not demonstrated by MRI but correlating with expressive language dysfunction and other developmental learning disabilities. - Editor. *Ped Neur Briefs* March 1990.

Frontal Lobe Function And Attention Deficits

The results of a psychological test battery administered to 54 clinic referred children aged 8 to 12 years with attention deficit disorders are reported from the Georgia Children's Center and the Department of Psychology, University of Oregon, Eugene, Oregon.

The patients were divided into three groups: 1) Those with attention deficit disorder with hyperactivity; 2) Attention deficit disorder without hyperactivity; and 3) Control group with internalizing disorders. The verbal and full scale IQ scores on the WISC-R were lower for both attention deficit disorder groups when compared with the control group. The groups did not differ significantly on any of the Nebraska clinical scales which include motor skills, tactile, visual, speech, language, writing, reading, arithmetic, memory and intelligence. Attention deficit disorder either with or without hyperactivity was not associated with neuropsychological dysfunction as measured by the Luria-Nebraska battery. (Schaughency EA et al, Neuropsychological test performance and the attention deficit disorders: Clinical utility of the Luria-Nebraska Neuropsychological Battery - Children's Revision. *J Consult Clin Psychol* 1989; *57*:112-116).

COMMENT. The authors admit that although these results failed to support the association of neuropsychological dysfunction with attention deficit disorders, a more focused assessment of frontal lobe development by alternative methods may have yielded different results. A neurological examination with attention to the occurrence of soft or subtle signs may have demonstrated differences in the groups tested and evidence of neurological dysfunction in the attention deficit hyperactivity disorder patients. (See *Ped Neur Briefs* May 1990; 4:40). - Editor. *Ped Neur Briefs* August 1990.

Risk Factors For Attention Deficit Disorder

Family-genetic and psychosocial risk factors for DSM-III attention deficit disorder (ADD) were evaluated among the 457 first degree relatives of clinically referred children and adolescents with ADD compared with psychiatric and normal controls at the Child Psychiatry Service, Massachusetts General Hospital, Harvard Medical School, Boston. Relatives of ADD probands had a higher risk for ADD, antisocial disorders and mood disorders than did relatives of psychiatric and normal controls. The findings could not be accounted for by low social class or family disruption. (Biederman J et al. Family-genetic and psychosocial risk factors in DSM-III attention deficit disorder. *J Am Acad Child Adolesc Psychiatry* July 1990; *29*:527-533).

COMMENT. These findings confirm that ADD is a highly familial disorder, and relatives of clinically referred ADD children and adolescents have a significantly increased risk for ADD.

Barkley RA et al (*J Am Acad Child Adolesc Psychiatry* July 1990; *29*:546-557) report an eight year prospective follow-up study of the adolescent outcome of hyperactive children diagnosed by research criteria. More than 80% of the hyperactive children had ADHD and 60% had either oppositional defiant disorder and/or conduct disorder at outcome. Antisocial acts, cigarette and marijuana use, and negative academic performance were considerably higher among hyperactives than normals. Conduct disorder accounted for many though not all of these adverse outcomes. There was considerably greater risk for family disturbance and negative academic and social outcomes in adolescents than previously reported.

In the pediatric and pediatric neurology examination of children with learning and behavior problems, the Pediatric Evaluation of Educational Readiness test (PEER) can assist in the developmental follow-up of children at risk for learning and behavior disorders. Observations of behavior including attention and activity correlated with test results obtained independently by a psychometrist. (Blackman JA, Bretthauer J. Examining high-risk children for learning problems in the health care setting. *Pediatrics* Sept 1990; *86*:398-404). - Editor. *Ped Neur Briefs* November 1990.

Cerebral Glucose Metabolism And ADHD

Whole brain and regional rates of glucose metabolism were assessed by PET scanning in 25 adults with hyperactivity of childhood onset at the Section on Clinical Brain Imaging and Child Psychiatry Branch, National Institute of Mental Health, Bethesda, MD. Global cerebral glucose metabolism was 8.1% lower in the adults with hyperactivity than in normal controls. The largest reductions in glucose metabolism were in the pre-motor cortex and the superior prefrontal cortex, areas of the brain shown to be involved in the control of attention and motor activity. No significant differences were found in global cerebral cortex metabolism between patients with hyperactivity who had current learning deficits and those who did not. (Zametkin AJ et al. Cerebral glucose metabolism in adults with hyperactivity of childhood onset. *N Engl J Med* Nov 15, 1990; *323*:1361-6).

> COMMENT. The frontal lobes are important in maintain-ing attention, and disorders of the prefrontal regions may result in inattentiveness, distractibility, and an inability to inhibit inappropriate responses, such as motor restlessness, calling out in class, verbal interruptions, and acting before thinking.

> Experimental neuroanatomical studies of hyperkinesia have been concerned with the effects of destruction of dif-ferent cortical and subcortical structures on locomotor activity. (Millichap JG. *Intern J Neurology* 1975; *10*:241-251). Bilateral removal of the prefrontal and frontal areas

in the monkey causes the greatest total increase in activity. (Kennard MA et al. *J Neurophysiol* 1941; *4*:512). Lesions in Walker's area 13 of the orbital surface produce the most extreme degree of hypermobility. Hyperactivity induced by parietal lobe lesions is not as marked as in frontal lobe lesions. Destruction of subcortical structures including the striatum, interpeduncular nucleus, and parts of the hypothalamus may also induce hyperactivity. Diffuse brain lesions have been thought to be a major cause of a large percentage of clinical cases of hyperactive behavior.

The correlation between functional and anatomical development and pathology is still unclear. Monaminergic transmitters such as norepinephrine are in high concentration in the frontal lobes and increase as the child grows older. (Njiokiktjien C. *Pediatric Behavioural Neurology* Suyi Publications, Amsterdam 1988). The hypometabolism in prefrontal areas noted in the above study might possibly extend to monaminergic metabolism and may explain the beneficial effects of methylphenidate which increases the neurotransmitters and activity of cortical inhibitory systems in hyperactive children. The efficacy of methylphenidate in hyperactive children has been related to the level of motor activity before treatment and the incidence of abnormal neurological signs and evidence of brain dysfunction. (Millichap 1975). It is apparent from these studies that ADHD must be distinguished diagnostically from behavioral disorders that may appear similar but are reactions to environmental crises or inappropriate school placement. (Weiss G. Hyperactivity in childhood. Editorial. *N Engl J Med* Nov 15, 1990; *323*:1413-1415). - Editor. *Ped Neur Briefs* November 1990.

DIET AND BEHAVIOR

Additives And Hyperkinetic Behavior

The authors studied 39 children with hyperkinetic and learning disorders in a summer camp setting. The behavior was monitored by videotape for 4-minute intervals at mealtimes. The Feingold Diet was administered for one week followed by a diet containing additives and preservatives for one week. Three observers who were blind to the respective diet periods rated the behavior for motor restlessness, disorganized behavior, and misbehavior. No significant differences were found in behavior during weeks one and two. The authors conclude that the Feingold Diet had no beneficial effect on most children with learning and hyperkinetic disorders. (Gross MD, Tofanelli RA, Butzirus SM, Snodgrass EW. *J Amer Acad Child Adol Psychiat* 1987; 26:53-55).

COMMENT. This study adds one more negative report regarding the Feingold Diet theory. The National Institutes of Health Consensus Development Panel on "Defined Diets in Childhood Hyperactivity" (1982) concluded that the Feingold Diet may be helpful for a small number of children with hyperkinesis but decreases in hyperactivity were not observed consistently.

The interest in the Feingold hypothesis, although waning in the U.S. is flourishing in England where consciousness about ecology and pure foods is growing. - Editor. *Ped Neur Briefs* June 1987.

Adverse Reactions To Food Additives

As part of a multicentre study of food additive intolerance commissioned by the UK Ministry of Agriculture, Fisheries and Food, the prevalence of reactions to food additive was studied in a survey population by the Depts of Dermatology and Community Medicine, Wycombe General Hospital, High Wycombe, Bucks, and St. Thomas' Campus, London University. Of

18,582 respondents to questionnaires, 7.4% had reactions to food additives, 15.6% had problems with foods, and 10% had symptoms related to aspirin. The incidence of a personal history of atopy reported in 28% of all respondents was significantly higher in those reacting to additives, food, and aspirin (50%, 47.5%, and 36% respectively). A preponderance of reactions occurred in children, boys more than girls. Older patients were affected less often and with a female preponderance.

Abnormal behavior and mood changes were mainly related to additives whereas headache was associated with foods more frequently than additives. Of 44 individuals (7% of 649 interviewed) who reported monosodium glutamate sensitivity, 13 (30%) suffered headache, and 8 (18%) had behavioral or mood changes. Headache was related to food intolerance in 14% of those interviewed but had not previously been regarded as migrainous in nature. Of 81 reactive subjects who completed an additive challenge with annatto or azo dye, only 3 showed consistent reactions. The authors estimated the prevalence of food additive intolerance in the study population at 0.01-0.23%. (Young E et al. *J Roy Coll Physicians London* 1987; *21*:241-247).

COMMENT. The debate in the UK on food additives and behavior waxes while in the USA interest wanes, with more attention being given to sugar and the effectiveness of stimulants in therapy (see *Ped Neur Briefs* 1987; *1*:5,22,38). In the same issue of the JRCP London, Pollock L and Warner JO at the Brompton Hospital report a follow-up of children with food additive intolerance showing that symptoms were mainly transient, 76% showing no reaction on rechallenge studies, and Lessof MH at Guy's Hospital reviews the literature and concludes that more reliable diagnostic tests and toxicological screening methods are needed. A food intolerance databank has been compiled at the Leatherhead Food Research Association, UK, that will provide constantly updated information on food product composition and brands free from ingredients most commonly associated with food intolerance (milk, egg, wheat, soya bean, cocoa, BHA and BHT, sulfur dioxide, benzoate, glutamate and azo colors). - Editor. *Ped Neur Briefs* November 1987.

Food Additives And Hyperactivity

Of 220 children referred to the Dept of Paediatrics, Royal Children's Hospital, Parkville, Victoria, Australia, because of suspected hyperactivity, 55 were included in a six week open trial of the Feingold Diet, 26 (47%) showed a placebo response, and 14 were identified as likely reactors. Of eight who subsequently completed a double-blind crossover study (utilizing each child as his own control), two demonstrated a significant dependent relationship between the challenge and ingestion of azo dye colorings (tartrazine and carmoisine 50 mg) and behavioral change. Extreme irritability, restlessness and sleep disturbance rather than attention deficit were the common behavioral patterns associated with the ingestion of food colorings, as described by the parents in this study. The authors conclude that the inclusion of children in trials on the basis of attention deficit alone may miss some reactors, and there is little place for use of a coloring-free diet in children with ADD unless the other behavioral features of irritability, restlessness and sleep disturbance are present. (Rowe KS. Synthetic food colourings and 'hyperactivity': A double-blind crossover study. *Aust Pediatr J* April 1988; *24*:143-147).

COMMENT. The phoenix of the Feingold Diet rises again with the suggestion that the treatment has been erroneously discarded because of inappropriate behavioral rating instruments and failure to identify specific reactors to food additives. In England, where the avoidance of all foods containing additives is widespread, the major problem is the level of public misinformation, occasionally leading to handicapping dietary restriction. (David TJ. *Arch Dis Child* 1988; *63*:582). - Editor. *Ped Neur Briefs* June 1988.

Serum Fatty Acids And Hyperactivity

Serum essential fatty acids (EFA) levels were measured in 44 hyperactive children and 45 age-and-sex-matched controls at the Dept. of Pediatrics and Psychiatry and Behavioral Science, Univ. of Auckland, New Zealand. Docasahexaenoic, dihomogrammalmolenic, and arachidonic acid levels were significantly lower in hyperactive children than controls. The hyperactive group of children had significantly *lower* birth weights than controls (3,058 and 3,410 g respectively; p 0.01), a greater incidence of learning difficulties and dyslexia, but no increase in asthma, eczema, or other allergies. In a double-blind placebo controlled, crossover study of evening primose oil in 31 hyperactive children, effects on behavior were modest and equivocal. (Mitchell EA et al. Clinical characteristics and serum essential fatty acid levels in hyperactive children. *Clin Pediat* 1987; *26*:406-411).

> COMMENT. The search for dietary related causes and treatments for hyperactive behavior continues and now involves fats in addition to food allergies, additives, preservatives, sugar and megavitamins. In support of fats, a beneficial effect of the ketogenic diet on the behavior of the epileptic child often complements its anticonvulsant properties in my experience. The present paper did not confirm previous reports of a high prevalence of allergy among hyperactive children and tends to minimize the possible importance of food allergy as an etiologic factor. - Editor. *Ped Neur Briefs* September 1987.

Sugar, Aspartame, And Behavior

The effects of glucose, sucrose, saccharin, and aspartame on aggression and motor activity in 30 boys, ages 2-6 years, were studied at the Child Psychiatry Branch and Laboratory of Developmental Psychology, NIMH, Bethesda, MD. Eighteen boys were recruited or selected as "sugar responders" and 12 male playmates were "non responders". Single doses of sucrose, 1.75 g/kg; glucose, 1.75 g/kg; aspartame, 30 mg/kg; or saccharine administered in a randomized, double-blind design produced no significant effect on aggression or on teacher ratings of behavior. Actometer counts for two hours after ingestion of aspartame were lower than those following other sweeteners. Parent ratings of activity and aggression after home challenges with sweeteners failed to show differences between substances for either the alleged "responders" or "non responders". Consistent with baseline measures, parents rated responders more hyperactive than playmates who were not believed to be sugar reactive. No parent differentiated between sugar and non-sugar trials. Mean daily sucrose intake and total sugar consumption correlated with duration of aggression against property for the alleged sugar responsive group but acute sugar loading did not increase aggression or activity in preschool children. (Krnesi MJP et al. Effects of sugar and aspartame on aggression and activity in children. *Am J Psychiatry* 1987; *144*:1487-1490).

COMMENT. Conners CK at the Children's Hospital, Washington, D.C. reports that deleterious effects of sugar on children with attention deficit may be demonstrated if the challenge follows a high carbohydrate breakfast but the effects are blocked or reversed by a protein load. The beneficial and protective effects of a protein diet are correlated with neuroendocrine changes and the prevention of the serotonergic effects of sugar on behavior and attention (personal communication and in *Diet and Behavior*, Lubbock, Texas Tech Univ Press). Diets low in protein and high in carbohydrates might be expected to cause increases in spontaneous activity, as demonstrated in animal studies, but these effects are not necessarily related to swings in blood sugar concentrations. For recent reviews of the effects of dietary nutrients and deficiencies on brain biochemistry and behavior see Yehuda S. *Intern J Neuroscience* 1987; *35*:21-36; and *Nutrition Reviews/Supplement* May 1986; *44*:1-250. - Editor. *Ped Neur Briefs* November 1987.

Aspartame And Learning And Behavior

The effects of aspartame on learning, behavior and mood of 9-10-year-old normal children were examined in the Department of Nutritional Sciences, University of Toronto, Ontario, Canada. Measures of associative learning, arithmetic calculation, activity level, social interaction and mood were unaffected by treatment with Kool-Aid containing 1.76 gram/kg of carbohydrate (polycose) plus either aspartame (34 mg/kg) or the equivalent sweetness as sodium cyclamate and amino acids as alanine. In a second experiment in which children received a drink of cold, unsweetened strawberry Kool-Aid containing either 1.75 gram/kg of sucrose or 9.7 mg/kg of aspartame, the frequency of minor and gross motor behaviors was significantly less after the consumption of sucrose than after aspartame treatment. (Saravis S et al. Aspartame: effects on learning, behavior and mood, *Pediatrics* July 1990; *86*: 75-83).

COMMENT. The authors concluded that the effects of aspartame on short-term behavior were more likely due to an "absence of metabolic consequences of providing sweetness rather than to neurochemical consequences related to its amino acid composition". The observed reduction in activity following sucrose ingestion is in agreement with some previous reports and adds to the controversy concerning hyperactivity and sugar. The tests in the above study that failed to show significant effects of aspartame included the Conditional Associative Learning Task, the Canadian Tests of Basic Skills, the Children's Depression Inventory and the State-Trait Anxiety Inventory for Children. The minor and gross motor behaviors which showed significant improvement with sucrose included the actometer measure, a modified self-winding wrist watch, and a video taped observation of behavior. The children in this study were normal and different responses may occur in patients with ADHD. - Editor. *Ped Neur Briefs* August 1990.

Sucrose, Motor Activity, And Learning

The effects of sugar (sucrose) on the behavior of 30 preschool children (20 boys and 10 girls, mean age 5 years 4 mos) and 15 elementary school children (6 boys and 9 girls, mean age 7 yrs 2 mos) were investigated by psychologists from Colorado State University, Fort Collins, CO, and the Univ of Mississippi Med Centr, Jackson, MS. Parents and teachers questioned before the study complained that the child was behaviorally sensitive to sugar in approximately 50% of subjects. Two preschool children had been considered hyperactive by the school director. A basic breakfast included a 4 oz orange flavored drink of high sucrose content (50 g), low-sugar (6.25 g) or aspartame (122 mg), randomly selected, five days on each, using a double-blind control design. The mean sucrose intakes for the high, low, and "control" aspartame conditions were 2.26, 0.28, and 0.00 g/kg, respectively, and the total carbohydrate contents of breakfast averaged 3.95, 1.88, and 1.54 g/kg, respectively.

On cognitive measures, girls made significantly more errors on a paired-associate learning task performed 20-30 min following a high-sugar content breakfast when compared to a low-sugar meal, whereas boys were unaffected. On global ratings, younger preschool children were affected differently than older children. On an Abbreviated Conners Teacher Rating Scale completed before lunch, both boys and girls were more active in behavior after the high sugar meal than that of low sugar content. Measures of behavior by observation for fidgetiness, change in activity, running, vocalization and aggressiveness, and other cognitive measures involving matching and academic tasks failed to demonstrate changes after sugar ingestion. (Rosen LA et al. Effects of sugar (sucrose) on children's behavior. *J Consulting Clin Psychol* 1988; *56(4)*:583-589).

COMMENT. Evidently, the effects of sugar on children's behavior is not yet resolved. This study demonstrates significant adverse effects although the authors conclude that these are minimal in degree. Certain limitations of the study design are admitted: 1) The sugar challenge dose was the same for all subjects and younger and smaller children, affected differently, received larger amounts than did older and larger children. The design was not adequate to pinpoint the amount of sugar that may cause deleterious effects. 2) The prior dietary history of the subjects was unknown, and those accustomed to consuming large amounts of sugar may have reacted differently from children who usually ate low sugar meals. 3) The assumption that aspartame used as a control is innocuous may not be correct (see *Ped Neur Briefs* Nov 1987; 1:45). Further work on possible behavioral effects of sucrose is clearly indicated. The only proven contraindication to excess sugar in a child's diet is that emphasized by the dental profession. - Editor. *Ped Neur Briefs* September 1988.

Elimination Diets
In Pre-School-Aged Hyperactive Boys

The effect of an experimental elimination diet was examined in 24 hyperactive boys aged 3.5 to 6 years at the Alberta Children's Hospital, and the Learning Center, Calgary, Alberta, Canada. The diet was broader than those studied previously in that it eliminated not only artificial colors and flavors but also chocolate, monosodium glutamate, preservatives, caffeine, and any substance that the families reported might affect the child. It was low in simple sugar (mono- and disaccharides) and dairy-free if an allergy to milk was suspected. A within-subject cross-over design was divided into 3 periods: a baseline of three weeks, a placebo-control period of three weeks, and an experimental diet period of four weeks. Approximately 42% (10) of the children showed 50% improvement in behavior on the elimination diet; an additional 16% (4) had lesser degrees of improvement (12%) with no placebo effect. Headache was less frequently reported during the diet period compared to placebo but not less than the baseline phase. Other nonbehavioral variables such as night awakenings and halitosis tended to improve during the dietary treatment phase. (Kaplan BJ et al. Dietary replacement in preschool-aged hyperactive boys. *Pediatrics* Jan 1989; *83*:7-17).

COMMENT. These results of replacement diets indicate larger response rates than challenge studies with specific items. Further studies of additive-free and hypoallergenic-sugar-restricted diets are warranted in the management of attention deficit disorders with hyperactivity, and headache and sleep disorders, particularly in preschool children. - Editor. *Ped Neur Briefs* March 1989.

School Breakfast Program And School Performance

The effects of participation in the school breakfast program by low income children on academic achievement and rates of absence and tardiness are reported from the Department of Pediatrics, Boston City Hospital, Boston, MA. The results in children grades 3-6 in the Lawrence, MA, public schools were compared with those children who also qualified but did not participate in the breakfast program. Participation in the program had a significant association with improvement in standardized achievement test scores and the rates of absence and tardiness. (Meyers AF et al. School breakfast program and school performance. *AJDC* Oct 1989; *143*:1234-1239).

COMMENT. Further study of this question is indicated, using prospective control designs as well as data regarding protein, fat and carbohydrate content of the meals. Conners has reported beneficial effects on behavior and learning of a sugar load following a protein breakfast whereas adverse effects were noted with sugar alone. (Personal communication). - Editor. *Ped Neur Briefs* October 1989.

DRUG TREATMENT OF ADHD

Attention Deficit Disorder And Methylphenidate

1) Members of the Departments of Social Ecology and Psychology at the University of California, Irvine 92717 and Los Angeles 90024 have investigated the effects of methylphenidate on the social behaviors of hyperactive children ages 6 to 11 during unstructured activities in an outdoor summer program. When a low dose of methylphenidate (0.3 mg/kg) was compared to placebo, 15 of 24 children treated showed medication-related decreases in negative behavior. The beneficial effects in younger children were greater than in older children and incremental improvements occurred between low and moderate dose levels (0.6 mg/kg). Neither low nor moderate doses of methylphenidate increased social withdrawal. (Whalen CK, Henker B et al. Natural social behaviors in hyperactive children: Dose effects of methylphenidate. *J Consult and Clin Psychol* 1987; *55*:187-193).

2) A psychologist, psychiatrist, and pediatric neurologist at the University of Rochester, Rochester, NY 14627 collaborated in a study of the effects of methylphenidate on 19 adolescents with a childhood history of attention deficit disorder. In a double-blind crossover trial of methylphenidate (40 mg/day) compared to placebo for three week periods, parents and teachers reported drug-induced improvement in attentiveness and behavioral compliance and lessened overactivity. Subjective ratings of dysphoria (sadness or unhappiness) were lower and heart rates were higher during stimulant therapy at this dose level. (Klorman R, Coons HW, Borgstedt AD. Effects of methylphenidate on adolescents with a childhood history of attention deficit disorder: I Clinical findings. *J Amer Acad Child Adol Psychiat* 1987; *26*:363-367).

COMMENT. These studies provide further evidence for the beneficial effects of methylphenidate in the treatment of children and adolescents with attention deficit disorders and hyperactivity. Those who favor the use of stimulants may be encouraged by the finding that disruptive behaviors were reduced successfully without affecting overall sociability.

The age at which treatment should be terminated is a debated question. Some authorities advocate medication only in young school-age children whereas others treat through adolescence to young adulthood. Contrary to popular belief, children with ADHD do not generally outgrow their symptoms at 12 years of age. An inefficient response to new problem-solving situations may persist through adolescence and may justify the continuation of stimulant therapy. - Editor. *Ped Neur Briefs* August 1987.

Sustained Release and Standard Methylphenidate Compared

The relative effects of sustained release (Ritalin [SR-207]) and standard methylphenidate (Ritalin 10 mg, BD) on cognitive and social behavior in 22 boys with ADD were investigated at a summer treatment program supervised by the Western Psychiatric Institute, Univ of Pittsburgh School of Medicine, PA. Group analyses of data showed that both drugs were effective but standard methylphenidate was superior to SR-20 on measures of disruptive behavior and SR-20 had a slower onset on a continuous performance task. Analyses of individual responsivity showed that most boys responded more positively to the standard compared to the sustained-release preparation of methylphenidate. The authors note that in contrast to advertising material, the effects of SR-20 and standard methylphenidate are not equivalent. They recommend pemoline or slow-release dextroamphetamine in preference to SR-20 if a single daily dose sustained effect is required. (Pelham WE Jr et al. Sustained release and standard methylphenidate effects on cognitive and social behavior in children with attention deficit disorder. *Pediatrics* 1987; *80*:491-501).

COMMENT. Stimulant medications used in the treatment of ADDH have different half lives: methylphenidate 2.6 hours on a dose of 0.60 mg/kg; dextroamphetamine 6.8 hours with 0.45 mg/kg; and pemoline 8.36 hours after doses up to 110 mg (see Zametkin AJ, Rapoport JL in *Ped Neur Briefs* 1987; 1(5):37. Clinical responses, however, are not always correlated with the half life of the drug or with plasma levels which may vary considerably from day to day in patients with a fixed dose. Previous studies have shown that time release Dexedrine may not act for longer time periods than the standard tablet form. These inconsistencies, together with the findings in the present study, suggest that standard methylphenidate or pemoline remain the treatments of choice in ADDH. - Editor. *Ped Neur Briefs* October 1987.

Methylphenidate In Hyperactive Autistic Children

Nine children, eight boys and one girl, ages 4 to 16 yrs, with a diagnosis of autism, were treated with methylphenidate (10-50 mg/day) as outpatients at Columbia Presbyterian Medical Center, Babies' Hospital Pediatric Psychiatric Clinic, NY. All were hyperactive, impulsive, and mentally retarded. All showed significant improvement on the Conner's Teacher and Parent Questionnaire scores during treatment with the stimulant. No significant side-effects were noted or worsening of stereotyped movements. (Birmaher B et al. Methylphenidate treatment of hyperactive autistic children. *J Am Acad Child Adolesc Psychiatry* March 1988; 27:248-251).

COMMENT. The beneficial effect of methylphenidate on the behavior of autistic children, at variance with many previous reports, is confirmed in a randomized trial of the drug in a 6-year-old autistic boy reported in the same journal from the Western Psychiatric Institute, Pittsburgh, PA (Strayhorn Jr. JM et al. *J Am Acad Child Adolesc Psychiatry* March 1988; 27:244). Negative effects on mood and tantrums were outweighed by positive effects on attention and activity, destructive behavior and stereotyped movements. These reports fail to support previous statements that stimulants are ineffective and contraindicated in hyperactive autistic children. Rutter M (*J Child Psychol Psychiatry* 1985; 26:193) writing on treatment refers to a basic cognitive deficit which underlies language and behavior problems in autistic children. Provided that methylphenidate does not exacerbate psychotic behavior, its known effects in promoting cognitive development could be beneficial. - Editor. *Ped Neur Briefs* April 1988.

Methylphenidate, Academic Performance, And Behavior

The effects of 0.3 mg/kg and 1.0 mg/kg of methylphenidate on the overt behavior and academic functioning of 12 children with ADDH are reported from the Department of Psychiatry Research, Hospital For Sick Children, Toronto, Ontario, Canada. A double blind placebo control crossover design was used and each child was tested four times in each drug condition. Methylphenidate enhanced academic functioning by increasing accurate productivity on academic tasks, as well as improving overt behavior. All 12 children were able to complete more work at all levels of the arithmetic task and the letter task without sacrificing accuracy. The majority showed more than a 25% increase in the number of problems completed correctly compared with placebo level performance. The beneficial effects on academic performance did not vary with dosage or task complexity. Behavioral and academic improvements produced by a dose of 0.3 mg/kg in the morning were no longer evident in the afternoon, but a morning dose of 1.0 mg/kg produced behavioral improvements that were clinically and statistically present in the afternoon although academic improvements had disappeared. An increase in pulse and blood pressure was observed one hour following 1.0 mg/kg methylphenidate. (Tannock R et al. Dose-response effects of methylphenidate on academic performance and overt behavior in hyperactive children. *Pediatrics* October 1989; *84*:648-657).

COMMENT. Sprague and Sleator reported differences in dose effects on learning and social behavior following treatment with methylphenidate (*Science* 1977; *198*:1274); cognitive performance was maximized at a dosage of 0.3 mg/kg and was impaired by dosages of 1.0 mg/kg or higher. The present study indicated that the larger dosage resulted in a leveling of academic performance and not a decline. The authors admit that the high dose may have enabled the children to sit still and be quiet thereby facilitating their cognitive functioning. In attempting to determine an optimal dose for each child it is essential that the physician notes the dose response and timed course of action on academic, cognitive, and behavioral performance. - Editor. *Ped Neur Briefs* October 1989.

Methylphenidate And Seizures

The effects of methylphenidate in ten children with attention deficit complicated by seizure disorders are reported from the Departments of Pediatrics and Neurology, Children's Hospital of Pittsburgh, PA. The seizure types were partial complex in five, generalized tonic-clonic in two, generalized atonic in two, and partial motor with secondary generalization in one. The seizures had been well controlled for at least three months preceding the study. Monotherapy consisted of carbamazepine in five, phenobarbital in two, valproic acid in two, and phenytoin sodium in one. Methylphenidate was administered 0.3 mg/kg/dose at 8 a.m. and 12 p.m. on school days only and the study design was a double blind medication-placebo crossover. There were significant improvements on the Conners' Teacher Rating Scale and on the finger tapping task. No seizures or changes in the EEG occurred during the study period. It was concluded that methylphenidate may be a safe and effective treatment for certain children with seizures controlled with anticonvulsant medication and complicated by attention deficit disorder. (Feldman H et al. Methylphenidate in children with seizures and attention-deficit disorder. *AJDC* September 1989; *143*:1081-1086).

COMMENT. The Physicians' Desk Reference includes a contraindication to the use of Ritalin as follows: "there is some clinical evidence that Ritalin may lower the convulsive threshold in patients with prior history of seizures, with prior EEG abnormalities in the absence of seizures, and, very rarely, in absence of history of seizures and no prior EEG evidence of seizures. Safe concomitant use of anticonvulsants and Ritalin has not been established. In the presence of seizures, the drug should be discontinued."

Based on the present study of ten patients and in a retrospective study of 23 patients (McBride MC et al. *Ann Neurol* 1986; *20*:428) there is some support for the use of Ritalin in the hyperactive patient with seizures controlled by anticonvulsant drugs. Phenobarbital is generally a poor choice as an anticonvulsant in children with attention deficit disorder and alternative medications are preferred. Pemoline (Cylert) is generally considered to have less tendency to lower seizure threshold than does methylphenidate. Some recommend that all patients considered for treatment with methylphenidate should first receive an electroencephalogram; those with a history of seizures and/or epileptiform discharges in the electroencephalogram should receive treatment with an anticonvulsant drug such as carbamazepine concomitantly with the CNS stimulant. In a study of the electroencephalogram in 100 consecutive children with attention deficit disorder and hyperactivity, 7% had Grade III dysrhythmias consisting of spike-and-wave, spike or sharp wave abnormalities indicative of seizure activity. (Millichap JG. The *Hyperactive Child with Minimal Brain Dysfunction.* Chicago, Yearbook Medical Publishers. 1975). The frequency of significant abnormalities in the EEG is sufficient to warrant testing before treatment with methylphenidate. - Editor. *Ped Neur Briefs* October 1989.

Stimulant Medication For ADHD

The use of stimulant medication by primary care physicians in treatment of attention deficit hyperactivity disorder was evaluated by a random national survey of family practitioners and direct screening of 457 patients in midwestern cities and is reported from the Division of Developmental Disabilities, Departments of Pediatrics and Preventive Medicine, University of Iowa, Iowa City and Department of Psychology, University of Kentucky, Lexington. In the national survey, methylphenidate was used by 85% of pediatricians, dextroamphetamine 11%, and pemoline 23%. Pediatricians used stimulant medication in preschool children and adolescents as well as children between 6 and 16 years of age. Drug holidays were employed by more than 2/3rds of physicians, but placebo trials were rarely used. Height and weight were monitored by three-quarters of the physicians. Timed or sustained release forms of methylphenidate were used by less than 50%. The Feingold diet and sugar restricted diets were employed by 10 and 15%, respectively, and behavior modification by 77%.

In the direct patient screening, the prevalence of ADHD diagnosis was 5.3% of all elementary school aged children screened, and 88% were treated with methylphenidate. Medication was considered effective by the parents of 85% of children and efficacy was unrelated to the accuracy of the diagnosis. When DSM-III-R criteria were used, only 72% of those assigned a diagnosis of ADHD by physicians would qualify on a psychiatric interview of the parents and only 53% on a teacher report of symptoms. Although physicians reported the use of behavioral treatments, parents reported infrequent use of behavior modification. (Wolraich ML et al. Stimulant medication use by primary care physicians in the treatment of attention deficit hyperactivity disorder. *Pediatrics* July 1990; *86*:95-101).

COMMENT. The authors concluded that systematic behavioral treatments were underused compared to medications and the accurate diagnosis of ADHD needs clarification by identification of subtypes. - Editor. *Ped Neur Briefs* July 1990.

Tricyclic Antidepressants And Attention Deficit Disorder

A review of the literature concerning imipramine and other tricyclics in the treatment of attention deficit disorder (ADD) is presented from the Dept Psychiatry, Univ. Texas Health Sci Centr, 7703 Floyd Carl Drive, San Antonio, TX 78284. Imipramine was the drug of choice in a subgroup of children with ADD who had higher levels of anxiety or depression or both. Methylphenidate was superior to imipramine in the treatment of ADD overall.

The author concludes that: 1) reports of imipramine as the drug of choice in ADD are unjustified, 2) stimulants are the first choice and imipramine second, 3) children with ADD complicated by anxiety and/or mood disturbance may respond better to imipramine than to methylphenidate, 4) small doses of imipramine are not superior to higher doses and 1 mg/kg/day is ineffective. (Pliszka SR. *J Amer Acad Child Adol Psychiat* 1987; *26*:127-132).

COMMENT. My own experience, without the benefit of double-blind controls, would place methylphenidate as the drug of choice in ADD with hyperactivity uncomplicated by anxiety. As a pediatric neurologist, I am reluctant to prescribe imipramine for ADD with anxiety or depression 1) because of the dangers of cardiac arrhythmia with accidental poisoning and 2) my inability to evaluate properly its effects on the associated psychiatric symptoms. It is my opinion that this treatment should be followed by our colleagues in child psychiatry. Since imipramine has fallen out of favor in the treatment of nocturnal enuresis which sometimes complicates ADD, I no longer use the drug in my practice. For those patients with ADD and secondary anxiety reactions, I prefer thioridazine (Mellaril) if medication is required.

Drugs in the management of ADD with hyperactivity are controversial and they play a larger role in the USA than in England, where dietary modification is in vogue. With increased awareness of the problem by educators and more individualized attention to associated learning disabilities, the need for medication has lessened appreciably. Behavior modification and other psychological approaches to deal with hyperactivity are often sufficient to deal with anxiety caused by frustration and to lessen the impulsivity.

The present article emphasizes the need to correctly classify children with ADD into groups with or without conduct and anxiety disorders when evaluating drug effects. Werry JS et al, writing in the same journal, find that the coexistence of ADD and conduct disorder increases the degree of disability and suggest that ADD with hyperactivity is a cognitive disorder, possibly of neurodevelopmental origin. (*J Amer Acad Child Adol Psychiat* 1987; *26*:133-143). - Editor. *Ped Neur Briefs* July 1987.

Teachers And Psychopharmacology

Educators at the UCLA Neuropsychiatric Hospital and Inpatient School, Los Angeles, CA, and the Division of Special Education, University of Iowa, IA, discuss the issues in child psychopharmacology that are of importance to teachers and stress the need for greater interdisciplinary collaboration between the medical profession and the schools. The beneficial and adverse classroom effects of four major classes of psychotropic medication are discussed: 1) CNS stimulants; 2) anticonvulsants; 3) neuroleptics or antipsychotics; and 4) antidepressants.

A so-called "metanalysis" of available research data by special educators involved 135 studies of stimulant medications used for treatment of hyperactivity. Benefits were demonstrated not only in attention and memory but also in academic performance. Children on stimulants gained the equivalent of a 15% rank increase in achievement while those treated with major tranquilizers for severe behavior disorders showed a 20% rank increase on various cognitive measures. Other metanalyses of certain classroom interventions such as perceptual motor training or diet treatments resulted in gains of only 5 or 6 percentile ranks. The authors allude to an antimedication bias and the application of different standards to drug studies compared to other classroom intervention techniques. Little systematic data on side-effects of medication were available in the studies analyzed.

Studies of antidepressants were limited and few had valid educational variables or measures suited to the classroom performance. One study demonstrated the importance of interpretation of behavior of children on medication in light of behavior of other untreated children in the classroom. What appeared to be significant effects of medication was actually a reflection of the overall disruptive or inattentive behavior of the whole classroom. (Forness SR, Kavale KA. Psychopharmacologic treatment. A note on classroom effects. *J Learn Disabilities* March 1988; *21*:144-147).

COMMENT. The pressures of clinical practice sometimes preclude physicians' visits to schools and close collaboration with patients' teachers. The point of this report is that as pediatricians, neurologist and psychiatrists increase their use of psychopharmacological agents, teachers must have increased access to information about the classroom effects and side-effects of these medications. Medical researchers are not always aware of the possible problems that drug treatments may present in classroom situations, and regular reports from teachers can provide valuable information regarding their overall effects. - Editor. *Ped Neur Briefs* April 1988.

FRAGILE X SYNDROME

Fragile X Syndrome And Infantile Autism

Japanese patients with infantile autism were studied cytogenetically for the occurrence of fragile X (fra(x)) syndrome at the Universities of Kurume and Nagasaki. Fra(X) chromosome was detected in 2 (siblings) of 39 boys and in none of 8 girls; a frequency of 2.6% (1/38) in the study population of male autistic children. (Matsuishi T et al. Fragile X syndrome in Japanese patients with infantile autism. *Pediatr Neurol* 1987; *3*:284-7).

> COMMENT. The fragile X syndrome is the most common familial form of mental retardation known, with an incidence of 1 in 1000 in the general population. The classical physical features in males are a long narrow face, large ears, and large testes. The pediatric neurologist may encounter cases referred because of large head circumference, hyperactive behavior and short attention span (ADD), and hand-flapping movement disorders. Poor eye contact and stereotyped movements have led to confusion with autism, reported in 5-53% of males with fragile X syndrome, and the classical manifestations have matched the DSM III diagnostic criteria for autism in some, as in the above study. For a comprehensive current overview of fragile X syndrome, see Hagerman RJ. *Curr Probl Pediatr* 1987; *17*:621-674. - Editor. *Ped Neur Briefs* November 1987.

Fragile X Syndrome And Epilepsy

A characteristic epileptogenic EEG pattern is described in five of 12 male subjects with fragile X syndrome evaluated at the Instituto Oasi, via C. Ruggero, Troina, Italy, and Clinica Neurologica, II Universita Roma and Bologna, Italy. Focal paroxysmal temporal spikes, at times multifocal, occurred in sleep in one non-epileptic and four epileptic patients with mental retardation and fragile X syndrome, but not in subjects with mental retardation, with or without epilepsy but without the fragile X chromosome. (Musumeci SA et al. Fragile-X syndrome: A particular epileptogenic EEG pattern. *Epilepsia* Jan/Feb 1988; *29*:41-7).

> COMMENT. The authors believe that epilepsy must be considered an important clinical feature of fragile X syndrome, occurring in an average of 26% of reported cases. Karyotyping is advised in mentally retarded patients with epilepsy, even in those without typical clinical features or positive family history and especially in children who frequently lack the characteristic facial dysmorphisms and macro-orchidism (see *Ped Neur Briefs* 1987; 1:41). - Editor. *Ped Neur Briefs* March 1988.

Fragile X Syndrome Recognition

The clinical characteristics of 20 children younger than 7-1/2 years of age with the fragile X syndrome were reviewed at the Cincinnati Center for Developmental Disorders, Children's Hospital Medical Center, University of Cincinnati College of Medicine, Cincinnati. The study was undertaken to establish guidelines that would aid the practicing physician in determining which children should have a chromosomal analysis. All children in the study were developmentally delayed: 95% had speech delays; and 50% or more had short attention span with hyperactivity, temper tantrums, mouthing of objects, autistic behaviors and poor gross motor coordination. The family history was positive for mental retardation in 65%, and 90% had a family history of at least one of the following: mental retardation, learning disabilities, or hyperactivity.

The most common physical findings included long and/or wide and/or protruding ears in 15 (75%), prominent jaw or long face in 14 (70%), high arched palate in 10 (50%), flattened nasal bridge in 10 (50%), macrocephaly in 8 (40%), hypertelorism 8 (40%), and epicanthic folds 8 (40%), and Simian creases of palms in 7 (35%). Only 17% had relative increase in testicular volume. The authors believe that a chromosomal test for fragile X is likely to be of diagnostic benefit in young children with developmental delay (particularly in speech), a maternal family history for mental retardation or developmental disabilities, and long and/or wide and/or protruding ears. (Simko A et al. Fragile X syndrome: Recognition in young children. *Pediatrics* April 1989; *83*:547-552).

COMMENT. Martin and Bell first showed the association of mental retardation with the X chromosome and the marker X, now known as the fragile X, was first described in 1969 by Lubs. Sutherland discovered the method to enhance expression of the fragile site on the human chromosomes, dependent on folic acid deficient tissue culture medium (1977). In the adult, the classical triad of physical findings in the fragile X syndrome consists of a long face with prominent jaw, large prominent ears and macroorchidism. A number of different minor nonspecific dysmorphic characteristics have been noted in the occasional affected female but no large group of young girls with fragile X syndrome has been described. - Editor. *Ped Neur Briefs* February 1989.

Psychopathology In Fragile X Syndrome

The physical and behavioral features of the fragile X syndrome are reviewed in a paper from the Child Development Unit and Behavioral Sciences Department, Children's Hospital, Denver. In the prepubertal child, macroorchidism means a testicular volume greater than 2 ml, documented in 39% of prepubertal fragile X males (Hagerman 1987). It is measured with an orchidometer, a string of ellipsoid shapes of known volume which can be matched for size next to the testicle. In the adult male, macroorchidism measures a testicular volume of approximately 30 ml or larger.

A broad spectrum of cognitive involvement occurs in both males and females affected by the fragile X syndrome. The majority of adult fragile X males are moderately retarded and function well in group homes and sheltered workshops; whereas the majority of prepubertal males are mildly retarded and 10% have IQs in the borderline or low normal range, associated with significant learning disabilities. Language deficits are seen in all affected fragile X males, even those with a normal IQ. Speech is described as jocular or staccato, in bursts which may include perseverations or repetition of words or phrases. Longitudinal IQ evaluations of fragile X males have shown that younger boys score higher cognitively than adults.

Heterozygous females may be completely unaffected by the syndrome or may have milder problems than those commonly seen in the males. Approximately 30% of heterozygotes have cognitive deficits ranging from a borderline IQ to more significant retardation. Heterozygotes with normal IQ (approximately 70%) have cognitive defects including a poor performance on arithmetic, digit span and block design subtest scales on the WISC. Physical features in the mildly affected heterozygotes include prominent ears, double jointed thumbs, hyperextensible finger joints, and elongated face or prominent jaw in older females. Typical fragile X facial features are reported in 55% of retarded heterozygotes and in 14% of normal IQ heterozygotes. Enlargement of ovaries has been noted by ultrasound studies. (Hagerman RJ and Sobesky WE. Psychopathology in fragile X syndrome. *Amer J Orthopsychiat* Jan 1989; *59*:142-152).

> COMMENT. This review article provides useful information about the clinical manifestations and psychopathology of heterozygous fragile X females. Careful examination will often reveal subtle physical features associated with the fragile X syndrome in females. Cognitive, social and emotional disorders are described. More detailed neuropsychological testing of heterozygotes has demonstrated learning disabilities in math, right left disorientation, constructional dyspraxia, and finger agnosia (Gerstmann's syndrome).

(Grigsby J et al. *Neuropsychologia* 1987; *25*:881). - Editor. *Ped Neur Briefs* February 1989.

Autistic Spectrum Disorder

In the second part of an excellent review of disorders of higher cerebral function, Dr. Isabelle Rapin, at the Albert Einstein College of Med, Bronx, NY, outlines the evaluation and management of preschool children with autism and inadequate communication skills. The core symptoms of the autistic spectrum disorder are listed as follows: 1) impaired socialization, 2) inadequately modulated affect, 3) language disorder always affecting communicative skills and comprehension, and 4) abnormal play with a narrow range of interests. There is a spectrum of autistic disorders, ranging from mute, withdrawn individuals with motor stereotypes to highly verbose persons with perseveration, insistence of routines and sameness, and overspecialized interests such as dictionaries, train schedules, and calendars. Autism usually denotes a static condition. The most efficient way to evaluate communication skills is to observe the child at play, to talk to him, and to ask questions about his play. Children who manipulate toys rather than play with them, who talk to themselves, or who are echolalic or perseverative are almost certainly abnormal. Hearing tests, speech and language evaluation, neuropsychological tests, and consultations with child neurologist and psychiatrist may be required before referral to a preschool specialized program. (Rapin I. Disorders of higher cerebral function in preschool children. *AJDC* Nov 1988; *142*:1178-1182).

COMMENT. Cerebellar hypoplasia and autism is discussed in the correspondence section of *N Engl J Med* Oct 17, 1988; *319*:1152-54). Patients with autism, mean age 20 yr, were reported to have a decrease in the size of cerebellar vermal lobules VI and VII on MRI scans. These findings were not confirmed in one study of 15 patients with autism (mean age 11.5 years) compared to 15 normal matched controls, but they were replicated in a study of

men with fragile X syndrome, a condition sometimes associated with autism. Investigations that include children as
well as adults would help to specify whether the observed
cerebellar changes on MRI are actually hypoplasia or atrophy occurring postnatally. - Editor. *Ped Neur Briefs*
October 1988.

Music And Adolescent Behavior

The role of music in the lives of adolescents and the use of
music preferences as clues to the emotional and mental health of
adolescents is reviewed from the Group on Science and
Technology, American Medical Association, Chicago, IL.
Between the 7th and 12th grades the average teenager listens to
10,500 hours of rock music. Unlike television viewing which
is often subject to family discussion and parental control, music
is largely uncensored. Music plays a large role in adolescent
socialization, as an information source about sexuality and alternative lifestyles, and as an introduction to political topics via various concerts organized for political causes. It is an important
symbol in the search for independence and autonomy. It may
provide an outlet for personal troubles or conflicts with parents.

Musical preferences may reflect different types of struggles
that adolescents face as they make the transition to adulthood.
Rock music has spawned many cultural accessories such as tee
shirts and dress styles. There may be a causal link between
school performance and music preference. A heavy involvement
in rock music by low achievers may be an adaptive reaction to
their failures as students and an expression of their alienation
from school and the learning experience. Successful students
exhibit a preference for mainstreamed music, less interest in
punk and rock music, and less involvement in peer groups.
Parent's groups have characterized many rock lyrics as sexually
explicit and violent, some even advocating suicide. Heavy metal
music glorifies hatred, abuse, sexual deviancy, and occasionally
satanism. An adult's interpretation of rock lyrics might be
entirely different from that of a teenager. Physicians can encour-

age parents to question their children about their interpretation of the music and what role it plays in their lives. The physician may also point out that so far there is no confirmation that this music has a deleterious effect on the behavior of adolescents. (Brown EF, Hende WR. Adolescents and their music. Insights into the health of adolescents. *JAMA* September 22/29, 1989; *262*:1659-1663).

COMMENT. It is apparent that theories regarding the influence of music on the behavior of adolescents are mainly conjectural and unproven. An adverse effect of this music not mentioned in this article is the incidence of nerve deafness. The inattention to the environment caused by the wearing of earphones while walking to school or work or bicycling may also contribute to an increased incidence of traffic accidents and injuries. - Editor. *Ped Neur Briefs* October 1989.

CHAPTER **4**

DYSLEXIA AND LANGUAGE DISORDERS

DYSLEXIA

GENETICS AND READING DISABILITIES

Psychologists and psychiatrists at the University of Surrey, Guildford, Surrey, and the Hospital for Sick Children, Great Ormond Street, London, UK studied the reading skills of 285 pairs of 13 year old twins using standardized measures of intelligence, reading and spelling ability and correlations in monozygotic and same-sex dizygotic twins. Genetic factors played only a moderate role in general reading backwardness and specific reading retardation whereas strong genetic influences for spelling disability were found. (Stevenson J, Graham P, Fredman G, McLoughlin V. A twin study of genetic influences on reading and spelling ability and disability. *J Child Psychol Psychiat* 1987; 28:229-247).

COMMENT. Of a total of 96 twin pairs reported in the literature, 36 (88%) monozygotic twins and only 16 (29%) dizygotic twins were concordant for dyslexia (Millichap JG, Millichap NM. *Dyslexia: As The Neurologist and Educator Read It.* Charles C. Thomas, Springfield, IL, USA, 1986). Between 25 and 50% of children with reading disability demonstrate transmission within families. Hallgren (1950) concluded that his data best fitted an autosomal dominant genetic mechanism and others have proposed alternative genetic models: autosomal dominant with reduced penetrance in females, and sex-linked recessive. These studies are at variance with the present authors' conclusions that emphasize the complexity of genetic influences on literacy skills and the importance of changes that occur with development in our understanding of the causation of reading difficulties. - Editor. *Ped Neur Briefs* June 1987.

Peripheral Vision In Dyslexics

Scientists from the Research Laboratory of Electronics and the Departments of Biology, Electrical Engineering, and Computer Science at MIT Cambridge, MA, have collaborated in an investigation of the peripheral and foveal (central) vision of 5 dyslexic adult subjects compared to 5 normal readers. Two letters, one at the fixation point and one at the periphery, at varying distances apart (eccentricities), were presented simultaneous and the scores for the correct identification of the single peripheral letters in the two groups were compared.

At 2.5° eccentricity (near central fixation point) the scores of normal readers were the higher. Correct identification fell off with increasing eccentricity (2.5 to 12.5°) in both groups but the falloff was slower in severe dyslexics than in normal readers. At 7.5° eccentricity (peripheral field vision), the scores of dyslexic subjects were higher than those of normal readers; i.e. they were better at perceiving briefly presented letters in the periphery.

When a string of three letters was substituted for the single letters in the periphery, the severe dyslexic could identify none of the letters at 2.5° eccentricity (near central vision) but at 5° and beyond (peripheral vision) his identification of letters was near normal. After a program of exercises involving spatial organization and eye-hand coordination and the use of a simple device to utilize his optimal peripheral vision in reading, the performance of the severe dyslexic subject showed improvement after four months up to a 10th grade level. (Geiger G, Lettvin JY. *N Engl J Med* 1987; *316*:1238).

COMMENT. These interesting findings and suggested treatments will undoubtedly bring joy to the optometrists and those who favor the Kephart and Frostig methods in the management of dyslexia. Kephart's three crucial perceptual skills to be mastered as prerequisites to reading are form perception, spatial discrimination, and ocular control. If these skills are underdeveloped, according to Kephart, the child will develop faulty intersensory integration abilities and concept formation. Frostig, similarly, maintains that adequate perceptual functioning in young children is the foundation on which later school success depends. Critics of these methods state that evidence from research studies does not support their value in reading remediation. However, several authors have emphasized abnormalities of eye movements, tracking, and visual fixations as a characteristic of dyslexics and further studies are needed.

The authors, Geiger and Lettvin, conclude that in dyslexics, there is an interaction between foveal and peripheral vision that degrades the normal ability to read in the foveal field. Dyslexics have masking or suppression of letter discrimination in the central foveal field and better than normal peripheral visual identification of letters. They suggest that dyslexics should be taught to read by use of their peripheral vision. Neurologists might argue alternative explanations for the findings based on changes in attention or cortical visual organization but the study offers a simple and practical method of treatment that is worthy of trial in a larger number of younger subjects. The results could be different in children from those in adults, aged 18-25, used in this study. - Editor. *Ped Neur Briefs* July 1987.

Zinc Deficiency And Dyslexia

An association between dyslexia and low concentrations of zinc in sweat has been demonstrated in a study of 26 children aged 6-14 yrs recruited from those attending the Dyslexia Institute, Staines, Middlesex, and the Hornsby Learning Centre, London. They were paired with their non-dyslexic school friends, who were matched for age and sex and had no obvious allergies, illnesses or behavior disorders. Sweat from the skin of the back and hair from the occipitonuchal region were collected for analyses of trace minerals at the Biolab Medical Unit, London W1N3FF (correspondence to Dr. Davies).

Zinc concentrations in sweat of dyslexic children (5.4 umol/l) was 66% that in controls (8.0 umol/l, P=.0001). Higher concentrations of copper, lead and cadmium and no differences in zinc concentrations were found in hair of dyslexics compared with controls. (Grant ECG et al. Zinc deficiency in children with dyslexia: concentrations of zinc and other minerals in sweat and hair. *Br Med J* 27 Feb 1988; *296*:607-9).

COMMENT. Zinc in sweat may be a more useful guide to clinical zinc deficiency than hair or serum concentrations (Davies S. *Sci Total Environ* 1985; *42*:45). The authors propose that zinc deficiency in parents may possibly predispose to familial dyslexia.

Zinc deficiency can be due to nutritional factors, inherited defects in zinc metabolism, and several disease states (Millichap JG. *Nutrition, Diet and Your Child's Behavior.* C C Thomas, Springfield, 1986). The high phytate content of protein and the fiber in certain cereals decrease the availability of zinc in persons who eat primarily cereals and little meat. Alcoholism, malabsorption, kidney disease, and sickle cell anemia predispose to zinc deficiency. The reported possible association of maternal zinc-deficient diets with developmental defects in fetal brain is of interest in relation to the brain malformations recorded on CT scans of occasional children with dyslexia (Galaburda AM et al. *Ann Neurol* 1985; *18*:222).

Hair zinc levels of urban toddlers were lower than rural toddlers, especially in summer and in those with frequent upper respiratory tract infections, in a study from North Rhine-Westphalia, Fed Rep Germany (Lombeck I et al. *Eur J Pediatr* Feb 1988; *147*:179). Environmental and seasonal factors and age, sex and infection affect the variability in zinc hair content in addition to dietary factors. Caution in the interpretation of hair analyses is stressed. - Editor. *Ped Neur Briefs* March 1988.

Drugs In Treatment Of Developmental Dyslexia

An acute 2 day trial of methylphenidate (10 mg) and of meclizine (12.5 mg) and a 6 month crossover placebo-controlled chronic trial of meclizine (12.5 mg) in children with developmental dyslexia are reported from the University of Calgary, Alberta, Canada. Oral reading fluency, coordination, and motor accuracy improved on methylphenidate, and clinical improvements of eye fixation and tracking were found with meclizine, in acute trials. Three of 6 children showing benefit from acute doses of meclizine also showed significant improvements in eye fixation stability after 3 months chronic administration of the drug (12.5 mg BD), but measures of reading skills including comprehension, phonetic analysis, structural analysis, achievement, and oral and silent reading rates, were not benefitted. (Fagan JE et al. The failure of antimotion sickness medication to improve reading in developmental dyslexia: results of a randomized trial. *J Dev Behav Pediatr* Dec 1988; *9*:359-367).

COMMENT. Levinson HN (*A Solution to the Riddle Dyslexia*. New York. Springer-Yerlag, 1980) has proposed a theory of cerebellar-vestibular dysfunction as the etiology of dyslexia and has claimed that treatment with antimotion sickness medications may result in improvement in reading in 77% of cases of dyslexia. The present study fails to confirm these results and suggests that antimotion sickness drug treatment of dyslexia is unjustified. The relationship between fixation error and impaired reading is not completely understood, however. Geiger and Lettvin have found that dyslexics have poor foveal vision, but when the target is moved into the peripheral visual field, their ability to identify letters is better than control nondyslexic subjects. Imperfect oculomotor control in the dyslexic may be accompanied by abnormalities of visual processing and cognitive difficulties that impede the acquisition of reading skills. Further work on this aspect of dyslexia seems justified. - Editor. *Ped Neur Briefs* December 1988.

Reading With One Hemisphere
The reading performance of two right-handed teenage girls who had undergone hemispherectomy for intractable epilepsy was examined at the MRC Applied Psychology Unit, Cambridge, the Department of Developmental Pediatrics, Institute of Child Health and Department of Psychological Medicine, Hospital for Sick Children, and the Neurosurgical Unit, Maudsley Hospital, London. Both subjects had developed normal language and reading capacities before the onset of their illness.

One patient, whose symptoms of left hemisphere abnormality commenced at the age of 13 years and whose left hemisphere was removed at the age of 15, was poor at virtually all aspects of reading; but her pattern of reading performance was not one of undifferentiated impairment. She was essentially perfect at recognizing letters, although not very successful at naming them and totally unable to give their sound equivalents. She was reasonably good at discriminating very common words from orthographically similar nonwords, but her lexical decision performance fell off quickly as word frequency declined. She could comprehend printed words as measured by matching two pictures, when those corresponded to common concrete objects but she occasionally made semantic errors in this task, and her success was dependent on maximal degrees of both word familiarity and concreteness. She also had some degree of success in oral reading of the most familiar and highly imageable words of the type that she could understand and had no means of translating a printed word into a phonological response except on the basis of its meaning. She could not read aloud nonsense words although she could repeat them perfectly. This patient's reading performance was identical in pattern though not in level to most cases of acquired deep dyslexia. There is a strong case for the equation of deep dyslexic reading with right hemisphere reading.

The reading performance of the second patient whose right hemisphere had been removed was not as advanced in level as that of a normal 17 year old but it showed no abnormality in any subcomponent or reading skill. The discrepancy between her chronological and reading ages could be entirely explained in terms of the five year history of preoperative illness. This patient's performance suggested that the right hemisphere plays no necessary role in supporting reading skills, at least of the type assessed in the study (mainly single word recognition, comprehension and pronunciation). (Patterson K et al. Reading with one hemisphere. *Brain* Feb 1989; *112*:39-63).

COMMENT. Although the right hemisphere appeared to play no necessary role in supporting reading skills, perhaps it is important both for reading acquisition and for mature efficient reading. In particular, the right hemisphere may be important for quick pattern recognition during speed reading and for semantic-thematic orientation to a situation or narrative. Loss of right hemisphere contribution to reading in adults would lead to subtle deficits in higher order reading which are rarely assessed in the neurological clinic. (Zaidel and Schweiger. *Cognitive Neuropsychology* 1984; *1*:351).

The normal acquisition of reading requires two functioning hemispheres and children with one hemisphere have difficulty learning to read whether it is the left or the right hemisphere that has been removed. The vast majority of right-handed people have left hemisphere dominance for language skills such as reading. It had been an unresolved question, however, whether the right hemisphere of a left hemisphere dominant individual also developed significant capacity for reading. Cases of hemispherectomy performed for neurological disease of late onset provide most convincing evidence regarding reading with one hemisphere. - Editor. *Ped Neur Briefs* April 1989.

Boder's Subtypes Of Dyslexia

The subtyping of dyslexic children proposed by Boder (1971, 1973) has been validated by quantitative neurophysiological techniques at the Gunderson Medical Foundation, LaCrosse, WI. Children were classified as being *dysphonetic* (auditory-phonetic disabilities), *dyseidetic* (visual spatial disabilities) or *mixed* (deficient in both processes). In one study of 21 dyslexic children between 7 and 10 years of age and six control children, there were significant differences between the dyslexic subgroups and between the dyslexic and control children on three of the six cognitive tasks (frustration level reading, spelling recognition, and drawing a clock). Significant differences occurred in EEG left temporal-parietal theta activity, and this difference occurred in the area of the angular gyrus, presumed to be important in phonetic decoding. This suggested that the reportedly normal phonetic skills of dyseidetic children may not be normal but rather a sign of overuse of a processing strategy associated with inefficiency of right hemisphere visual gestalt abilities. Additional support for an overuse theory in dyseidetic dyslexia came from the behavior of the children during reading tasks. The dyseidetic children audibly decoded many words whereas dysphonetic and mixed dyslexics skipped unknown words or substituted words with the same beginning sound.

On a second study involving 33 eight and nine year old dyslexic children and 31 controls, the results of two of seven cognitive tasks confirmed subtype differences. Significant differences in left temporal-parietal theta activity in the electroencephalograms of the dyseidetic children suggested that their reading disabilities may be the result of overuse of linguistic abilities rather than deficient visual spatial skills. (Flynn JM, Deering WM. Subtypes of dyslexia: Investigation of Boder's system using quantitative neurophysiology. *Dev Med Child Neur* 1989; *31*:215-223).

COMMENT. A diagnostic screening test for subtypes of reading disability, the *Boder Test of Reading Spelling Patterns*, is published by the Psychological Corporation, San Antonio, TX. The Boder Test is easily administered and identifies four subtypes of reading disability on the basis of reading and spelling performance. The test is based on the premise that dyslexic readers have characteristic patterns of strengths and weaknesses in two distinct cognitive components of the reading process: 1) the *visual gestalt function* and 2) the *auditory analytic function*. The visual gestalt function underlies the ability to develop a sight vocabulary. The auditory analytic function underlies the ability to develop phonic word-analysis skills. These two cognitive functions are basic to the two standard methods of initial reading instruction: 1) the *whole word method* and 2) the *phonics method*. The Boder test provides a diagnosis that is meaningful to the educator in the choice of remediation methods. This *matching method* or *neuropsychological approach* to reading remediation involves matching the learning strengths with a teaching strategy designed to exploit these strengths. It is favored by Johnson and

Mykelbust who recognize two main subtypes of dyslexia, "visual dyslexia and auditory dyslexia" and also by Mattis who identified language, dyscoordination, and visuospatial subtypes.

The validation of Boder's neuropsychological approach and classification of dyslexic subtypes is an important advance in the evaluation of reading remediation methods. The Boder method, matching learning strengths to teaching methods, appears to be theoretically sound and much preferred to techniques based on deficit remediation which involve the training or retraining of damaged or dysfunctional areas of the brain. (Millichap JG, Millichap NM. *Dyslexia: As the Neurologist and Educator Read It.* Springfield, IL. Charles C. Thomas, Publisher 1986). - Editor. *Ped Neur Briefs* July 1989.

Alexia, Agraphia, And Frontal Lobe Damage
The case history of a right-handed woman who developed severe and stable alexia and agraphia following a circumscribed surgical lesion in the left premotor cortex is reported from the Department of Neurology, Division of Behavioral Neurology and Cognitive Neuroscience, University of Iowa College of Medicine, Iowa City, Iowa. The lesion was above Broca's area in Exner's area. Her visual perception, intellect, memory, oral spelling, and drawing were normal and she was not aphasic or hemiparetic. She was unable to read sentences and her reading of single words and letters was severely impaired. She could not write recognizable letters or words. By contrast she was able to write numbers and perform written calculations without difficulty. These dissociations of function provide evidence of specificity of cognitive and neural representation. (Anderson SW, Demasio AR, Demasio H. Troubled letters but not numbers. Domain specific cognitive impairments following focal damage in frontal cortex. *Brain* June 1990; *113*:749-766).

COMMENT. The isolated simultaneous occurrence of alexia and agraphia is rare. In this case the anatomical lesion within the left frontal lobe was unusually circumscribed. The sector of association cortex in the frontal lobe, known as Exner's area, appears to be related to the ability to read and write. The pathology of the small lesion removed surgically was a single metastasis from an adenocarcinoma of the lung. Neurological evaluation was normal except for the cognitive defect described. The neuroanatomical basis of developmental dyslexia has been debated since this hypothesis was proposed by Orton in 1937.

Patterns of task related slow-brain potentials have been investigated in six dyslexic youths by Landwehrmeyer B et al (*Arch Neurol* July 1990; 47:791-797). Whereas control subjects revealed greater left hemisphere negativity during linguistic tasks, the reverse was found with dyslexics. The authors, working at the Neurologische Universitatsklinik, Freiburg, West Germany, concluded that dyslexia is associated with changes in the lateral distribution of cortical activity during certain types of language processing. - Editor. *Ped Neur Briefs* August 1990.

LANGUAGE DISORDERS

Crossed Aphasia
A case of crossed aphasia with persistent language disturbances in a right-handed boy aged 5 yr 9 mos is reported from the Centre Hospitalier Universitaire Vaudois, Lausanne, France. An acute left hemiplegia resulted from occlusion of the internal carotid siphon of undetermined cause and demonstrated by arteriography. The boy was mute, his auditory comprehension impaired, and tongue and facial movements apraxic. His first intelligible words (maman and non) were pronounced at 2 months after the onset. The language remained agrammatic and

the vocabulary and comprehension poor but the tongue apraxia resolved. Twelve years later, language disturbances were still present although his IQ on the WAIS was 100 full scale, 86 verbal (information 6, comprehension 6, digit memory 5, vocabulary 7, arithmetic 8) and 116 performance scale.

The CT scan showed an atrophic right hemisphere and dilated lateral ventricle with cortical and subcortical low densities involving the base of the 3rd frontal, supramarginal, insular and middle part of 1st temporal convolutions, the lenticular and caudate nuclei and the anterior limb of the internal capsule. (Assal G. Aphasie croisee chez un enfant. *Rev Neurol* (Paris) 1987; *143*:532-535).

> COMMENT. Crossed aphasia is the combination of right hemiparesis with aphasia in a left-handed patient or left hemiparesis and aphasia in a right-handed patient. It is rare in dextrals, only 9 cases cited in a review article by Brown JW and Hecaen H (*Neurology* 1976; *26*:183). Diagnosis requires the following: a pathologic lesion limited to the right hemisphere, absence of early childhood brain damage, strong right-handedness, and a negative family history of left-handedness. These criteria were satisfied in the author's case. A state of incomplete left lateralization is suggested to explain crossed aphasia in a right-handed patient. Although recovery of fluency is quicker and more extensive than in adults, later academic problems are common in children with aphasia even with those caused by left hemisphere lesions. (Cranberg LD et al. *Neurology* 1987; *37*:1165). - Editor. *Ped Neur Briefs* October 1987.

Language Disorders And Attention Deficit Disorders (ADD)

The prevalence rates of speech and language disorders and ADD in 116 children referred for psychiatric services were determined at the Ontario Association of Children's Mental Health Centres and the Dept of Psychiatry, Hospital for Sick Children,

Toronto, Canada. Speech and language disorders were diagnosed in 65% and ADD in 73%. Only 16% had speech and language disorders alone and only 25% had ADD alone. The overall prevalence for the dual diagnosis was 48%. Three-quarters of those with language disorders also had ADD and two-thirds with ADD also had language disorders. The average age at evaluation was 5 yrs. Boys outnumbered girls for language disorders with or without ADD. The presence of language disorder was correlated with intact family status in lower socioeconomic classes, single-child families, and serious parent/child problems. (Love AJ, Thompson MGG. Language disorders and attention deficit disorders in young children referred for psychiatric services: analysis of prevalence and a conceptual synthesis. *Amer J Orthopsychiat* Jan 1988; *58(1)*:52-64).

COMMENT. This study suggests that pre-school children referred for psychiatric outpatient services are at high risk for language disorders. Failure to develop oral language on schedule is among the earliest concerns voiced by parents of children who later are identified as ADD or learning disabled. Speech and language evaluations should be included in any comprehensive examination of a child with ADD. - Editor. *Ped Neur Briefs* February 1988.

Language Development And Otitis Media

The effects of otitis media on early language development assessed at 1 year of age in 46 high-risk and low birthweight infants and 19 healthy full-term babies were examined in the R.F. Kennedy Center's Clinical Research Center for Communicative Disorders, Albert Einstein College of Medicine, Bronx, NY. Patients were largely of Hispanic background but subjects were recruited from English speaking families. By pneumatic otoscopy examination, 15 were otitis free and 12 were bilaterally otitis positive. The Bayley Scales of Infant Development and the Sequenced Inventory of Communication Development (SICD) Receptive scale showed no significant differences in the 2 groups, but the SICD Expressive language scores were significantly lower in the otitis positive group. Full-term infants with frequent episodes of bilateral otitis media performed no better than high risk infants with otitis media. (Wallace IF et al. Otitis media and language development at 1 year of age. *J Speech and Hearing Disorders* Aug 1988; 53:245-251).

COMMENT. Infants who suffer repeated episodes of bilateral otitis media during the first year of life are at risk for expressive language difficulties. These findings are important in the evaluation of infants who have experienced perinatal insults such as asphyxia and are late in acquiring expressive language. The delay may be caused by peripheral factors as much as damage to cerebral language centers.

Disorders of higher cerebral function including developmental language are reviewed by Dr. Isabelle Rapin at the Albert Einstein College of Medicine, Bronx, NY (*AJDC* Oct 1988; *142*:1119-1124). Included under the differential diagnosis of language delay are the following: hearing loss, mental deficiency, dysphasia, autism, mutism, dysarthria and structural respiratory tract abnormalities. No meaningful words by age 18 months or no meaningful phrases by age 24 months should be cause for concern and the use of language intervention programs. - Editor. *Ped Neur Briefs* September 1988.

Oromotor Dyspraxia In Benign Childhood Epilepsy

A six year old right handed boy with prolonged intermittent drooling, oromotor dyspraxia, and benign childhood epilepsy with centrotemporal spikes is reported from the Departments of Pediatrics and Neurology, Centre Hospitalier, Universitaire Vaudois, Lausanne, Switzerland. Seizures began on the third day of life and were controlled with phenobarbital. Febrile seizures began at eight months and recurred 12 times up to six years of age. At first the seizures were generalized but after four years of age they were partial motor, involving the face and sometimes the right arm. The drooling probably resulted from hypersalivation and oromotor dyspraxia. The fluctuant course of the symptoms and correlation with intensity of the paroxysmal discharges on EEG were consistent with an epileptic dysfunction located in the lower rolandic fissure. No lesion was demonstrated by MRI. (Roulet E, Deonna T, Despland PA. Prolonged intermittent drooling and oromotor dyspraxia in benign childhood epilepsy with centrotemporal spikes. *Epilepsia* October 1989, *30*:564-568).

COMMENT. This case provides evidence that a continuous epileptic dysfunction can occur in benign childhood epilepsy with centrotemporal spikes. The case resembles the acquired aphasia epilepsy syndrome of Landau-Kleffner. - Editor. *Ped Neur Briefs* November 1989.

Landau-Kleffner (Aphasia-Epilepsy) Syndrome And Neurocysticercosis

A seven year old right-handed boy with a one year history of language disorder associated with clinical seizures and paroxysmal EEG is reported from the Division de Neurologia, Instituto Nacional de Neurologia Y Neurocirugia, Mexico, D.F. He had normal speech and comprehension up to age six when he developed several brief episodes of loss of awareness and unresponsiveness associated with automatic movements of the hands, recurring more than 20 times a day. Two months later he did not respond to calls and did not comprehend stories read to him. His speech became telegraphic. CT and MRI revealed a small cysticercus deep in the left Sylvian fissure. An EEG showed sharp and slow wave complexes over the left centrotemporal regions with spread to the right side. Treatment with the anticysticercal drug Albendazole resulted in reduction in size of the cyst, valproate controlled the seizures, and the language disorder improved. Follow-up at six months showed no recurrence. (Otero E et al. Acquired epileptic aphasia (the Landau-Kleffner syndrome) due to neurocysticercosis. *Epilepsia* October 1989; *30*:569-572).

COMMENT. Deonna T and associates from the Pediatric Department, Lausanne, Switzerland, report an adult follow-up study of seven patients with acquired aphasia-epilepsy syndrome beginning in childhood (*Neuropediatrics*, August 1989, *20*:132-138). One man had recovered completely, one had normal oral language but was severely dyslexic, one recovered normal comprehension but had severe expressive language problems, four had absent language comprehension and lack of expressive speech. Only one had learned and is using sign language with some efficiency, and none had developed functional written language. Attempts to offer a substitutive language to children with acquired aphasia-epilepsy syndrome were not very successful. Isolated reports of improvement with anticonvulsant drug treatment justified further trials.

Ansink BJJ et al from the Saint Lucas Ziekenhuis, Amsterdam, the Netherlands, report a child who developed seizures with fever at 20 months of age. The fever was caused by pneumonia. Four months later she had fever and status epilepticus which were followed by abnormal behavior and aphasia. (*Neuropediatrics*, August 1989, *20*:139). The aphasia was complicated by visual agnosia and spatial disturbances. The EEG showed multifocal epileptic activity. Treatment with valproic acid controlled the seizures and language functions recovered slowly.

At the 1989 annual meeting of the American Epilepsy Society there were two papers on the Landau-Kleffner syndrome: 1) Marescaux C et al from Strasbourg, France and Liege, Belgium described two patients with a syndrome of continuous spike wave discharges during sleep associated with aphasia; and 2) Morrell F et al from Rush Medical College, Chicago, reported four patients with the syndrome who were treated successfully by subpial transection. - Editor. *Ped Neur Briefs* November 1989.

Developmental Dysphasia Subtypes

The syndromes of developmental dysphasia and their remediation are outlined in the selected proceedings of the Fourth
International Child Neurology Congress held in Jerusalem,
Israel, March 16-20, 1986. Six dysphasic syndromes are identified through the combined psycholinguistic/ aphasiology
model: 1) Verbal dyspraxia, 2) phonological production deficit,
3) verbal auditory agnosia, 4) phonologic-syntactic deficit, 5)
lexical-syntactic deficit, and 6) semantic pragmatic deficit.

In subtypes 1 and 2 impairment is in the expressive system
with comprehension relatively intact. *Verbal dyspraxia* is a
severe expressive disorder in which the child is extremely nonflu-
ent and may be mute. *Phonological production deficit* is characterized by fluency but nonetheless unintelligibility. In both syndromes the production of consonants is more difficult than of
vowels. Apraxia of speech and developmental misarticulation
are terms sometimes applied to these expressive dysphasias. All
dyspraxic dysphasias are difficult to treat and many require
speech and language therapy beyond the preschool years. Many
need to be introduced to a visual-manual system such as reading
and writing at an early age, and some severe cases require formal
sign language in conjunction with verbalization. Subtype 3 *verbal auditory agnosia*, commonly called word deafness, is an
inability to decode spoken language at the level of phonology.
Despite normal peripheral hearing the individual is unable to
derive any meaning from the sounds he or she hears. These
children comprehend virtually nothing and are essentially mute.
Naming an object, drawing a picture of the object, and naming
the picture with a printed label facilitates vocabulary building
and the labels can then be used to make requests. Subtype 4
phonologic-syntactic deficit is a mixed receptive expressive deficit
and results in telegraphic speech with omission of prepositions,
verbs, and the endings on nouns and verbs. The use of gestures,
communication boards and written words to supplement oral
language are encouraged. In dysphasia subtype 5, *lexical syntac-
tic deficit*, syntax or the arrangement of words is immature and

comprehension of abstract language may be poor. Language is dysfluent with multiple hesitations, false starts and self-corrections. The syndrome is seen in both autistic and nonautistic children. Dysphasia subtype 6, *semantic pragmatic deficits* with hyperverbal or loquacious speech but their communicative intent and semantic content are limited and superficial. Jargon, neologisms, paraphasias, and circumlocutions are common. Speech is quite rapid and "cluttered". The subtyping of dysphasic children permits the design of specific interventions for the particular language needs of the children in each group. (Allen DA, Mendelson L, Rapin I. Syndrome specific remediation in preschool developmental dysphasia. In *Child Neurology and Developmental Disabilities*, edited by French JH, Harel S, Casaer P. Baltimore, London, Sydney, Toronto. Paul H. Brookes Publishing Company, 1989).

COMMENT. These attempts to subtype dysphasic children are helpful in the definition of pathogenesis and brain localization and they allow the development of specific intervention strategies. The neurologic bases of developmental dysphasias are probably multiple. Some syndromes may result from genetic abnormalities in brain development while early focal or multifocal acquired brain pathology may be responsible for others. The differentiation of developmental and acquired aphasias in young children may be difficult and subtle cerebral abnormalities may be uncovered by the MRI in children who have otherwise normal neurologic findings. The authors of this article hypothesize that in the course of providing sound therapeutic intervention at an early age they may be able to enhance brain reorganization through the development of alternative pathways. For example, providing dysphasic children of subtype verbal auditory agnosia with a visual language system may promote a bypass of areas of auditory dysfunction and enable the children to acquire verbal language that would have been inaccessible through the auditory channel alone. Failure to show improvement after intensive remediation may be explained by bilateral brain abnormalities that prohibit reorganization. Autistic children who exhibit severe social attentional and behavioral deficits have the most guarded prognosis. - Editor. *Ped Neur Briefs* July 1989.

Prognosis Of Expressive Language Delay

The rate of improvement and its predictive factors have been studied in 26 two year old children with expressive language disorder at the Departments of Pediatrics and Psychology, State University of New York at Stony Brook, and Department of Child Development and Family Relations, University of North Carolina-Greensboro. After a five month follow-up, improvement in expressive language was variable, with approximately 1/3 of the children showing no improvement, 1/3 with mild improvement, and 1/3 in the normal range. Three variables measured by the pretest evaluation could be used to predict improvement within the five month period: 1) The size of the child's vocabulary with a cutoff score of 8; 2) whether the child was reported as eating regular meals; and 3) the extent that the child engaged in quiet "other" behaviors during the mother-child interaction. The more vocabulary the child had used at home, the more improvement in expressive language was seen. If the child was characterized as not eating three regular meals a day, the less improvement in expressive language was seen. Children who engaged in more periods of quiet non-interactive activity during play and cleanup situations were more likely to improve in expressive language. The reported vocabulary size was 81% accurate in identifying children's improvement and the prediction of improvement in growth of language. (Fischel, JE et al. Language growth in children with expressive language delay. *Pediatrics* February 1989; *83*:218-227).

COMMENT. Expressive language delay is not self-correcting in a short term period of five months for many two year old children. A pediatrician or other professional who routinely advises parents of two year old children with expressive language delay to wait for spontaneous improvement would be wrong 39% of the time. However, these authors found that improvement in expressive skill was not related to a child's involvement in intervention services and the results were not encouraging with regard to the effectiveness of early childhood intervention programs. These findings agree with other reports that early intervention efforts did not reduce the frequency of later problems during the school years.

The lack of validation of many early intervention efforts noted in the literature places the concerned pediatrician or other professional in a quandary. Apparently, he can use the parent's report of the child's vocabulary size to advise the parent with a high degree of accuracy as to whether the child's expressive language skills will improve in the next few months. However, if the parent wants advice about seeking treatment the basis of action is not clear. The parents should probably be advised of the importance of careful assessment and differential diagnosis in any child with a severe expressive delay and intervention should certainly be considered if the problem persists beyond the third birthday, even given the uncertain effects of intervention techniques.

The more accurate diagnosis of subtypes of language delay or dysphasia might lead to more specific intervention techniques as described in the previous article and the beneficial effects of treatment may become more apparent. The early language milestones scale (ELM) has been found a reliable tool to base referral of a child showing evidence of language delay when the test is applied between 25-36 months of age. In the 12 month and younger age groups the test is of no value, and for infants between 13 and 24 months of age there is moderately good agreement between the ELM and the more direct testing with a sequenced inventory of communication development

(SICD). (Walker D et al. Early language milestone scale and language screening of young children. *Pediatrics* Feb 1989; *83*:284-288). - Editor. *Ped Neur Briefs* July 1989.

Developmental Dysphasia And Cerebral Pathology

The neuropathological findings in a seven year old girl with developmental dysphasia who died of complications of infectious mononucleosis are reported from the Departments of Neurology and Pediatrics and the Department of Pathology, Medical College of Georgia, Augusta, GA. The child had been followed for developmental dysphasia and attention disorder with hyperactivity and had been treated with methylphenidate and behavior modification. Her birth was normal, she walked at 17 months and language milestones were significantly delayed with first words at two years and short phrases at four years of age. Her six year old brother had developmental dyslexia of the dysphonetic subtype. Speech and language evaluations at 2 yrs 10 mos showed no expressive language and wishes were communicated through pointing or gesturing. Receptive language function was at an 18 month level and play audiometry revealed normal hearing. The neurological examination showed inconstant asymmetry of deep tendon reflexes and a questionable Babinski on the left side. The head circumference was at the 20th percentile. Her intelligence level by the "WPPSI" was 70, expressive vocabulary 70 and receptive vocabulary 72. In addition to the language disorder she had a dysfunction in short term auditory memory and short term visual memory. In contrast her visual spatial perception and construction were relatively strong. At six years of age she did not have number or letter recognition and was unable to write her name. Arithmetically, she could count to four by rote and demonstrated number concepts to two. Academically a global learning disability was present.

The neuropathological studies revealed atypical symmetry of the plana temporale and a dysplastic gyrus on the inferior surface of the left frontal cortex along the inferior surface of the

Sylvian fissure. The authors proposed that these anomalies are likely related to midgestation, the period of neuronal migration from the germinal matrix to the cerebral cortex and are consistent with a neurodevelopmental cause of developmental dysphasia. (Cohen M et al. Neuropathological abnormalities in developmental dysphasia. *Ann Neurol* June 1989; *25*: 567-570).

> COMMENT. The Child Neurology Society Task Force on the nosology of disorders of higher cerebral function in children (1981) defined developmental dysphasia as a delayed, and usually aberrant, acquisition of language for communicative use, provided the delay is not accounted for by deafness or by severe mental retardation. It must be distinguished from acquired aphasia as a result of focal pathological lesions usually affecting the left hemisphere. In the present case report there was no evidence of an acquired insult or disease process although the patient did have a delay in walking. The language disorder was associated with oromotor apraxia, anomia and the use of gesture. The assumed developmental basis for the dysphasia was correlated with subtle developmental brain anomalies characterized by symmetry of the plana temporale similar to that reported in cases of dyslexia. (Galaburda AM et al. *Ann Neurol* 1985; *18*:222). - Editor. *Ped Neur Briefs* July 1989.

Handedness, Stuttering And Allergies

The relationship of left-handedness to allergic disorders and stuttering using epidemiological data of two French samples, is reported from L'Institut National de la Sante et de la Recherche Medicale, Villejuif, France. A higher frequency of stuttering, but not of allergic disorders, occured in left-handers. Extreme right-handedness was significantly associated with a lower frequency of allergic disorders. The Geschwind-Galaburda theory of cerebral dominance was not supported by these findings. Any significant association of allergic disorders with handedness disappeared after the exclusion of the extreme right-handers. On the contrary, stuttering was associated with left-handedness even after exclusion of extreme handedness. (Dellatolas G et al. An epidemiological reconsideration of the Geschwind-Galaburda theory of cerebral lateralization. *Arch Neurol* July 1990; *47*:778-782).

COMMENT. The Geschwind-Galaburda theory of cerebral dominance invokes in utero testosterone-induced-immune disorders and left-handedness by effects on the thymus and the brain. Their clinical observations showed a higher frequency of immune diseases, migraine, and developmental learning disorders in left-handed individuals and their families. - Editor. *Ped Neur Briefs* August 1990.

CHAPTER **5**

TOURETTE SYNDROME AND OTHER MOVEMENT DISORDERS

Transient Tics And Tourette's Syndrome

The relation of transient tic disorder (TTD - motor or vocal tics lasting less than 1 year) to Tourette's syndrome (TS - multiple motor and vocal tics lasting longer than 1 year) has been evaluated in two Canadian Mennonite families at the Dept of Neurology, Univ of Rochester Sch of Med, NY. One girl aged 9 yrs experienced frequent repetitive throat clearing and eye blinking episodes that resolved after several months (TTD). Her father and brother had TS and 2 siblings had chronic tic disorder (CTC - motor or vocal tics, but not both, with duration more than 1 year). A boy aged 12 yrs had frequent head jerks resolving over several months (TTD). His father had TS and sibling had CTD. In adulthood, the patient had 3 children, one with TS. (Kurlan R et al. Transient tic disorder and the spectrum of Tourette's syndrome. *Arch Neurol* Nov 1988; *45*:1200-1201).

COMMENT. Transient tic disorder may be an expression of the TS gene that may be transmitted to offspring as an autosomal dominant. The frequency of transient tics in childhood is quoted at 4-16%. The observations in this study suggest that TS and related tic disorders are more prevalent than generally appreciated. - Editor. *Ped Neur Briefs* October 1988.

Tourette's Syndrome Prevalence

The prevalence of Gilles de la Tourette's syndrome (TS) in school children from Monroe County, NY, was examined in the Depts of Psychiatry, Neurology and Pediatrics, University of Rochester Medical Center, Rochester, NY. Forty-one TS patients were detected with an estimated prevalence of 28.7 per 100,000. Twenty (50%) of the 41 children had obsessive ideas or ritualistic motor behaviors associated with obsessive ideas. These included rituals to make sure the body was symmetrical or balanced, mental arithmetic games, touching of objects to ward off bad luck, or repetitively placing objects. Only 3 had a diagnosable obsessive-compulsive disorder. Eleven children had attention deficit disorder with hyperactivity (ADDH); of 10 who had received methylphenidate, one developed tics after 18 months of therapy and movements almost completely ceased when drug was discontinued. Eleven had insomnia and seven had self-harming behaviors, including lip biting, sticking pins in the skin, and burning fingers on hot objects. Twenty patients had complex vocalizations including coprolalia, echolalia, and stuttering. On neurologic examination, 12 showed subtle abnormalities or soft signs including synkinesis, impaired rapid alternating movements, and inability to hop, and one had significant postural and motor defects associated with microcephaly and growth retardation. Thirty-seven were male and four were female. Fifty-six percent had a positive family history of TS or tics. TS was a mild disorder requiring no drug treatment in 23 (56%) patients. Thirteen of those who received haloperidol (0.5-2.5 mg daily) were benefitted and 5 patients were uncontrolled. (Caine ED et al. Tourette's syndrome in Monroe County school children. *Neurology* March 1988; *88*:472-5).

COMMENT. Tourette's syndrome is manifested by the onset of recurrent multiple motor tics and involuntary vocal tics in childhood. The incidence of reported cases was low until the 1960s and the condition was generally omitted from the index of textbooks of neurology. Increased public awareness of the disorder and recognition of organic in addition to functional psychiatric causes have led to an increase in apparent prevalence. Formerly, the combination of tics, coprolalia and barking were required for diagnosis whereas recently, patients with simple habit spasms are sometimes included in collected series. The exact etiology is unknown although organic factors are suspected. About 10% have a history of previous head injury or neonatal asphyxia (Erenberg G et al. *Cleve Clin Q* 1986; *53*:127). Many have learning problems and behavior disorders for which psychostimulant medication may be indicated. Methylphenidate should be withheld or used with caution at lower dose levels in children with tics or a family history of Tourette's syndrome. - Editor. *Ped Neur Briefs* March 1988.

Behavioral Problems In Tourette Syndrome

Behavioral and emotional difficulties in 78 males, 6-16 years of age, with Tourette syndrome were examined at the Departments of Neurology, Pediatrics, Psychiatry, and Education at Johns Hopkins University School of Medicine and School of Continuing Studies, Baltimore, Maryland. Symptoms most often identified included obsessive compulsive behavior, aggressiveness, hyperactivity, immaturity, withdrawal and somatic complaints.

Results were divided into two age groups, 6-11 years, (21 patients) and 12-16 years (30 patients). Scores were abnormal in 24% of children and 43% of adolescents. In the younger age group, somatic complaints and obsessive compulsive scales were abnormal in 43%, whereas in the older group more than 40% were described as being uncommunicative, obsessive compulsive, aggressive, hyperactive, immature and having hostile withdrawal. Delinquency, aggressiveness and hyperactive behavior were significantly increased in the older age group and abnormal behavioral profiles were more frequent in this age group. Tic severity was not a statistically significant predictor of behavioral disturbance, although a suggestive relationship between tic severity and behavioral disturbance was observed in the 12-16 year old group. Hyperactivity did not demonstrate an increased frequency of additional behavior problems. The authors emphasize the relative frequency of psychopathology in Tourette syndrome and the need for a comprehensive approach to this syndrome. (Singer HS, Rosenberg LA. Development of behavioral and emotional problems in Tourette syndrome. *Pediatr Neurol* Jan-Feb 1989; 5:41-44).

COMMENT. The demonstration in this study that there is a relationship between age and psychopathology in Tourette syndrome differs from a previous study which failed to reveal a relationship to age. Behavior and emotional problems were greater in the adolescent. In previous studies, the severity of motor and phonic tics have been claimed to be a predictor of behavioral disturbances in Tourette syndrome. This study corroborates previous reports and the original description by Gilles de la Tourette (1885) describing obsessive compulsive behavior as common in Tourette syndrome. Further studies are required to define the effect of attention deficit disorder with hyperactivity on the development of psychopathology in Tourette syndrome children. - Editor. *Ped Neur Briefs* February 1989.

Tourette Syndrome Diagnostic Criteria

The current concepts of Tourette syndrome, including research diagnostic criteria formulated by a workshop sponsored by the Tourette Syndrome Association, are reviewed from the Department of Neurology, University of Rochester School of Medicine, Rochester, NY. The author concludes that Tourette syndrome is a common, hereditary, neurobehavioral disorder with heterogeneous clinical manifestations. Chronic multiple motor or phonic tic disorder and transient tic disorder represent milder variants of the same illness. Behavioral disorders such as obsessive compulsive disorder and attention deficit disorder with hyperactivity occur in 50% of patients and may represent the predominant or only clinical manifestation of the illness. Diagnostic criteria for Tourette syndrome in the DSM-IIIR include 1) multiple motor tics, 2) one or more vocal tics, 3) onset before 21 years of age, and 4) duration more than one year.

The Tourette Syndrome Association Workshop participants divided tic disorders into 11 categories: 1) definite Tourette syndrome, 2) Tourette syndrome by history, 3) definite chronic multiple motor or phonic tic disorder, 4) chronic multiple motor or phonic tic disorder by history, 5) chronic single motor or phonic tic disorder by history, 6) definite transient tic disorder, 7) transient tic disorder by history, 8) definite nonspecific tic disorder, 9) nonspecific tic disorder by history, 10) definite tic disorder diagnosis deferred until followed for one year, 11) probable Tourette syndrome. Causes of associated school problems in Tourette syndrome are as follows: 1) primary Tourette syndrome symptoms, 2) obsessive compulsive behaviors, 3) attention deficit hyperactivity disorder, 4) general behavioral disturbances, 5) associated learning disabilities, 6) poor socialization, 7) low self-esteem, and 8) medication side effects.

Genetic factors in etiology are recognized and striatal dopamine receptor supersensitivity is suggested as the likely mechanism for tics. Pharmacotherapy should be considered only when symptoms of Tourette syndrome are functionally disabling and not remediable by nondrug interventions. Most patients with Tourette syndrome can probably be managed well without drug therapy and by educating the patients, family members, and school personnel concerning the nature of Tourette syndrome, restructuring the school environment (one on one tutoring) and supportive therapy. Haloperidol is the most commonly prescribed medication for Tourette syndrome but the "reflex" prescribing of this medication at diagnosis of Tourette syndrome should be avoided. (Kurlan R. Tourette's syndrome: Current concepts. *Neurology* December 1989; *39*:1625-1630).

> COMMENT. The author correctly notes that the accurate assessment of drug effectiveness in Tourette syndrome is hampered by the natural waxing and waning course of tics and the strong placebo effect of medications. The author's condoning of a combination of haloperidol and methylphenidate in selected patients with attention deficit disorder complicated by tics, a view shared by his colleague from the same institution (Roddy SM. *Contemporary Pediatrics.* November 1989; *6*:22-36) may not receive universal acceptance. - Editor. *Ped Neur Briefs* December 1989.

Therapy For Tourette Syndrome

A 12 year old male with Tourette Syndrome whose symptoms improved with gum chewing is reported from the Division of Pediatric Neurology, Hahnemann University, Philadelphia, PA. With onset at 3 years of age, symptoms had included blinking, head nodding, neck twisting, shoulder shrugs, snorting, sniffing and blowing, and coprolalia. Haloperidol controlled tics but was associated with excessive drowsiness. Clonidine was of some benefit. After chewing gum, using 2-3 sticks to make a large wad, the urge to move and vocalize was decreased and jaw movements made noise-making more difficult. The author recommends gum chewing as an adjunct therapy in Tourette Syndrome to decrease stress, facial movements, and particularly vocalizations. (Brill CB. Gum chewing as therapy for Tourette syndrome. *Pediatr Neurol* April 1988; *4*:128).

> COMMENT. Provided that teachers and parents are tolerant of gum chewing, this form of therapy might be recommended. The prevalence of Tourette syndrome was discussed in a previous issue (*Ped Neur Briefs* March 1988; 2:24). Tics were controlled by haloperidol in 13 of 18 children requiring treatment; the disorder was mild and treat-

ment was unnecessary in 23 (56%) patients. (*Neurology* 1988; *88*:472). - Editor. *Ped Neur Briefs* May 1988.

Sydenham's Chorea Carbamazepine Therapy

Five patients with chorea successfully treated with carbamazepine at plasma levels of 6.5-8.8 mcg/ml are reported from the Dept of Pediatrics, Child Neurology and EEG Service, Hospital Infantil Vall d'Hebron, Autonomous University, Barcelona, Spain. The cause of the chorea was streptococcal infection in 2, post-head injury (1), and unknown in 2. Therapy was continued for 3 to 36 months; it was discontinued in 1 because of an allergic cutaneous rash. (Roig M et al. Carbamazepine: An alternative drug for the treatment of non-hereditary chorea. *Pediatrics* Sept 1988; *82*(pt2):492-495).

COMMENT. Prednisone has also been advocated in the treatment of Sydenham's chorea. Kelts and Harrison, reporting at the recent 17th annual meeting Child Neurology Society in Halifax, found prednisone beneficial in 9 cases; an initial average dose of 1.8 mg/kg/day begun within 2 weeks of onset of chorea was tapered over 2 to 6 months.

Despite the self-limiting nature of the involuntary movements, they are frequently incapacitating and warrant treatment. If low to moderate doses of phenobarbital are ineffective, a trial of carbamazepine appears to be worthwhile, and prednisone in resistant cases. Paradoxically, choreoathetosis or dystonia may occur as a side-effect of carbamazepine treatment in epileptic patients. - Editor. *Ped Neur Briefs* September 1988.

Dystonia And Biopterin Deficiency

Five patients with childhood dystonia associated with reduced CSF biopterin, responsive to levodopa, and characterized by diurnal and exertional variation are reported from the Developmental and Metabolic Neurology Branch, National

Institute of Neurological and Communicative Disorders and Stroke, Bethesda, MD. Of 4 familial cases of dystonia with biopterin deficiency limited to the CNS and of unknown etiology, 2 brothers were more severely affected than 2 sisters, and the dystonia was complicated by hyperreflexia and extensor plantar responses indicative of associated pyramidal tract involvement. The fifth patient had a systemic deficiency of biopterin with hyperphenylalanemia and atypical phenylketonuria, and his dystonic rigidity was purely extrapyramidal and without spasticity. Patients were least symptomatic in the early morning or after a nap and became progressively weak, rigid and dystonic during the day with complete immobility in the afternoon or evening, and often unable to speak or to swallow. Improvement following Sinemet 10/100 began within 36 hours and benefit has been sustained during treatment of 18 months in 4 patients and 6 years in one, with apparent development of drug tolerance. (Fink JK et al. Dystonia with marked diurnal variation associated with biopterin deficiency. *Neurology* May 1988; *38*:707-711).

> COMMENT. The familial cases described here are similar to those with hereditary progressive dystonia reported by Segawa et al and characterized by diurnal variation and extreme sensitivity to levodopa. (*Adv Neurol* 1976; *14*:215). Response to levodopa is generally seen in only 10% of patients with dystonia. - Editor. *Ped Neur Briefs* May 1988.

Dystonia And Hypoparathyroidism

Recurrent attacks of flexion of the right hand and arm and bowing of the head initiated by sudden movement were associated with idiopathic hypoparathyroidism in a 12 yr old boy seen at the Children's Hospital of Philadelphia, PA. An EEG showed a right frontal spike wave focus, and attacks were initially controlled by phenytoin. The boy later developed massive myoclonic spasms of the legs. CT scan revealed calcification of the basal ganglia, frontal lobes, and the right cerebellar hemisphere. The serum calcium was 5.6 and phosphorus 11 mg/dl.

The spasms responded to ergocalciferon, 25,000 units twice daily, and calcium lactate. The authors propose this association of "paroxysmal dystonic choreoathetosis and hypoparathyroidism" as a syndrome distinct from "familial paroxysmal choreoathetosis without hypocalcemia" and "movement reflex epilepsy". They cite 2 similar cases in the literature. (Barabas G. Tucker SM. Idiopathic hypoparathyroidism and paroxysmal dystonic choreoathetosis. *Ann Neurol* Oct 1988; *24*:585).

COMMENT. In the differential diagnosis of dystonia, a CT scan showing calcification in the basal ganglia lead to tests for hypoparathyroidism whereas an MRI may be helpful in the diagnosis of Hallervorden-Spatz disease. Dystonia and striking MRI abnormalities in the globus pallidus ("eye-of-the-tiger" sign) are described in 2 patients with Hallervorden-Spatz syndrome (Sethi KD et al. *Ann Neurol* Nov 1988; *24*:692). One patient developed arching of the body backward and a diagnosis of dystonia at 14 years. She slowly deteriorated and at age 20 had progressive difficulty with mouth closure and at 32 years, frequent falling. CT scan of the head was normal whereas the MRI T2-weighted images showed a low-signal area surrounding a relatively circumscribed region of high signal in the globus pallidus. The "eye-of-the-tiger" sign is an appropriate name for this abnormality. The second patient, a 20-year-old woman, had a 1-year history of progressive difficulty with night vision and repeated forceful eye closure aggravated by sudden noise and attempted eye opening. The neurological findings were frequent blepharospasm, repetitive slow tongue protrusion, and tapetoretinal degeneration. Slow deterioration occurred over the next 2 years and reexamination showed facial grimacing, severe blepharospasm, tongue protrusion, resting tremor of hands, tongue, and jaw, and cogwheel rigidity of arms. CT scan was normal and the MRI showed the "eye-of-the-tiger" sign in the globus pallidus. - Editor. *Ped Neur Briefs* October 1988.

Idiopathic Dystonia: Natural History

The natural history of early onset idiopathic torsion dystonia in 30 young patients is reported from the Instituto Neurologico "C. Besta", Milan, Italy. Twenty-one were sporadic and nine familial. Of the familial cases, eight had an autosomal recessive hereditary pattern and one an autosomal dominant pattern. All were of European origin and none was of Jewish origin. Quantitative criteria and a dystonic severity scale were used. Drug trials in eight patients were without benefit and stereotactic thalamotomy in ten patients relieved a unilateral action tremor. Age at onset ranged between one and ten years, maximum between five and ten years. An abnormality of gait was the presenting sign in 12. The disease became generalized in 17 and remained localized in 13. Early onset was characterized by a spontaneous tendency towards a stabilization of the motor disability following aggravation of the disability during the first seven years of the disease. Most retained functional independence and none showed mental deterioration, mood alteration or personality disturbance. The mean IQ in familial cases was 73.4 compared to 94.9 in sporadic cases. (Angelini L et al. Idiopathic dystonia with onset in childhood. *J Neurol* September 1989; *263*:319-321).

> COMMENT. In the majority of childhood cases the dystonia is generalized, in some segmental, involving more than one body part, but none is focal and restricted to a single body part. Focal dystonia occurs only in those with adult onset. The observation of spontaneous stabilization in the patients of this study is of interest and the long term prognosis was relatively good. - Editor. *Ped Neur Briefs* September 1989.

Huntington's Disease: PET Findings

The positron-emission tomography (PET) findings in a seven year old girl with the juvenile form of Huntington's disease are described from the Department of Neurology and Neurosurgery, Montreal Neurological Institute and Hospital, Montreal, Canada.

The birth and early development were normal and at three years of age she could dance and ice skate. By 3-1/2 years she had difficulties in dancing and by four to five years of age she had developed an awkward stiff gait, she became socially withdrawn in personality, had frequent nightmares, speech was dysarthric, and she began to fall frequently and to have problems controlling her hands. Swallowing, chewing and speech progressively deteriorated. She was hypertonic and had exaggerated deep tendon reflexes. Her father had Huntington disease. Her EEG showed bilateral epileptic foci but she had no clinical seizures. PET showed marked reduction in cerebral glucose metabolism in the posterior nuclei of the thalamus, a finding that differs from adults with the disease who show normal or increased rates of thalamic glucose metabolism. These metabolic findings were consistent with previously recognized postmortem pathologic differences between juvenile and adult forms of the disease. (Matthews PM et al. Regional cerebral glucose metabolism differs in adult and rigid juvenile forms of Huntington disease. *Pediatr Neurol* Nov-Dec 1989; 5:353-356).

COMMENT. The juvenile form of Huntington disease has a more rapid progression than the adult form and is manifested by rigidity rather than chorea. In children, the globus pallidus and thalamus reveal marked degeneration and unlike the adult form, the cerebellum and cortex are also involved. - Editor. *Ped Neur Briefs* December 1989.

Botulinum Toxin-A In Dystonia

A report of the Therapeutics and Technology Assessment Subcommittee of the American Academy of Neurology concludes that local injection of type A botulinum toxin (Botox) is proven as a safe and efficacious modality for the treatment of blepharospasm, cervical dystonia, and hemifacial spasm. The literature is reviewed in detail and 62 references are provided. Botox causes muscle paralysis by acting at peripheral nerve endings to block the release of acetylcholine. The effectiveness of the injections is transient lasting on the average four months.

Side effects are transient, well tolerated, and amenable to treatment when indicated. (Van den Noort S et al. Assessment: The clinical usefulness of botulinum toxin-A in treating neurologic disorders. *Neurology* Sept 1990; *40*:1332-1336).

COMMENT. Efficacy of this treatment in children parallels that in adults but safety has not been studied. Use during pregnancy or lactation is not recommended. FDA approval for the use of Botox has been obtained for the treatment of strabismus and blepharospasm associated with dystonia in patients 12 years of age and older.

Snow BJ et al report a beneficial effect of botulinum toxin on focal spasticity of leg adductors in nine patients with multiple sclerosis. (*Ann Neurol* Oct 1990; *28*:512-515). - Editor. *Ped Neur Briefs* October 1990.

Psychogenic Tremors

The clinical presentations and criteria for diagnosis of psychogenic tremor in 24 patients are reported from the Department of Neurology, Kansas University Medical Center, Kansas City, KS. Two were adolescents and the remainder were adults; nine men and 15 women. The tremors were complex (resting, postural, and kinetic), and of abrupt onset with a variable course. The clinical characteristics included spontaneous remissions, clinical inconsistencies, changing tremors, unresponsiveness to drugs, exacerbation by attention, improvement with distractibility, responsiveness to placebo, absence of other neurologic signs, and remission with psychotherapy. Other medical factors suggesting a psychogenic etiology included multiple undiagnosed conditions, unwitnessed paroxysmal disorders, employment in allied health professions, litigation or compensation pending, secondary gain, psychiatric disease, and functional disturbances in the past. (Koller W et al. Psychogenic tremors. *Neurology* August 1989; *39*:1094-1099).

COMMENT. Despite these clearly defined clinical features the diagnosis of psychogenic tremor is often difficult. Psychogenic and organic diseases may coexist and psychogenic tremor is usually a diagnosis of exclusion. In Pediatric Neurology practice, tremor is a frequent complication of valproate therapy for seizures and iatrogenic causes must be remembered in the differential diagnosis. The majority of patients with torsion dystonia in childhood are first diagnosed as hysteria. Acute dystonia is reported with cocaine withdrawal. - Editor. *Ped Neur Briefs* September 1989.

CHAPTER **6**

NEUROMUSCULAR DISORDERS

NEONATAL DISORDERS

Neonatal Guillain-Barre Syndrome

A term female infant presenting with generalized hypotonia, paucity of lower limb movements, and diminished DTRs was diagnosed as a case of Guillain-Barre syndrome at the Hospital for Sick Children, University of Toronto, Canada. At three weeks of age, motor nerve conduction studies showed slowed velocities and decreased action potentials, and the CSF protein was elevated with normal cells. Clinical improvement began at age two weeks and examination was normal at 22 weeks. (Al-Qudah AA et al. Neonatal Guillain-Barre syndrome. *Pediatr Neurol* Aug 1988; 4:255-6).

Neonatal Myasthenia Gravis

The advantages of electrodiagnosis in a premature infant with neonatal myasthenia gravis are proposed by the Dept of

Rehabilitation Medicine, Children's Hospital and Medical Center, Univ of Washington School of Medicine, Seattle, WA. The infant, born to a mother with myasthenia, suffered hypoxia and subependymal hemorrhage which probably contributed to the hypotonia and poor respiratory effort. Testing with edrophonium, 0.1 mg/kg IV, demonstrated no clinical improvement, whereas repetitive motor nerve stimulation testing showed a significant decremental response consistent with a diagnosis of neonatal myasthenia gravis. The decremental response was corrected following IV infusion of edrophonium 0.15 mg/kg. Pyridostigmine in a dose of 8 mg/kg/day resulted in clinical improvement of respiratory and muscular activity, and the infant was weaned from assisted ventilation at 27 days of age. He was discharged at 41 days of age on pyridostigmine therapy. The authors conclude that repetitive motor nerve stimulation may be a more reliable diagnostic procedure than edrophonium IV in the newborn with suspected myasthenia gravis. (Hays RM, Michaud LJ. Neonatal myasthenia gravis: Specific advantages of repetitive stimulation over edrophonium testing. *Pediatr Neurol* Aug 1988; 4:245-7).

COMMENT. The value of electrodiagnostic tests in the differential diagnosis of the hypotonic infant is demonstrated in these two case reports. Neonatology texts often recommend edrophonium as the test of choice in neonatal myasthenia gravis. The above experience indicates that the pharmacological test alone may not be as sensitive as repetitive nerve stimulation in the newborn with multiple problems. Ultrasonography is an additional technique of potential value in the work-up of the hypotonic infant. Heckmatt JZ and Dubowitz V of Hammersmith Hospital, London, have introduced the method for the differentiation of congenital muscular dystrophy and non-neuromuscular cases of hypotonia. (*J Child Neurol* 1987; 2:205). - Editor. *Ped Neur Briefs* September 1988.

Congenital Myotonic Dystrophy

Ten infants with congenital myotonic dystrophy admitted to the Dept Pediatrics and Neonatal Medicine, Royal Postgraduate Medical School, Hammersmith Hospital, London, 1982-86, were investigated by ultrasonography or CT brain scans between 1 day and 2 months of age. The infants presented with generalized hypotonia, facial diplegia, and respiratory and feeding difficulties, and the diagnosis was confirmed by demonstrating maternal myotonia.

Cerebral ventricular dilation was demonstrated in 8 (80%) infants, and 3 were scanned on the first day of life. Neonatal asphyxia occurred in 7, associated with intraventricular hemorrhage (IVH) in 2. One had subarachnoid hemorrhage and one showed infarcts in the white matter. The pathogenesis of ventricular dilation in congenital myotonic dystrophy was probably IVH in 2, but a developmental anomaly during fetal life was the more likely explanation in the remainder. The authors note that mental retardation in 70% of cases can be related to the ventricular dilation which may be progressive and require surgical treatment. (Regev R, Dubovitz V et al. Cerebral ventricular dilation in congenital myotonic dystrophy. *J Pediatr* 1987; *111*:372-6).

COMMENT. It may be impolite to shake hands with a lady! But a handshake for a mother of a floppy baby with respiratory distress may be diagnostic of myotonia and is good clinical practice. Dr. Koh of Hope Hosp, Salford, England, asks the question "Do you shake hands with mothers of floppy babies?" as the title to his article on congenital myotonic dystrophy (*Br Med J* 1984; *289*:485). - Editor. *Ped Neur Briefs* September 1987.

Congenital Myotonic Dystrophy And Pleural Effusion

Two infants with congenital myotonic dystrophy complicated by pleural effusions and hydrops fetalis are reported from the Valley Children's Hospital, Fresno, CA, and the Royal Alexandra Hospitals, University of Alberta, Edmonton, Alberta,

Canada. The mothers had myotonic dystrophy diagnosed at or after the delivery. The pregnancies were complicated by polyhydramnios, and the infants were delivered by cesarean section because of breech presentation. Infant 1 was areflexic, profoundly hypotonic, failed to breath spontaneously, and died at 3 days of age. Muscle biopsy at autopsy revealed extreme muscle immaturity with poor type I/II fiber differentiation, type I and type IIc fibers, and central nucleation. Infant 2 died 25 minutes after delivery despite aggressive resuscitation. The authors cite 6 other cases of congenital myotonic dystrophy with fetal hydrops and 2 with pleural effusions. Fetal hydrops may obscure the diagnosis, especially if the mother is asymptomatic. (Curr CJR et al. Hydrops and pleural effusions in congenital myotonic dystrophy. *J Pediatr* Sept 1988; *113*:555-557).

COMMENT. Chromosomal defects, cardiac abnormalities, and genetic syndromes are described with fetal hydrops but congenital myotonic dystrophy has been associated infrequently. When a mother is known to have myotonic dystrophy, the fetus should be monitored for abnormal breathing patterns and pleural effusions. A hypotonic infant born with pleural effusion or hydrops should alert the examiner to check for myotonia in the mother. (See *Ped Neur Briefs* Sept 1987; *1*:29-30). - Editor. *Ped Neur Briefs* September 1988.

Neonatal Rhabdomyolysis And Dystrophy

A boy, aged 2 years, presenting at birth as a case of rhabdomyolysis and later shown to have an x-linked recessive dystrophy, is reported from the Section of Child Neurology, St. Christopher's Hospital for Children, Philadelphia, PA, and the Child Neurology A.I. Dupont Institute, Wilmington, DE. Palpation of upper and lower extremities on newborn examination revealed stiff, indurated large muscle groups. The birth was a cephalic presentation without forceps. The CK at 2 days of age was 156,000 IU/l, and a benzidene dipstick for heme and myoglobinuria was negative at 4 days. Repeat CK determinations at 6 days and between 5 weeks and 14 months were approximately 12,000 and 6,000-9,000 IU/l, respectively. Percutaneous needle biopsy of the quadriceps at 1 year demonstrated many degenerating fibers, marked variation of fiber size, and increase in endomysial and perimysial connective tissue and fat. DNA analysis showed a partial X chromosome deletion adjacent to the Duchenne/Becker locus. On clinical examination the infant was developmentally delayed at 11 months and had speech delay, proximal lower extremity weakness, and calf pseudohypertrophy at 24 months. (Breningstall GN et al. Neonatal rhabdomyolysis as a presentation of muscular dystrophy. *Neurology* Aug 1988; *38*:1271-1272).

COMMENT. Rhabdomyolysis is an acute muscle necrosis usually accompanied by myoglobinuria which may complicate muscular dystrophy in association with malignant hyperthermia or anesthetic induced cardiac arrest. This patient had neither myoglobinuria nor hyperthermia. A neonatal presentation of Duchenne muscular dystrophy is exceptional, signs usually appearing when the patient becomes ambulant. - Editor. *Ped Neur Briefs* September 1988.

Congenital Myopathy, Cleft Palate, And Malignant Hyperthermia

Six children with congenital ptosis, generalized weakness, hypotonia, cleft palate, and susceptibility to malignant hyperthermia with anesthesia, are reported in Lumbee Indians from Duke University Medical Center, Durham, NC. All patients were members of the same ethnic group, 3 were related, and inheritance was probably autosomal recessive. Surgery for cleft palate at 14 months and for ptosis at 27 months, using halothane anesthesia, was complicated by malignant hyperthermia in one child. This syndrome showed some resemblance to *King syndrome*, characterized by multiple congenital facial and skeletal abnormalities along with slowly progressive myopathy and susceptibility to malignant hyperthermia. (Stewart CR et al.

Congenital myopathy with cleft palate and increased susceptibility to malignant hyperthermia: King syndrome? *Pediatr Neurol* Nov/Dec 1988; 4:371-4).

COMMENT. Clinicians, especially surgeons and anesthesiologists, should be aware of the risk of malignant hyperthermia in children with this syndrome and other myopathies, including Duchenne muscular dystrophy, myotonia congenita, and central core disease. Malignant hyperthermia is manifested by muscle rigidity, rapid elevation of temperature, metabolic acidosis, and rhabdomyolysis. Anesthetic agents most frequently invoked are halothane and succinylcholine. Screening of susceptible patients and their families by CK determinations is advised. - Editor. *Ped Neur Briefs* January 1989.

Congenital Myopathy In Lowe Syndrome

Congenital fiber type disproportion myopathy is described in two brothers with oculo-cerebro-renal syndrome of Lowe from the Department of Pediatrics, Tsuchiura Kyoudou Hospital, Ibaraki; Tsukuba University; Tokyo Medical and Dental University; and National Institute of Neuroscience, Kodaira, Japan. Both brothers had congenital cataracts, they were floppy as infants and psychomotor development was delayed. Both suffered febrile tonic seizures and one was hyperkinetic and had stereotypic hand movements. There was generalized muscle hypotonia, deep tendon reflexes were absent and serum creatine kinase activity was elevated. There was nystagmus in all directions of gaze. Biopsies of the biceps and brachia muscles showed selective type I fiber atrophy and mild type I fiber predominance similar to that observed in congenital fiber type disproportion myopathy. (Kohyama J et al. Congenital fiber type disproportion myopathy in Lowe syndrome. *Pediatr Neurol* Nov-Dec 1989; 5:373-376).

COMMENT. Selective type I muscle atrophy is uncommon and occurs in congenital nonprogressive myopathies, including nemaline myopathy, myotubular myopathy, central core disease, and congenital fiber type disproportion. In association with type I fiber predominance it is observed in Pompe disease, Krabbe leukodystrophy and multiple sulfatase deficiency in which peripheral nerves are involved. The oculo-cerebro-renal syndrome of Lowe is characterized by mental retardation, glaucoma, congenital cataracts, and renal impairment. The elevated CPK led to the muscle biopsies in the present patients. - Editor. *Ped Neur Briefs* February 1990.

Congenital Inflammatory Myopathy

Three patients with congenital inflammatory myopathy are reported from the Montreal Children's Hospital and Neurological Institute, McGill University, Montreal, Canada. Seven additional cases are reviewed from the literature. The essential criteria for diagnosis were 1) antenatal or neonatal presentation with decreased fetal movements, muscular hypotonia and weakness with or without arthrogryposis, and 2) muscle biopsy evidence for inflammatory cell infiltrate and muscle fiber damage. CPK is elevated and the EMG is myopathic. CNS involvement was present in six of the patients. Two died, one at nine months and the other at five years. Treatment with steroids was used in 7 of the 10 patients with variable results. Possible etiologies included intrauterine viral infection or an autoimmune process. (Shevell M et al. Congenital inflammatory myopathy. *Neurology* July 1990; *40*:1111-1114).

COMMENT. Congenital inflammatory myopathy is a rare cause of the "floppy infant syndrome", and the differential diagnosis includes a congenital muscular dystrophy syndrome of Fukuyama or Walker-Warburg. Fukuyama's congenital muscular dystrophy includes hydrocephalus, ocular manifestations and mental retardation and Walker-Warburg's syndrome is characterized by lissencephaly and retinal abnormalities. Treatment of the cases of congenital inflammatory myopathy with steroids may improve motor development but does not result in intellectual improvement. - Editor. *Ped Neur Briefs* July 1990.

Congenital Myasthenia And Facial Malformations

A new genetic syndrome of congenital myasthenia with distinctive ethnic clustering and associated facial malformations transmitted as an autosomal recessive disorder is reported from the Departments of Neurology and Medical Genetics, Chaim Sheba Medical Center, Tel Hashomer, Sackler School of Medicine, Tel Aviv University, Israel. The syndrome was demonstrated in 14 Jewish patients from ten families of Iraqi or Iranian origin. All patients had bilateral ptosis and predominant facial muscle weakness, 11 had weak masticatory muscles, and 12 had easy fatiguability on prolonged speech. Very mild limb muscle involvement was present in only three cases. The facial malformations included an elongated face, mandibular prognathism with malocclusion and a high arched palate. The course was mild and nonprogressive, the electromyogram showed a decremental response on repetitive stimulation of either the accessory or the facial nerve but myopathic changes were not seen. Antibodies to acetylcholine receptor were absent and all patients had a response to cholinesterase inhibitors and a positive Tensilon test. There was clinical improvement with pyridostigmine. In seven of ten families there was close parental consanguinity. (Goldhammer Y et al. Congenital myasthenia associated with facial malformations in Iraqi and Iranian Jews. *Brain* Oct 1990; *113*:1291-1306).

COMMENT. The distribution of muscle weakness in congenital myasthenia in these cases is compatible with previous reports where extraocular and facial muscle involvement have predominated (Millichap JG, Dodge PR. *Neurology* 1960; *10*:1007). The authors postulated that the facial abnormalities were secondary to the neuromuscular defect. Congenital myasthenia has been described in association with arthrogryposis, the subject of the following article. - Editor. *Ped Neur Briefs* December 1990.

Arthrogryposis Congenita
And Hepatorenal Abnormalities

Arthrogryposis multiplex congenita with renal and hepatic abnormalities, demonstrated at autopsy in a two month old child of consanguineous parents, is reported from the Pediatric Hospital, Coimbra, Portugal. Three brothers and eight first cousins had died within the first month, all with jaundice. The brothers of the proband had limb abnormalities and one had polyuria, glucosuria, and metabolic acidosis. The patient was born with flexed knees and joint limitation, cubital deviation of the hands with clenched fingers, and muscular atrophy. During the second week of life the infant became jaundiced and on day 18 she was admitted with cholestatic jaundice and hepatomegaly. Electromyography and muscle biopsy were compatible with neuropathic muscular atrophy. There was hypercalcemia with increased density of the base of the skull, renal tubular degeneration, and biliary stasis with pigmentary deposits. The family pedigree suggested an autosomal recessive inheritance. (Saraiva JM et al. Arthrogryposis multiplex congenita with renal and hepatic abnormalities in a female infant. *J Pediatr* Nov 1990; *117*:761-763).

COMMENT. This syndrome was first described by Nezelhof C et al (*J Pediatr* 1979; *94*:258) who reported four patients with these findings. As found in this case report, arthrogryposis is most commonly associated with neuropathic muscular atrophy. The underlying lesion may be found in the anterior horn cells of the spinal cord, the peripheral nerves, the neuromyal junction, the muscle, and sometimes in the brain. - Editor. *Ped Neur Briefs* December 1990.

Congenital Arthrogryposis And Maternal Myasthenia

An infant with arthrogryposis multiplex and other malformations born to a mother who presented with myasthenia gravis immediately following cesarean section is reported from the Depts Neonatology and Obstetrics, Hasharon Hospital, Petah-

Tiqva, Tel Aviv Univ Med Sch, Israel. The baby had hypotonia, absent suck, weak cry, and incomplete Moro. Multiple malformations included craniofacial dysmorphism, kyphoscoliosis, eventration of the diaphragm, and flexion contractures of the limbs. A Tensilon test at 7 days was negative and treatment with Mestinon for 3 weeks was without benefit, the infant dying at 5 weeks of age. Cytogenetic studies on infant and mother were normal. The authors suggest that the failure to recognize and treat the myasthenia gravis during pregnancy may be causally related to the infant's multiple malformations and fatal outcome. (Dulitzky F et al. An infant with multiple deformations born to a myasthenic mother. *Helv paediat Acta* Dec 1987; *42*:173-176).

> COMMENT. Electromyography and nerve conduction studies, muscle biopsy and serum CPK may assist in determination of the site and nature of the pathology in cases of arthrogryposis. These tests were apparently not performed in the present case and the underlying cause of the hypotonia was not defined, except to rule out a transient neonatal form of myasthenia. A fetal form of spinal muscular atrophy, as described originally by Beevor CE (*Brain* 1902; *25*:85). and later by Brandt S (*Acta paediat* 1947; *34*:365), in association with arthrogryposis multiplex congenita, seems a more likely explanation for the fatal outcome than the maternal myasthenia. - Editor. *Ped Neur Briefs* February 1988.

Congenital Amyelinating Neuropathy And Arthrogryposis

A case of severe neurogenic arthrogryposis multiplex congenita caused by absence of peripheral nerve myelin in an infant who died at age 31 days of aspiration pneumonia is described from the Dept of Neurology, Neuromuscular Division, Johns Hopkin University School of Medicine, Baltimore, MD. The infant, delivered by Cesarean section, had Apgar scores of one at 1 and 5 minutes, and examination revealed multiple fixed joints, small chin and triangular face, bilateral extraocular and facial pareses, diffuse hypotonia, muscle atrophy, and areflexia. Absence of myelin in the peripheral nerves at autopsy reflected an arrest in the differentiation or maturation of Schwann cells at the stages of elongation and longitudinal growth of the mesaxon. The authors refer to serial ultrasonography to assess fetal movement after the 18th week, the time of onset of peripheral nerve myelination, as an antenatal diagnostic technique in such families, and as suggested by Miskin M et al. (Charnas L et al. Congenital absence of peripheral myelin: Abnormal Schwann cell development causes lethal arthrogryposis multiplex congenita. *Neurology* June 1988; *38*:966-974).

COMMENT. The most common cause of arthrogryposis multiplex congenita is probably an amyoplasia due to anterior horn cell maldevelopment and associated muscle atrophy. Other causes include anterior horn cell degeneration, congenital myopathies, mechanical interference with fetal movement, and peripheral neuropathy. Paralysis of fetal movement is the common link in all forms of the disorder. For a comprehensive account of arthrogryposis, the reader should refer to *Clinical Orthopedics* April 1985; *194*, an issue developed entirely to the topic. A long-term follow-up study showed that 17 of 34 patients examined at 16 years of age or older were able to walk independently and 9 others walked with the aid of crutches or braces. The prognosis is obviously hopeful in a majority of cases with nonprogressive underlying causes, and appropriate orthopedic procedures can achieve correction and relative independence at an early age. - Editor. *Ped Neur Briefs* June 1988.

Congenital Contractural Arachnodactyly

An infant girl with arachnodactyly and spontaneously resolving contractures who died in cardiac failure is reported from the Paediatric Unit, Northern General Hospital and Department of Ophthalmology, Royal Hallamshire Hospital, Sheffield, England. In addition to the arachnodactyly the infant had dolichostenomelia, iridodonesis, and mitral and tricuspid incompetence. There was no evidence of lens subluxation on slit lamp biomicroscopy. Chromosome studies and urinary homocystine were normal. (Huggon IC et al. Contractural arachnodactyly with mitral regurgitation and iridodonesis. *Arch Dis Childhood* March 1990; *65*:317-319).

> COMMENT. Congenital contractural arachnodactyly has been described as an autosomal dominant syndrome distinct from classical Marfan's syndrome and usually unassociated with serious ocular and cardiovascular complications. This case report questions this distinction and emphasizes the importance of cardiovascular and ophthalmic assessment of patients with contractural arachnodactyly. As an editorial comment from Springfield, Illinois, I cannot omit the frequent reference to President Abraham Lincoln and Marfan's syndrome. - Editor. *Ped Neur Briefs* April 1990.

NEUROPATHIES

Hereditary Motor And Sensory Neuropathy (HMSN)

Thirteen affected males and 25 obligate or probable heterozygous females with X-linked HMSN are reported from the Depts Neurology and Pathology, Duke Univ Med Centr, Durham, NC and Dept Neurology, Univ of Pennsylvania, Philadelphia, PA. The German family ancestry was traced back to a female born in 1819 with 2 affected brothers. In 9 generations there were 34 affected males and 54 heterozygous females. No son of an affected male had symptoms or signs of neuropathy. Intelligence and cranial nerves were normal and peripheral nerves were not hypertrophied. The affected or heterozygous patients had at least one of the following: 1) symmetrical distal> proximal weakness and/or atrophy; 2) symmetrical distal sensory loss, 3) hyporeflexia, 4) pes cavus, 5) abnormal NCVs, 6) obligate heterozygote (i.e. mother of a patient or daughter of an affected male). Affected males suffered from a progressive crippling neuropathy with onset in childhood or adolescence and female carriers were minimally affected or normal. DNA probes placed the gene in the DXYSI-p58-1 region of the X-chromosome. (Rozear MP, Pericak-Vance MA, Fischbeck K et al. *Neurology* 1987; *37*:1460-1465).

COMMENT. In a child presenting at the age of 5-10 years with a progressively clumsy gait, pes cavus, depressed ankle jerks, and weakness and loss of sensation in the hands and feet, the diagnosis of hereditary motor sensory neuropathy (Charcot-Marie-Tooth disease) must be suspected and nerve conduction and electromyography studies ordered. Ask the parents to remove their shoes and examine them also for pes cavus and absent ankle jerks, if the hereditary nature of the gait disorder has not already been established. Some may have autosomal dominant and others an X-linked inheritance, as in this family. With no documented male-to-male transmission in a family, both autosomal dominant and X-linked forms are possible and need to be considered in counseling.

Of 205 patients referred to the Mayo Clinic with undiagnosed peripheral neuropathy, 42% had inherited disorders, most commonly HMSN. (Dyck PJ, Oviatt KF, Lambert EH. *Ann Neurol* 1981; *10*:222). Sural nerve biopsy showing demyelination was occasionally useful. Leg cramps were more common and paresthesiae less troublesome in inherited neuropathies than in inflammatory or other acquired neuropathies. - Editor. *Ped Neur Briefs* October 1987.

Central Motor Conduction In HMSN

Transcranial magnetic brain stimulation was used to study central motor conduction (CMCT) to small hand muscles in patients with peroneal muscular atrophy (HMSN) and hereditary spastic paraplegia (HSP) at the National Hospital and Institute of Neurology, Queen Square and the Department of

Neurological Science, Royal Free Hospital, London, UK. Proximal motor roots were excited at the intervertebral foramina, the stimulating cathode placed at C7-T1 and the anode 6 centimeters laterally on the ipsilateral side. Central motor conduction time was estimated by subtracting the latency of this potential from that of the response to brain stimuli. CMCT was normal in HSMN I, HSMN II, and HSP. In patients with HSMN I with pyramidal signs, central motor conduction time was greatly prolonged bilaterally. The results reflected an involvement of the central motor pathways. (Claus D et al. Hereditary motor and sensory neuropathies and hereditary spastic paraplegia: A magnetic stimulation study. Ann Neurol July 1990; 28:43-49).

COMMENT. Dyck PJ and Lambert EH (*Arch Neurol* 1968; *18*:603-625) subdivided patients with HSMN into two main groups: HSMN I, with demyelination in peripheral nerves and HSMN II, without demyelination. Patients with HSMN who had pyramidal signs were designated type V. Pyramidal signs may occur as a regular feature in some families but do not reflect disease severity. The authors of the above study found no correlation between the degree of general disability and the occurrence of abnormal CMCT. - Editor. *Ped Neur Briefs* July 1990.

Peripheral Neurolopathy In Xeroderma Pigmentosum

The peripheral nerve pathology in two autopsied cases of group A xeroderma pigmentosum (*De Sanctis Cacchione syndrome*) is reported from the Tokyo Medical and Dental University, Tokyo Metropolitan Neurological Hospital, and Tokyo Metropolitan Kita Medical and Rehabilitation Center, Tokyo, Japan. One patient died at 19 years of age because of intractable respiratory tract infection and acute renal failure and the other died aged 23 due to choking. The diagnosis of xeroderma pigmentosum had been made in early infancy because of prominent light sensitivity. Neurological symptoms had developed in childhood and included slurring of speech, ataxia, and mental retardation. The patients were bedridden at age 15 and 22.

Examination revealed microcephaly, short stature, and hyperpigmentation of the skin exposed to sunlight. There was severe muscle atrophy in all limbs, contractures of joints, and fasciculation of the tongue. Tendon reflexes were absent and plantar responses were extensor. Evoked muscle action potentials and sensory action potentials were absent on stimulation of peripheral nerve trunks. Pathologic changes in the nerves suggested a neuronopathy with loss of myelinated nerve fibers and endoneurial fibrosis. Changes in the spinal cord included a severe decrease in anterior horn cells, reduction in lateral columns and severe depletion of dorsal root ganglion cells. The brains were small and showed widespread sclerotic leucoencephalopathy and severe neuronal loss in the cerebral cortex, thalamus, substantium nigra and cerebellar cortex. (Kanda T et al. Peripheral neuropathy in xeroderma pigmentosum. *Brain* August 1990; *113*:1025-1044).

COMMENT. Xeroderma pigmentosum is a group of autosomal recessive disorders related to a defect in the mechanism of DNA repair. The findings in the peripheral nerves are similar to those reported in ataxia telangiectasia, another disorder which shows defective DNA repair. The authors suggest a common pathogenic mechanism. - Editor. *Ped Neur Briefs* October 1990.

Peripheral Neuropathy In Ataxia-Telangiectasia

EMG examinations performed on 32 children aged three to 13 years with ataxia-telangiectasia are reported from the Neurological Department of the Child Health Centre, Warsaw, Poland. Four main EMG patterns were distinguished: 1) normal, 2) increased polyphasia of motor unit potentials, 3) neurogenic lesions with denervation activity, 4) denervation, fasciculations, and a picture characteristic of advanced motor neuron disease. The severity of the neurogenic lesions increased from the proximal arm muscles to the distal leg muscles. An EMG pattern resembling motor neuron disease was seen most often in the extensor digitorum brevis. Nerve conduction studies showed a decrease in motor response amplitude in the older children and a reduction in sensory nerve action potentials in median and sural nerves of all children older than seven years. The authors consider that a generalized slowly progressive sensory system degeneration together with neurogenic amyotrophy affecting distal parts of the lower limbs is a constant feature of ataxia telangiectasia and can be taken to be one of the diagnostic characteristics. (Kwast O, Ignotowicz R. Progressive peripheral neuron degeneration in ataxia-telangiectasia: An electrophysiological study in children. *Dev Med Child Neurol* September 1990; *32*:800-807).

COMMENT. The clinical diagnosis of ataxia-telangiectasia is based on a progressive cerebellar ataxia, ocular telangiectasia, and immunological abnormalities. Muscle weakness progresses with age and atrophy affects especially the distal leg muscles. The child is confined to a wheelchair after the 9th to the 12th year. EMG and nerve conduction studies are important in the diagnosis. - Editor. *Ped Neur Briefs* October 1990.

Immunoglobulin For Polyneuropathy

The value of high-dose intravenous immunoglobulin in the treatment of chronic inflammatory demyelinating polyneuropathy was studied in a double-blind, placebo controlled, crossover investigation at the Department of Neurology, University Hospital Rotterdam-Dijkzigt, the Department of Immunohematology and Bloodbank, University Hospital Leiden, and the Central Laboratory of the Netherlands, Red Cross Blood Transfusion Service, Amsterdam, The Netherlands. Of seven patients treated two were children aged 10 and 7 and five were adults. At initial diagnosis one child was severely disabled and the other moderately disabled (Rankin score 5 and 3, respectively). All patients had weakness of both legs, areflexia, slowed nerve conduction velocities, and elevated CSF protein level. All had responded to treatment with IVIg, 0.4 g/kg bodyweight/2 weeks. All patients showed deterioration after IVIg was discontinued. The patients were then randomized to IVIg or placebo (albumin treatment) in a double-blind crossover study. Those treated with IVIg improved by day eight after the onset of treatment whereas those treated with placebo showed no improvement. The time lapse between discontinuation of the IVIg treatment until deterioration was 6.4 weeks. After placebo the time lapse in weeks until clinical deterioration was 1.3 weeks. (van Doorn PA et al. High-dose intravenous immunoglobulin treatment in chronic inflammatory demyelinating polyneuropathy: A double-blind, placebo-controlled, crossover study. *Neurology* Feb 1990; *40*:209-212).

COMMENT. Chronic inflammatory demyelinating polyneuropathy may fluctuate in severity or show deterioration over many months or years and the course and prognosis differs from Guillain-Barre syndrome. Improvement has followed treatment with prednisone, plasmapheresis, and IV gamma globulin (Cook JD et al. *Neurology* 1987; *37*(suppl 1):253). High dose intravenous immunoglobulin is more convenient than plasma exchange and has less long-term side effects than corticosteroids. It was also of value in the treatment of two patients with demyelinating neuropathy associated with monoclonal gammopathy. (Cook D et al. *Neurology* Feb 1990; *40*:212). Dyck PJ in an editorial comments that the processing of Ig is sufficiently rigorous that HIV or hepatitis should not be transmitted by IVIg and there are no other known complications from this treatment. The major drawback was the high cost, $750-1000/treatment. - Editor. *Ped Neur Briefs* February 1990.

Plasmapheresis In Childhood Guillain-Barre Syndrome

The role of plasmapheresis in childhood Guillain-Barre syndrome was examined by retrospective analysis of children admitted to the Children's Hospital of Philadelphia, University of Pennsylvania School of Medicine, Philadelphia, PA. Of 23 patients included in the study nine had been treated with plasmapheresis and 14 served as control subjects. Therapeutic plasma exchanges were performed on an alternate day schedule. The mean age was 8.8 years and the duration of the illness prior to admission was 5.9 days. The plasmapheresis treated group recovered to the stage of independent ambulation significantly faster than the control group, 24 versus 60 days, respectively. By six months after discharge all children in both groups were ambulating independently. Plasmapheresis diminished morbidity by shortening the interval until recovery of independent ambulation, but this treatment cannot be routinely advocated for all patients until well designed prospective studies comparing plasmapheresis and IV gamma globulin have been performed in children (Epstein M A, Sladky, J T. The role of plasmapheresis in childhood Guillain-Barre Syndrome. *Ann Neurol* July 1990; *28*:65-69).

COMMENT. The proceedings of a symposium on "Autoimmune Neuropathies: Guillain-Barre Syndrome" sponsored by the National Institutes of Health are published in the Annals of Neurology Supplement to Volume 27, 1990. Plasmapheresis was the accepted therapy for Guillain-Barre syndrome, particularly in adults, but other approaches are being explored. One is the infusion of immunoglobulins and another is the use of high dose steroids early in the disease. Controlled studies are in progress, but results are not yet available. (McKhann GM. Guillain-Barre Syndrome: Clinical and therapeutic observations. *Ann Neurol* 1990; *27* (Supplement): S13-S16). - Editor. *Ped Neur Briefs* July 1990.

SPINAL MUSCULAR ATROPHIES

Acute Infantile Spinal Muscular Atrophy
Massive muscle cell elimination by apoptosis in an infant who died eight weeks after birth from acute infantile spinal muscular atrophy is described from the Department of Neurology,

Medical Academy, Warsaw, Poland, and the Division of Neuropathology, University of Mainz, Mainz, FRG. The classical morphological changes of ISMA included degeneration and loss of motor neurons in the spinal cord, loss of large myelinated fibers in anterior roots, and neurogenic atrophy in muscle. Ultrastructural findings in the muscle showed membrane bound muscle cell fragments or apoptotic bodies. Numerous immature muscle fibers were also observed suggesting a failure in muscle maturation. The authors speculate that in growth retarded muscle the process of muscle apoptosis may also be prolonged or repeated. The resulting protracted muscle cell death may lead to a greater reduction in the number and size of muscle fibers. The removal of the peripheral target of anterior horn cells then results in secondary death of motor neurons. (Fidzianska A et al. Acute infantile spinal muscular atrophy. Muscle apoptosis as a proposed pathogenetic mechanism. *Brain* April 1990; *113*:433-445).

COMMENT. Death of muscle cells by apoptosis has not been demonstrated in infants with SMA previously. The term "apoptosis" was proposed by Kerr et al (1972) for cell death which plays a role in the regulation of animal cell populations. This form of cell death differs from that caused by coagulative necrosis. Apoptosis is responsible for the focal elimination of cells during embryonic development and metamorphosis. The final number of motor neurons in the spinal cord following fetal development depends on input from muscle for survival. Naturally occurring death of motor neurons is accentuated by the removal of the target muscle. The findings in this case report suggest that motor neuron death in infantile spinal muscular atrophy may be secondary to muscle cell apoptosis. - Editor. *Ped Neur Briefs* May 1990.

Spinal Muscular Atrophy In Twins

Juvenile chronic segmental spinal muscular atrophy of Hirayama is described in two adult identical twins from the

Department of Neurology, University of Vermont College of Medicine, Burlington, VT. In both patients examined at 69 years of age, the weakness was first noticed in the right hand at age 16 and within six months there was similar weakness of the left hand and atrophy of muscles in both hands. The disability progressed over the next four years but after age 21, further decline was barely noticeable. Examination at age 69 showed marked atrophy and weakness of the intrinsic muscles of both hands, the ulnar half of the forearm flexors, and of the brachio-radialis muscles more on the right side. Occasional fasciculations were noted in involved muscles. The triceps and Achilles reflexes were decreased in one patient and the tendon reflexes were otherwise normal. Nerve conduction studies showed reduced amplitude of the ulnar and median compound muscle action potential, mildly slow conduction in upper and lower extremity motor nerves, and mild prolongation of the F-wave latencies. EMG showed no fibrillations, positive waves or fasciculations. The motor units in the upper extremity muscles showed neurogenic features. Based on the identical sex, phenotypes, blood groups, and HLA typing in the two brothers there was a 98.8% calculated chance that these twins were identical. (Tandan R et al. Chronic segmental spinal muscular atrophy of upper extremities in identical twins. *Neurology* Feb 1990; *40*:236-239).

> COMMENT. Hirayama, the first to describe this disease, reported 38 cases and one autopsy report, showing loss of motor neurons and astrogliosis in C7/C8 anterior horns. A genetic cause for the disease is supported by its occurrence in identical twins. - Editor. *Ped Neur Briefs* February 1990.

Juvenile Amyotrophic Lateral Sclerosis

Forty-three patients with hereditary motor system diseases belonging to 17 families were studied at the Institut National de Neurologie, La Rabta, Tunis, Tunisia. The mean age of onset was 12 years; the range was three to 25 years. Progression was very slow. Inheritance was autosomal recessive. Patients were subdivided into three groups: 1) Upper limb amyotrophy and pyramidal syndrome (17 patients); 2) spastic paraplegia and peroneal muscular atrophy (14); and 3) spastic pseudobulbar form (12). Nerve and muscle biopsies showed neurogenic atrophy in the peroneus brevis muscle and minor changes in the superficial peroneal nerve. Infantile and juvenile ALS is usually rare and the frequency in Tunisia may be explained by the high incidence of consanguinity. (Ben Hamida M et al. Hereditary motor system diseases (chronic juvenile amyotrophic lateral sclerosis). Conditions combining a bilateral pyramidal syndrome with limb and bulbar amyotrophy. *Brain* April 1990; *113*:347-363).

COMMENT. Ford FR, in his *Diseases of the Nervous System in Infancy, Childhood, and Adolescence,* refers to his own experience with hereditary amyotrophic lateral sclerosis as small, but unlike the cases described in the present study, Ford's cases showed a more rapid progression. The hereditary factor in juvenile ALS distinguishes this type from classical ALS or Charcot's disease, which develops in late middle age and which is usually neither hereditary nor familial. Both Ford and the present authors refer to articles by Holmes in 1905 and an autopsy report by Mass in 1911 on a child who had nystagmus in addition to the characteristic features, including degeneration of the pyramidal tracts and the motor cells of the anterior horns. The earliest report of an infantile amyotrophic lateral sclerosis of the familial type was by Brown CH (*J Nerv and Ment Dis* 1894; 21:707). - Editor. *Ped Neur Briefs* May 1990.

MUSCULAR DYSTROPHIES

Duchenne Muscular Dystrophy

The clinical progression and effects of therapy in 283 boys with Duchenne dystrophy and ten with Becker dystrophy followed for up to ten years in a collaborative study are reported from the Departments of Neurology and Biostatistics,

Washington University School of Medicine, St. Louis, MO; the Departments of Neurology, Vanderbilt University, Nashville, TN; Ohio State University, Columbus, Ohio; and University of Rochester, Rochester, New York. The protocol measured function, strength, contractures, and scoliosis. A series of milestones allowed the severity of the disease to be defined in an individual boy. After age 11, 89 of 120 patients developed a scoliosis. The use of a body jacket to control a progressive scoliosis was ineffective but back surgery was beneficial if carried out before the forced vital capacity was less than 1.5 litres. The average age at the time of surgery was 14.6 years and patients with a curve exceeding 35° were considered to be candidates for surgery. No correlation could be detected between the use of passive joint stretching exercises and joint contractures but there was a significant correlation between the use of leg braces and the prevention of contractures of the heel cords, knee extensors, and iliotibial bands. There were 25 deaths while the boys were enrolled in the protocol. Most deaths occurred from respiratory failure, often after repetitive bouts of pneumonia, or from cardiac failure. Weaker patients died from respiratory failure whereas those whose muscles were stronger were more likely to die from a cardiomyopathy. (Brooke MH, Fenischel GM et al. Duchenne muscular dystrophy: Patterns of clinical progression and effects of supportive therapy. *Neurology* April 1989; *39*:475-481).

COMMENT. In the same issue of Neurology, genetic abnormalities in Duchenne and Becker dystrophies with clinical correlations (Medori R et al) and molecular and clinical correlations of deletions leading to Duchenne and Becker muscular dystrophies (Baumbach LL et al) are reported. Duchenne muscular dystrophy (DMD) and Becker muscular dystrophy (BMD) are two allelic forms of an x-linked muscle disorder with phenotypic heterogeneity. Of 32 DMD patients, 14 had an internal deletion in the same region of the gene and 7 of 11 patients with a mild DMD or BMD phenotype showed deletions at the 5' end of the gene. Patients with classic DMD who had a detectable deletion had a milder clinical course than those without. BMD patients may be genetically different from boys with classic DMD. There was no correlation between the extent of a deletion, its location, and clinical severity of the associated disease. Duchenne muscular dystrophy is a severe x-linked disease with an incidence of 1 in 3500 males; approximately one-third result from a new mutation. Becker muscular dystrophy is a clinically similar but less severe form of dystrophy affecting 1 in 30,000 males. The application of recombinant DNA technology to the diagnosis of DMD has resulted in the development of more accurate tests which supplement the serum CPK, muscle biopsy and EMG. - Editor. *Ped Neur Briefs* May 1989.

Selenium And Muscular Dystrophy

Selenium metabolism and supplementation in patients with Duchenne muscular dystrophy was studied at the Muscle Research Center, Department of Medicine, University of Liverpool, and the Universitat Klinik Mainz, Mainz, FRG. Plasma selenium concentrations measured in seven Duchenne muscular dystrophy patients and in 11 age matched normal boys showed no significant difference after two months of sodium selenite supplementation (1 mg selenium daily). All patients demonstrated a rise in plasma selenium concentration as did all but one of the normal subjects. The studies did not confirm any abnormality of selenium metabolism in patients with muscular dystrophy, and there was no evidence that high dose selenium supplementation influenced the activity of the selenium dependent enzyme glutathione peroxidase in skeletal muscle. An elevation of thiobarbituric acid-reacting substances in the muscle of patients with Duchenne muscular dystrophy was unaffected by selenium supplementation. (Jackson MJ et al. Selenium metabolism and supplementation in patients with muscular dystrophy. *Neurology* May 1989; *39*:655-659).

COMMENT. The present finding of normal plasma selenium concentrations in Duchenne muscular dystrophy patients differs from reports from Finland where selenium in soils and indigenous food stuffs is naturally low in concentration. The increase in thiobarbituric acid-reacting substances in dystrophic muscle confirms previous reports but the elevated levels in patients with Duchenne muscular dystrophy contrasted with normal levels in patients with other forms of muscular dystrophy and in control subjects. - Editor. *Ped Neur Briefs* May 1989.

Sleep Breathing Patterns And Muscular Dystrophy

The breathing patterns and $HbSaO_2$ changes during nocturnal sleep were monitored in 11 chair-bound Duchenne muscular dystrophy patients at the Institutes of Neurology and Respiratory Diseases, University of Pavia, Italy. Nocturnal sleep had no significant adverse effects on the nighttime polygraphic sleep recordings and respiration. Infrequent central apneas occurring in six patients were associated with falls in $HbSaO_2$ greater than normal and correlated with functional residual capacity values. The blood oxygen balance was relatively preserved but unstable during nocturnal non-REM and REM sleep in patients with Duchenne muscular dystrophy, mean age 15 years (range 10-21) even in advanced stages of the illness. (Manni R et al. Breathing patterns and $HbSaO_2$ changes during nocturnal sleep in patients with Duchenne muscular dystrophy. *J Neurol* October 1989; *236*:391-394).

> COMMENT. Acute respiratory failure is an important factor contributing to death in most patients with Duchenne muscular dystrophy. During the later stages of the illness, a restrictive lung disease related to the progressive inspiratory muscle weakness and rib cage deformities develops. In this study, nocturnal sleep did not seem to have a significant adverse effect on respiration and no pathological breathing patterns were observed. Unimpaired diaphragmatic function might account for the relatively preserved arterial oxyhemoglobin desaturation during REM sleep in the population studied. - Editor. *Ped Neur Briefs* November 1989.

Becker's Dystrophy

Two brothers affected with Becker's muscular dystrophy in whom the disease followed completely different courses are reported from the Departments of Neurology/Neurosurgery and Genetics, Washington University Medical School, St. Louis, MO. The oldest sibling died at 37 following many years of severe disability whereas the younger sibling, now 26, has normal muscle strength. Symptoms began between 10 and 12 years of age in both patients. Analysis of the DNA from each revealed a similar deletion at the 5' end of the dystrophin gene. The younger brother had epilepsy from age 13 and had been treated with phenytoin continuously for 13 years. (Medori R, Brooke MH, Waterston RH. Two dissimilar brothers with Becker's dystrophy have an identical genetic defect. *Neurology* November 1989; *39*:1493-1496).

COMMENT. The long term treatment with phenytoin from the onset of the muscle symptoms may have influenced the clinical course of the younger brother. The authors suggest that the action of a membrane stabilizer such as phenytoin may prevent the degeneration of the muscle fibers lacking dystrophin. - Editor. *Ped Neur Briefs* November 1989.

Genetics Of Duchenne And Becker Dystrophies

The molecular basis for Duchenne and Becker muscular dystrophies is reviewed from the Department of Pediatric Neurology, Floating Hospital for Infants and Children, New England Medical Center Hospitals and Tufts University, Boston, Mass. Until recently the diagnosis of DMD or BMD depended on clinical signs and symptoms, serum creatine kinase, EMG and muscle biopsy. The isolation of the gene defective in DMD and BMD and the identification of dystrophin have revolutionized the diagnostic issues. The mutated gene causing Duchenne and its allelic milder Becker phenotype has been assigned to band P21 of the short arm of the X chromosome (Xp21). Dystrophin has been characterized by DNA sequencing and by immunologic studies. When the family history is negative for DMD and BMD the Western Blot assay of protein derived from a specimen can confirm the clinical diagnosis of DMD or BMD and can be used to predict the severity of the disease. If the dystrophin assay result is abnormal DNA analysis should be performed. Detection of a dystrophin gene deletion will facilitate carrier detection and prenatal diagnosis in the proband's family. If no deletion or duplication is found, linkage analysis may be attempted for prenatal diagnosis and carrier detection. Peripheral blood DNA may be used for Southern Blot testing if a muscle biopsy specimen is not available and may confirm the diagnosis in more than 65% of the cases. In typical cases of DMD or BMD with a family history of X linked muscular dystrophy, linkage analysis is unnecessary if the clinical diagnosis has been confirmed in an affected family member by analysis of dystrophin or DNA or both. The less invasive polymerase chain reaction test may be used if the diagnosis has not been confirmed by dystrophin or DNA analysis in other family members. Muscle biopsy for dystrophin analysis will be required in families without a clear cut X linked pattern of inheritance or in families with both male and female siblings affected, suggesting an autosomal recessive form of MD (Darras BT. Molecular genetics of Duchenne and Becker muscular dystrophy. *J Pediat* July 1990; *117*:1-15).

COMMENT. Gross abnormalities of the dystrophin gene may still result in a partially functional dystrophin protein and a relatively mild clinical progression, compatible with a diagnosis of Becker muscular dystrophy. Angelini C et al. (*Neurology* May 1990; *40*:808) describe a patient with a duplication of more than 400,000 bp of the dystrophin gene, the largest characterized to date. The propositus a 13 year old boy presented at age 4 with myalgia and cramps after exercise or running in the cold. The CK ranged from 1400 to 8630 U/l, the EMG showed small polyphasic motor units, and the muscle biopsy revealed a mild myopathic picture with scattered atrophic and hypertrophic muscle fibers, a few degenerating fibers and a mild inflammatory reaction. Electronmicroscopy showed hypertrophic ring fibers. Leg muscle ultrasound revealed scattered fibrosis. He was treated for five months with prednisone at 50 mg/d followed by two months at 50 mg on alternating days. The CK levels declined and the child had less muscle pain. - Editor. *Ped Neur Briefs* July 1990.

Early Development In Duchenne Muscular Dystrophy

The early development of 33 boys with Duchenne muscular dystrophy (DMD) was assessed at the Institute of Medical Genetics, University of Wales College of Medicine, Heath Park, Cardiff, Wales. The average age of entry into the study was 3.4 years (range 0.8 to 6.7). The Griffiths Developmental Scales, The Reynell Language Scales and the British Picture Vocabulary Scales were used at three evaluations at 6 monthly intervals over a one year period. Compared to a control group the boys with DMD showed developmental delay which was most severe in the locomotor and language areas. Locomotor quotients deteriorated over time and behavior problems were probably secondary to the developmental delay. (Smith RA et al. Early development of boys with Duchenne muscular dystrophy. *Dev Med Child Neurol* June 1990; 32:519-527).

COMMENT. Unexplained developmental delays should prompt a neurological evaluation to exclude Duchenne muscular dystrophy in boys. Young children with DMD have significant problems with motor, speech and behavioral disorders before muscle weakness becomes an obvious clinical sign.

The etiology of intellectual impairment in Duchenne muscular dystrophy was investigated by MRI studies at Jordan University, Amman, Jordan (Al-Qudah AA et al. *Pediatr Neurol* 1990; 6:57-59). Four DMD patients were studied prospectively by cranial MRI, DNA deletion analysis, clinical evaluation and IQ testing. There was no significant correlation between verbal IQ and MRI findings,

DNA deletion or the clinical severity of the disease. Other than mild atrophy in two patients, no significant anatomical brain lesion was discovered. Previous reports have attributed intellectual impairment in DMD to anatomic brain changes, abnormal dendritic development, and migrational lesions. Others have described a direct relation between the severity of clinical disease and impairment of IQ. (Rosman NP. *Brain* 1966 *89*:769). - Editor. *Ped Neur Briefs* July 1990.

Dystrophin Analysis And
Diagnosis Of Muscular Dystrophy

The value of dystrophin analysis in the early diagnosis of two patients with childhood autosomal recessive muscular dystrophy is reported from the Department of Pediatrics, Sapporo Medical College, Sapporo, Japan. The first patient, a five year old boy referred because of an elevated serum CK had developed normally until two years of age when an abnormal gait was observed. He had slight proximal muscle weakness without enlargement of calf muscles or involvement of facial muscles. Gower's sign was negative. The deep tendon reflexes in the lower limbs were slightly decreased. A muscle biopsy from the biceps showed marked variation in fiber size and a number of necrotic and regenerating fibers with proliferating connective tissue characteristic of muscular dystrophy. Dystrophin was demonstrated in all sarcolemma after immunocytochemical staining using antidystrophin antibody. The second patient, a seven year old boy with rubella, was found to have an elevated serum CK. His motor milestones of development were normal and neither muscular weakness nor atrophy were observed. There was no enlargement of calf muscles or involvement of facial muscles. Deep tendon reflexes were slightly hypoactive. The serum CK was 4250 IU. From seven to 11 years of age the clinical course was static. Muscle biopsies from the rectus femoris and biceps brachii showed a marked variation in fiber size and degenerating and regenerating fibers with proliferated connective tissue indicative of muscular dystrophy. By immunocytochemical staining with antidystrophin antibody the dystrophin was located in the sarcolemma. Both patients were diagnosed as having childhood autosomal recessive muscular dystrophy. There was neither consanguinity nor any history of neuromuscular disorder in the families. (Tachi N et al. Dystrophin analysis in the differential diagnosis of autosomal recessive muscular dystrophy of childhood and Duchenne muscular dystrophy. *Pediatr Neurol* July-August 1990; *6*:265-268).

COMMENT. In boys with a muscular dystrophy that develops in early childhood the early differentiation of Duchenne, Becker, and the autosomal recessive limb-girdle dystrophies is important. The onset of limb-girdle dystrophy is more commonly between 10 and 20 years of age but it may present in the first decade and sometimes as early as two years of age. The course is variable but occasionally progression is as rapid as with Duchenne muscular dystrophy. - Editor. *Ped Neur Briefs* October 1990.

Dr. Stephen D. Rioux, Maine Medical Center, Portland, ME, comments that without Western Blot analysis of the dystrophin molecule or DNA genetic analysis, Duchenne and Becker muscular dystrophy cannot be ruled out. Normal amounts of sub-sarcolemmal dystrophin can be seen in Becker dystrophy, using the immunochemical staining method employed in this report. The presumed diagnosis of autosomal recessive muscular dystrophy and differentiation from Duchenne and Becker dystrophies are not proven by the immunochemical analysis alone. (Letter to the Editor. *Ped Neur Briefs* November 1990).

POLYMYOSITIS

Diagnosis Of Polymyositis

The criteria for the diagnosis of polymyositis, the differential diagnosis, and treatment are reported from the Division of

Rheumatology and Internal Medicine, Mayo Clinic, Rochester, MN. A muscle biopsy is considered the standard diagnostic procedure for polymyositis but it is not infallible. Characteristic features are inflammatory mononuclear cell infiltration, degenerating and regenerating muscle fibers, and central nuclei. Electromyographic findings are characteristic but not specific. They include insertional activity, fibrillation potentials, motor unit potentials of increased frequency and decreased duration, and normal conduction velocity in nerves. The most useful blood test in polymyositis is a serum CK determination but this may be normal in about 2% of patients. The MM fraction constitutes the majority of the CK in polymyositis; the MB fraction may be increased because of skeletal muscle regeneration and less often because of myocarditis. Treatment with high dose corticosteroids is administered as early as possible in the course of the disease. The longer the delay before diagnosis and appropriate treatment, the worse the prognosis. The best known dermatological change is Gottron's sign, an erythema over the knuckles. Gottron's rash is a scaly, violaceous rash on various areas of the body including the hands, elbows, and knees as well as a heliotrope rash on the eyelids. Calcinosis occurs in 13% of childhood cases but in less than 5% of adult cases of polymyositis. No therapy has proved effective for calcinosis and occasionally, surgical excision of painful calcific areas has been necessary. When polymyositis develops during pregnancy the incidence of fetal loss is 32%. Women with a history of inactive polymyositis should be warned that pregnancy might exacerbate the disease. Myositis has been reported with human immune deficiency virus infection and may closely mimic the myopathic changes seen in polymyositis. (Bunch TW. Polymyositis: A case history approach to the differential diagnosis and treatment. *Mayo Clin Proc* Nov 1990; *65*:1480-1497).

COMMENT. A good review of polymyositis and dermatomyositis in children is provided by Pachman LM (Juvenile dermatomyositis. *Pediatr Clin North Am* 1986; *33*:1097-1117). An edited summary of a combined clinical staff conference at the NIH (Plotz PH et al. Current concepts in the idiopathic inflammatory myopathies: Polymyositis, dermatomyositis, and related disorders. *Ann Intern Med* July 1989; *111*:143-156) provides an excellent review of biopsy findings, causes, pathogenesis, studies on humoral immunity, and treatment. - Editor. *Ped Neur Briefs* December 1990.

MRI In Childhood Dermatomyositis

The demonstration of muscle involvement using the MRI in four patients with dermatomyositis is reported from the Departments of Radiology and Pediatrics, University of Michigan Hospitals, Ann Arbor, MI. Ages ranged from 4-1/2 to 18 years (median 8 years). The affected muscles had increased signal intensity on the T2 weighted images and normal appearance on the T1 weighted sequence. The mean intensity ratio for the patients with dermatomyositis differed significantly from that of four normal control children. Muscle groups with higher intensity ratios had lower scores on functional testing. Follow-up MRI scans demonstrated normal findings after treatment, coincident with progressive clinical improvement. (Hernandez RJ et al. Magnetic resonance imaging appearance of the muscles in childhood dermatomyositis. *J Pediatr* Oct 1990; *117*:546-50).

COMMENT. The authors concluded that the MRI may be useful in the evaluation of dermatomyositis in children because it 1) is noninvasive, 2) has clear signal changes in affected muscle, 3) shows positive results at an early stage, 4) is a guide for biopsy, and 5) may assist in monitoring of the disease progress. The MRI appearances of muscles affected by hypotonic syndromes and muscular dystrophies differ from those of muscles affected by dermatomyositis. Ultrasound has been used in the diagnosis of patients with muscular dystrophy. - Editor. *Ped Neur Briefs* December 1990.

OTHER MYOPATHIES

Mitochondrial Myopathy And Cardiomyopathy

Two siblings with infantile lactic acidosis and mitochondrial myopathy are reported from the Department of Pediatrics, Goteborg University, Ostra Hospital, Goteborg, Sweden. The first child, a girl, appeared healthy during the first four months of life. She was admitted at five months of age with feeding difficulties, vomiting and weight loss and muscular hypotonia. Her serum lactate concentration rose to 20 mmol/L (n:0.8-1.8 mmol/L), she developed edema, became comatose and died of circulatory failure eight days after admission. At autopsy, the heart was slightly enlarged and the pleurae and pericardium showed clear yellowish fluid. The second patient, the younger brother of patient one, had congenital lactic acidosis but no other symptoms until six months of age when he developed progressive muscle weakness. Treatment with dichloroacetate lowered the serum lactic acid level but did not affect his clinical condition. Cardiomyopathy was diagnosed at 13 months of age and he died of circulatory failure at 29 months. Both patients had mitochondrial myopathy with changes in skeletal muscle and the myocardium. Biochemical investigations of skeletal muscle mitochondria showed deficiencies in cytochrome c oxidase and NADH ferricyanide reductase. (Tulinius MH et al. Mitochondrial myopathy and cardiomyopathy in siblings. *Pediatr Neurol* May/June 1989; 5:182-188).

> COMMENT. Patients with mitochondrial myopathies or cytopathies show marked heterogeneity in clinical manifestations and system involvement. Two major variants of mitochondrial myopathy and cytochrome c oxidase deficiency in infancy have been described. Most cases are rapidly progressive and fatal and are associated with renal dysfunction; occasionally the course is milder and reversible. In the present study, the heterogeneity in the mitochondrial cytochrome c oxidase activity provided clinical symptoms in proportion to the fraction of damaged

mitochondria, thus explaining the different clinical course in the siblings. - Editor. *Ped Neur Briefs* June 1989.

Nemaline Myopathy

A boy, five years of age, with nemaline myopathy complicated by respiratory failure and hypertrophic cardiomyopathy is reported from the Albany Medical College, Albany, NY. He presented at two months of age with failure-to-thrive, diminished suck, and hypotonia. CK was normal and EMG showed rare fibrillations and fasciculations. Muscle biopsy demonstrated variation in fiber size and electron-dense nemaline rods. He walked late at three years, fell frequently and required a walker outdoors. At 5-1/2 years, during an upper respiratory tract infection, respiratory distress necessitated intubation. Neurologic examination revealed hypotonia, proximal muscle weakness, mild facial weakness, and absent deep tendon reflexes. Echocardiography disclosed a thickened ventricular septum consistent with hypertrophic cardiomyopathy. Because of chronic nocturnal hypoventilation, tracheostomy and assisted ventilation were required. The authors recommend routine cardiac and pulmonary function evaluations in patients with nemaline myopathy. (Van Antwerpen CL et al. Nemaline myopathy associated with hypertrophic cardiomyopathy. *Pediatr Neurol* Oct 1988; 4:306-8).

COMMENT. Sleep hypoventilation, a rare complication of Nemaline myopathy, has been attributed to central nervous system CO2 unresponsiveness. Cardiomyopathy has not been reported previously in a child with nemaline myopathy and the authors found only 2 other references, both in adults. Neurologic conditions associated with hypertrophic cardiomyopathy include Leigh disease, Kearn-Sayre syndrome, Friedreich ataxia, neurofibromatosis, and Pompe disease. - Editor. *Ped Neur Briefs* November 1988.

McArdle's Disease

Muscle biopsy specimens from 48 patients with biochemically proven phosphorylase deficiency (McArdle's disease) have been analyzed by gel electrophoresis (SCS-PAGE), immunoblotting, and immunotitration (ELISA) at Columbia University College of Physicians and Surgeons, New York, NY. The majority had no detectable enzyme protein, six had markedly decreased phosphorylase protein, and only one had a normal amount of protein. The presence or absence of enzyme protein was not correlated with the clinical presentation or muscle glycogen concentration. In four patients tested, messenger RNA was normal in two, abnormally short in one, and absent in one, suggesting heterogeneity of the molecular lesion in McArdle's disease. (Servidei S, DiMauro S et al. McArdle's disease: biochemical and molecular genetic studies. *Ann Neurol* Dec 1988; *24*:774-781).

COMMENT. McArdle's disease (muscle phosphorylase deficiency; glycogenosis type V) is manifested by exercise intolerance with myalgia, early fatigue, and muscle stiffness relieved by rest. Strenuous exercise is accompanied by acute muscle necrosis and myoglobinuria. Patients presenting in infancy or childhood may have a mild congenital muscle weakness, tiredness or poor stamina without cramps or myoglobinuria, or severe, rapidly progressive weakness soon after birth that results in respiratory failure and death in infancy. The various types of myophosphorylase protein and messenger RNA observed in the above patient population were consistent with at least five different mutations that give rise to McArdle's disease. - Editor. *Ped Neur Briefs* November 1988.

Familial Myopathy With Thrombocytopenia

Three cases of a familial myopathy with thrombocytopenia in three generations of a family are reported from the Royal Manchester Children's Hospital, Withington Hospital, and University of Manchester Medical School, England. The family showed autosomal dominant inheritance of both myopathy and thrombocytopenia. The myopathy presented in early childhood with an abnormal gait noted by the age of 4 years and an asymmetric limb girdle weakness diagnosed in the proband by 8 years. By puberty, distal upper limb weakness had developed, and the myopathy was slowly progressive as evidenced by increasing disability in the mother and wheelchair confinement in the grandfather. The asymmetrical myopathic findings became generalized with increasing age. The CK was elevated in all 3 patients (800, 600, and 524 IU/l). EMG obtained in 2 patients was normal in the son at 9 years, and showed a high amplitude motor unit with a slightly diminished interference pattern in the mother at 32 years of age. The bleeding disorder manifested by easy bruising and prolonged bleeding following injury was fully expressed in the proband when first examined at 8 years and the platelet disorder showed no progression with age. Muscle biopsies from mother and son showed type I fiber preponderance and hypertrophy, and type II fiber atrophy and rimmed vacuoles. Electron-microscopy revealed tubular aggregates in both cases. (Mahon M et al. Familial myopathy associated with thrombocytopenia: a clinical and histomorphometric study. *J Neurol Sci* Dec 1988; *88*:55-67).

COMMENT. Limb girdle dystrophy is not a single entity and should prompt examination of the blood for platelet abnormalities. This appears to be the first recorded family with defects of both muscle and platelets in the same patients. - Editor. *Ped Neur Briefs* January 1989.

Familial Myopathy With Inclusion Body Myositis

Five male siblings affected by a progressive myopathy, inclusion body myositis, and periventricular leukoencephalopathy are reported as a new syndrome from the Montreal Neurological Hospital and Institute, Canada. Patient 1, the first of twins, examined at 35 years of age, walked at 18 months but was never able to run. Muscle weakness, mainly proximal, progressed slowly during adolescence, and a cane was required to walk by 26 years. At 35 years, he had genu recurvatum and excess lumbar lordosis, proximal weakness with minimal wasting, and absent tendon jerks in the upper limbs, reduced at the knees, and preserved at the ankles. He required crutches to walk, and he had a waddling gait. His mentation, cranial nerves, sensation, and coordination were normal. The four siblings had similar histories and findings. CK was elevated, EMG showed small polyphasic motor units, fibrillation, and positive sharp waves; NCV showed minimal slowing; CSF protein was 0.56-0.68 g/l; and muscle biopsies revealed fiber loss, rimmed vacuoles, variability of fiber calibre, and some necrosis, and abnormal cytoplasmic filamentous inclusions. CT white matter hypodensities and MRI high signal intensities were compatible with leukodystrophy, yet the patients had no symptoms of white matter dysfunction. The authors conclude that this constellation of familial myopathy with muscle cytoplasmic inclusions and cerebral white matter changes represents a hitherto undescribed syndrome. (Cole AJ et al. Familial myopathy with changes resembling inclusion body myositis and periventricular leucoencephalopathy. *Brain* Oct 1988; *111*:1025-1037).

COMMENT. Familial cases of inclusion body myositis have been reported in younger patients but none associated with cerebral white matter changes as described above. In contrast to those myopathies sometimes associated with CNS dysfunction (e.g. Duchenne muscular dystrophy, myotonic dystrophy, congenital muscular dystrophy of Fukuyama and others, and Kearns-Sayre-Shy syndrome) the white matter changes in the present cases were asymptomatic. The mode of inheritance could not be determined with certainty. Limb girdle dystrophy presents in yet another form and should prompt examination not only of blood platelets but also CT and MRI for white matter changes. CT findings were not included in the report from Manchester and blood platelet counts were not indicated in the Montreal syndrome. - Editor. *Ped Neur Briefs* January 1989.

CHAPTER 7

HYDROCEPHALUS AND OTHER CONGENITAL MALFORMATIONS

HYDROCEPHALUS

Congenital Hydrocephalus

Intrauterine intraventricular hemorrhage occurring about 2 weeks or more prior to birth was the cause of congenital hydrocephalus in 4 newborn infants reported from the Abteilung Neonatologie, Universitats-Kinderklinik, Rumelinstrasse 23; D-7400 Tubingen, FR Germany. Multiple pregnancy was an associated risk factor in 2 cases and a hemorrhagic diathesis was present or suspected in 2. Intrauterine diagnosis of subependymal/intraventricular hemorrhage may be made by sonography of the fetal brain when indicated, especially in multiple pregnancy, hemorrhagic diathesis by history, fetal growth retardation, and signs of distress. Postnatally, cerebral ultrasound, CT and examination of the CSF for siderophages may be confirmatory. (Leidig E et al. Intrauterine development of posthemorrhagic hydrocephalus. *Eur J Pediat* Jan 1988; *147*:26-29).

COMMENT. Congenital hydrocephalus occurs in 0.5-1.8/1000 births. Subarachnoid hemorrhage at the time of birth has long been invoked as a cause of hydrocephalus (Paine RS. In *Pediatric Neurology*, Ed. Millichap JG, *Ped Clin N Amer* 1967; *14*:779), but the intrauterine development of posthemorrhagic hydrocephalus has been reported only recently. The authors encountered their 4 cases in a period of 2 years so that the incidence may be higher than the literature suggests. - Editor. *Ped Neur Briefs* February 1988.

Progressive Hydrocephalus: Symptoms And Signs

The etiologies and clinical features of progressive hydrocephalus in 107 children, 56 with and 51 without shunts, were analyzed retrospectively at the Department of Neurology, Royal Hospital for Sick Children, Edinburgh, Scotland. Patients with arrested hydrocephalus, or with ventriculomegaly resulting from atrophic or ischemic brain damage or tumor were excluded. Intracranial pressure was measured percutaneously or through ventriculostomy reservoirs, using a Gaeltec miniature strain gauge transducer. Etiologies included spina bifida (54%), idiopathic (15%), hemorrhage (13%), and meningitis (10%). In those with malfunctioning shunts, symptoms were vomiting, drowsiness, headache, behavioral change, and anorexia; and signs were absent in 25% and included decreased level of consciousness in 18%, acute strabismus (18%), neck retraction (11%), and distended retinal veins (11%). Patients without shunts were asymptomatic in 49%; headache occurred in 33%, and vomiting in 16%. Signs in the nonshunted group included abnormal head growth in 76%, tense fontanel (65%), scalp vein distention (33%), setting sun sign or absent upward gaze (22%), and neck rigidity (14%). Unusual clinical features included neurogenic pulmonary edema, profuse sweating, macular rash, ptosis, autonomic dysfunction, and neurogenic stridor. Papilledema occurred in only eight cases (8%). The authors emphasize the variability, unreliability, unusual nature, and even absence of clinical symptoms and signs of hydrocephalus with raised intracranial pressure. CT or MRI may not be diagnostic, and direct measurement of intracranial pressure is essential in patients with unexplained clinical features. (Kirkpatrick M, Engleman H, Minns RA. Symptoms and signs of progressive hydrocephalus. *Arch Dis Child* Jan 1989; *64*:124-128).

COMMENT. The infant referred because of a large head is a fairly common problem in pediatric neurology practice. This instructive article points out that we may be relying too frequently on our colleagues in neuroradiology for diagnostic help and neglecting the much simpler and more economical method of direct measurement of intracranial pressure. The finding that one-half the infantile cases of hydrocephalus were without symptoms is disturbing. - Editor. *Ped Neur Briefs* February 1989.

Management Of Hydrocephalus
With IC Pressure Monitor

Thirteen premature infants with posthemorrhagic hydrocephalus were treated by repeated aspiration of cerebrospinal fluid using a subcutaneous ventricular catheter reservoir at the Departments of Paediatrics and Neurosurgery, University of Heidelberg, Federal Republic of Germany. Criteria for the insertion of the catheter and reservoir were as follows: 1) Increase in head circumference of more than 1 cm/week; 2) Progressive ventricular dilatation on ultrasound scan; 3) Failure of lumbar puncture route of fluid removal; or 4) Bradycardia or apneic complications of lumbar puncture. Hydrocephalus was controlled by aspiration of fluid (median 6 ml) one to four times a day for an average of 40 days. Clinical signs (tense fontanel and increasing head size) and ultrasound were unreliable indicators of the amount and frequency of fluid removal. Direct intracranial pressure measurements made through the reservoir increased the efficacy and safety of the method. Complications included skin breakdown in one, red blood cells in the cerebrospinal fluid in one, hyponatremia in eight, and hypoproteinemia in two.   The authors suggest that shunting should be performed if resolution of the posthemorrhagic hydrocephalus has not occurred in an infant weight 2000 grams and if spinal fluid protein is low. (Leonhardt A et al. Management of posthaemorrhagic hydrocephalus with a subcutaneous ventricular catheter reservoir in premature infants. *Arch Dis Child* Jan 1989; *64*:24-28).

COMMENT. C. Bannister, Consultant Paediatric Neurosurgeon, Manchester, England, comments that the reservoir allows easy repeated removal of cerebrospinal fluid from the lateral ventricles and is a convenient monitor of intracranial pressure. The disadvantages include risk of infection, skin breakdown, intraventricular bleeding from rapid aspiration and pressure fluctuations, and local cortical damage secondary to catheter insertion. - Editor. *Ped Neur Briefs* February 1989.

Hydrocephalus And Shunt Infections

In the 10-year period, 1973-82, 431 children underwent cerebrospinal fluid shunt insertion for hydrocephalus at Children's Memorial Hospital, Chicago. The authors, now in Verona, Italy (Casella Postale 401.1-37100), have studied the relationship between the etiology of hydrocephalus, age at the time of shunt placement, and infection rate. Meningomyelocele was present in 40%, congenital communicating or obstructive hydrocephalus in 34%, and tumors in 18%. Intraventricular hemorrhage and meningitis were the causes in 5% and 3%, respectively. The age at surgery was less than 1 year in 83% and 1 week or younger in 18%. Each patient had an average of 3 procedures. Infections occurred as a complication of the shunt in 96 patients at rates of 22% per patient and 6% per procedure. Younger patients and those with meningomyelocele were most susceptible to infection. In the meningomyelocele group, infection occurred less often when shunted at 2 weeks of age or later, compared to 1 week or earlier, when the rate was 48%. (Ammirati M, Raimondi AJ. Cerebrospinal fluid shunt infections in children. *Child's Nerv Syst* 1987; *4*:106-109).

COMMENT. The rate of operative shunt infection reported in this study is high, and the authors are able to cite similar statistics from two other centers. Attempts to reduce the incidence of infection by perioperative antibiotics or a surgical isolator had not been successful. If a rate of infection of 20% or more per patient is the rule with the operative treatment of hydrocephalus, a reappraisal of techniques and indications for surgery would seem to be a necessity. - Editor. *Ped Neur Briefs* September 1987.

Trapped Ventricle And Shunted Hydrocephalus

Occluded fourth ventricle (trapped ventricle) is reported in eight of 47 children (17%) receiving repeated shunt revisions for hydrocephalus at the Stritch School of Medicine, Loyola University of Chicago, Maywood, IL. The hydrocephalus was caused by intraventricular hemorrhage but the fourth ventricular enlargement developed only after shunting. Massive dilatation of the ventricle occurred in four, three developed a progressive spastic quadriparesis, and two had increased intracranial pressure with lethargy and vomiting. Two children underwent a fourth ventricular shunt; one became more alert and less quadriparetic, and the other showed gradual improvement in motor function. (Coker SB and Anderson, CL. Occluded fourth ventricle after multiple shunt revisions for hydrocephalus. *Pediatrics* June 1989; *83*:981-985).

COMMENT. Trapped ventricle following repeated shunting may be manifested by headache, lethargy, vomiting, ataxia, spastic quadriparesis, cranial nerve palsies and head tilt. This complication appears to be common among children with intraventricular hemorrhage who have received ventricular peritoneal shunting. Progressive fourth ventricular enlargement may be silent and diagnosis requires post shunt neural imaging and brain stem auditory evoked responses. Shunting of the fourth ventricle results in clinical improvement. - Editor. *Ped Neur Briefs* June 1989.

Shunts For Posthemorrhagic Hydrocephalus

The outcome of 19 infants who underwent cerebrospinal shunting for posthemorrhagic ventricular dilatation is reported from the Department of Pediatrics and Neonatal Medicine, Hammersmith Hospital, London W12. Periventricular hemorrhages were diagnosed by ultrasound scanning, and surgery was considered necessary if the hydrocephalus could not be controlled by intermittent lumbar or ventricular tapping and the CSF pressure was above 6 mmHg. Complications of ventriculoperitoneal shunts included seizures at the time of the surgery in 8 infants, postoperative infection in 12 of 58 (20%) procedures and blockage of 29 shunts. Shunt infection with Staphylococcal epidermidis occurred in almost half the patients in spite of prophylactic antibiotics. Shunt blockage occurring in 70% of infants was less frequent in those over 2.5 kg and with CSF protein below 1 g/l. Long-term outcome was poor: 3 died, 4 were quadriplegic and mentally retarded, and only 4 (20%) were developmentally normal. Outcome was correlated with preoperative parenchymal brain lesions diagnosed by ultrasound scans. (Hislop JE et al. Outcome of infants shunted for post-haemorrhagic ventricular dilation. *Dev Med Child Neurol* August 1988; *30*:451-456).

COMMENT. Assessment and therapeutic management of neonatal posthemorrhagic hydrocephalus is also reported from the Universitats-Kinderklinik Mannheim (Arnold D et al. *Klin Padiatr* July-August 1988; *200*:299-306). In this series, 40 of 135 neonates with intraventricular hemorrhage developed hydrocephalus. Treatment was by serial lumbar puncture in 70% and only 40% required a shunt. Acetazolamide and furosemide were used in 10%. At follow-up in 25 children, 40% were normal or had mild developmental delay, and 60% were seriously handicapped. As in the study from Hammersmith, poor outcome was related to severe hemorrhage and preoperative brain damage. Cerebral damage may occur without an increase in intracranial pressure, and normal fontanelle and head circumference do not rule out the development of hydrocephalus. - Editor. *Ped Neur Briefs* August 1988.

Sequelae Of Posthmorrhagic Hydrocephalus

The neurologic and developmental outcome of 33 low birth weight neonates with ventriculomegaly and in 39 with no ventriculomegaly after hemorrhage were evaluated prospectively in the Departments of Pediatrics and Neurosurgery, Wayne State University School of Medicine and Children's Hospital of Michigan, Detroit. Ventriculoperitoneal shunts were inserted in 23 of the 33 ventriculomegaly (VM) group infants at a mean age of 26 days. Shunt revisions were performed in 18 of the 23 children for obstruction (71) or infection (11). The total group of 72 children were followed to a mean age of 50 months. More children in the VM group had neurologic sequelae and microcephaly in comparison with the children in the non-VM group. Mild abnormalities included hypotonia and moderate and severe sequelae included spastic quadriplegia in 12 children and right hemiplegia in two children. Visual, language and hearing impairments were significantly increased in the VM group and included strabismus, myopia, nystagmus, and blindness. Developmental delay occurred in 19 patients in the VM group and in only eight in the non-VM group. Among the children with shunts, a higher incidence of sequelae occurred when lack of ventricular decompression was noted immediately after shunt insertion and when shunt infections occurred. The most important predictor of mental and motor outcome in the group with shunts was lack of ventricular decompression immediately after shunt insertion. The authors speculate that in some infants loss of brain tissue, cerebral atrophy or both may occur before insertion of the ventriculoperitoneal shunt even when the shunt is inserted early. (Shankaran S et al. Outcome after posthemorrhagic ventriculomegaly in comparison with mild hemorrhage without ventriculomegaly. *J Pediatr* Jan 1989; *114*:109-114).

COMMENT. There was no delay in the initial ventriculoperitoneal shunt insertion in this group; shunt infection and obstruction appeared to be responsible for the poor neurodevelopmental outcome. - Editor. *Ped Neur Briefs* February 1989.

Electroencephalogram In Pre-Shunt Hydrocephalus

The EEG findings in 105 hydrocephalic children with proven ventriculomegaly and increased intracranial pressure are reported prior to initial shunt treatment in the Department of Pediatrics, University of Oulu, Finland. Abnormal EEGs were seen in 98%. Paroxysmal slow wave activity, generalized or posterior, was present in 37 (35%) recordings and focal slow waves in 28 (27%) patients. Spike or sharp wave activity was recorded focally or generally in 45 (43%). The prevalence of spikes and sharp waves became less with increasing age and only generalized spikes occurred after seven years of age. The etiologies of the hydrocephalus were perinatal hemorrhage (20), infection (10), tumor (22), and malformations (64). Of 45 patients studied between one month and one year of age five had hypsarrhythmia. (Saukkonen A. Electroencephalographic findings in hydrocephalic children prior to initial shunting. *Child's Nerv Syst* Dec 1988; 4:339-343).

COMMENT. It is important to study the electroencephalogram of infants with hydrocephalus prior to shunting so that effects of increased intracranial pressure and malformations can be distinguished from those secondary to the shunt and possible infection. Spikes and sharp waves in the EEG of hydrocephalics are predictive of the prognosis and the probable occurrence of epilepsy. (Watanabe K et al. *Clin electroencephalogr* 1984; 15:22). - Editor. *Ped Neur Briefs* May 1989.

EEG And Slit Ventricle Syndrome (SLV)

The EEG changes and the frequency and type of epilepsy in patients with slit ventricles has been analyzed in 113 shunt-treated hydrocephalic children reported from the Department of Pediatrics, University of Oulu, Finland, and the Regional

Pediatric Habilitation Center, Gothenburg, Sweden. Slit ventricles are caused by overdrainage of the cerebrospinal fluid and collapse of the ventricles following shunting of hydrocephalus. The incidence was 56% in this group of patients followed for a mean of 8.9 years. In patients who developed SLV the age at initial shunting was significantly lower (1.2 years) than for those who did not (2.7 years). Spike and sharp wave activity in the EEG developed more frequently in patients with SLV (81%) than in those without (54%). The severe generalized spike wave activity disappeared from the EEG after treatment of the slit ventricles. Epileptic seizures appeared after initial shunting in 44% of patients who developed SLV but in only 6% of the non-SLV group. Treatment of the SLVs reduced the frequency of epilepsy to the level corresponding with the non-SLV group. (Saukkonen A et al. Electroencephalographic findings and epilepsy in the slit ventricle syndrome of shunt-treated hydrocephalic children. *Child's Nerv Syst* Dec 1988; 4:344-347).

COMMENT. This study demonstrates the value of repeated EEGs in shunt treated patients. If EEG abnormality appears after the initial shunting and especially severe spike wave activity, a shunt malfunction and overdrainage of the CSF should be suspected. The slit ventricle syndrome should be prevented or at least treated early to avoid permanent brain damage and long-term psychomotor retardation. Epileptic seizures have been reported in 10-40% of shunted hydrocephalic children. The position of the shunt, the frequency of the shunt revisions and epileptic seizures have been correlated in the present study. The ventricular size is also correlated with the frequency of epileptic seizures.

Six patients suffering from West and Lennox syndromes associated with slit ventricle syndrome showed dramatic improvement and became asymptomatic after treatment for the slit ventricle syndrome. Anticonvulsant prophylactic therapy is warranted for at least a year after shunting and particularly in patients who develop slit ventricles. Raimondi AJ provides an editorial comment on shunts, indications, problems, and characteristics (*Child's Nerv Syst* Dec 1988; 4:321). - Editor. *Ped Neur Briefs* May 1989.

Baers In Congenital Hydrocephalus

Brainstem auditory evoked responses were studied in 20 children with congenital hydrocephalus before and after shunt surgery at the Departments of Neurosurgery and Neurology, National Institute of Mental Health and Neurosciences, Bangalore, India. Ninety-five percent showed abnormal responses preoperatively. Prolonged wave V latency was the most common abnormality, followed by increased interwave latencies. Absence of evoked responses was more common in children with communicating hydrocephalus. Following shunt surgery 50% of the responses returned to normal and 20% showed a significant improvement. The ages of the patients ranged from 2-30 months (mean 8.5). The duration of neurological symptoms ranged from 1-12 months (mean 3.9). A progressive increase in head size was the chief sign on presentation. Twelve of the children had congenital hydrocephalus alone and 8 had hydrocephalus and an associated meningomyelocele. BAER abnormalities were similar in the two groups. Postoperative BAER changes correlated well with reduction in ventricular size as determined by CT. The worsening of BAER postoperatively in 4 patients (20%) correlated with an abnormality in the postoperative CT scan, which showed progression of hydrocephalus due to shunt block and slipped shunt tube and subdural hematoma (2). BAER abnormalities referable to dysfunction of the rostral brainstem recovered later than those localized to the caudal brainstem. The proximity of the upper brainstem to the enlarged ventricular system could be responsible for pathological changes such as compression, distortion or displacement leading to associated persistent edema and more prolonged BAER abnormalities. (Venkataramana N K et al. Evaluation of brainstem auditory evoked responses in congenital hydrocephalus. *Child's Nerv Syst* Dec 1988; 4:334-338).

COMMENT. The study of BAER is useful for identifying physiological brainstem abnormalities in hydrocephalic children and promises to be a sensitive, noninvasive, diagnostic tool for the detection of complications of shunt surgery other than those secondary to infection. Causes of dysfunction in the brainstem associated with congenital hydrocephalus include distortion and displacement, raised intracranial pressure, and developmental anomalies of the brainstem and auditory pathways. In 20% of the cases in this study, worsening of BAER postoperatively was correlated with complications such as subdural hematoma and raised intracranial pressure. - Editor. *Ped Neur Briefs* April 1989.

Baer In Posthemorrhagic Ventricular Dilatation

Nineteen infants with posthemorrhagic ventricular dilatation were studied with serial auditory brainstem responses at the Department of Paediatrics and Neonatal Medicine, Hammersmith Hospital, London. The cerebrospinal fluid pressure was measured in 9 of the 19 infants directly during lumbar or ventricular taps with a Gaeltic pressure transducer. No correlation was found between cerebrospinal fluid pressure and prolonged interpeak intervals on the BAER. Improvement occurred in 3 patients when cerebrospinal fluid was withdrawn. In one full term infant, improvement in BAER occurred one week after shunting. The lack of correlation between the I-V interpeak interval and the intracranial pressure in preterm infants was probably due to better adaptation of the immature brain to increased intracranial pressure. (Lary S, Dubowitz V et al. *Arch Dis Child* Jan 1989; *64*:17-23).

COMMENT. Abnormalities in auditory brainstem responses in premature infants may resolve irrespective of the persistence of progression of ventricular dilatation. Improvements in BAER, especially of the amplitude, could occur after drainage of cerebrospinal fluid in some cases. The responses in full term infants may differ from those of preterm infants. - Editor. *Ped Neur Briefs* April 1989.

CHIARI MALFORMATIONS

Arnold-Chiari With Myelomeningocele

The outcome of 19 infants with complications of Arnold-Chiari malformation and meningomyelocele was reviewed at the Depts of Pediatrics, Pathology, and Neurosurgery, University of Pennsylvania School of Medicine and the Children's Hospital of Philadelphia. Vocal cord paralysis and inspiratory stridor alone occurred in 10 (grade I), apnea was an additional symptom in 4 (grade II), and cyanotic spells and dysphagia were associated in 5 (grade III).

Ventricular shunt was performed in 14 infants, with resolution of symptoms in 7 (in 5 of 8 with grade I, 2 of 4 with grade II, and none of 2 with grade III symptoms). Of 10 with posterior fossa decompressions, symptoms resolved in only 2 (in 1 of 4 with grade I, one of 2 with grade II, and none of 4 with grade III symptoms). Within 6 months after symptoms began, one infant with grade II and 3 with grade III died. No deaths occurred with the grade I group. Infants with grade II or III symptoms have more extensive brain stem damage, such as hemorrhage, infarction and necrosis, and carry a poor prognosis whereas those with grade I symptoms often improve after neurosurgical procedures. (Charney EB et al. Management of Chiari II complications in infants with myelomeningocele. *J Pediatr* 1987; *111*:364-71).

COMMENT. The grading of cases according to complications is useful in investigation, treatment and prognosis. In a previous study from the University of Toronto (Park TS et al. *Neurosurgery* 1983; *13*:147), decompression was recommended before rapid neurologic deterioration takes place, even if a functioning shunt is present. Of 45 infants with surgical decompression of the Chiari malformation, 28 survived and showed improved neurologic function and in 24 of these, recovery was complete. About 71% of patients died among those who developed cardiorespiratory arrest, vocal cord paralysis, or arm weakness within 2 weeks before decompression, compared with 22% of those with more gradual neurologic deterioration. - Editor. *Ped Neur Briefs* September 1987.

Chiari Type I Malformation And Ataxia

A 13-year-old girl with posttraumatic cerebellar ataxia, transient upper extremity weakness, and lower cranial nerve dysfunction was found to have a Type I Chiari malformation on MRI at the Depts of Neurosurgery and Neurology, San Francisco General Hospital, CA. She lost consciousness and had a cardiopulmonary arrest after hitting her neck and head on the windshield in an automobile accident. On the 2nd day, her right upper limb was paralyzed; on day 4 she had upbeating nystagmus and was unable to swallow, phonate, or protrude her tongue; and on day 12 right vocal cord paralysis was noted which recovered by day 15. She continued to have improvement of the lower cranial nerve weakness but the ataxia persisted at the time of discharge. It was thought that the initial cardiopulmonary arrest after trauma and the brain stem dysfunction and ataxia were causally related to the Type I Chiari malformation. The continued improvement argued against surgical decompression. (Mampalam TJ et al. Presentation of Type I Chiari malformation after head trauma. *Neurosurgery* 1988; *23*:760-762).

COMMENT. This sudden manifestation of symptoms and signs of Chiari I malformation after head and neck trauma is unusual. Previously reported cases include a 3-year-old child who died 48 hours after a mild head injury, a 2-1/2 year-old boy who developed acute paraparesis after a fall, and a 17-year-old girl who developed hemianesthesia, nystagmus, dysarthria, and tongue deviation 1 week after chiropractic manipulations, and acquired torticollis after endotracheal anesthesia for tonsillectomy. All cases were found to have Chiari I malformation; only one had an associated syringomyelia. The diagnosis of Chiari I malformation has been facilitated by the use of MRI and asymptomatic cases are being uncovered by this imaging technique. - Editor. *Ped Neur Briefs* December 1988.

Chiari II Malformation

The theories of the basic embryological defect hat lead to the Chiari II malformation are reviewed and a unified theory proposed from the Division of Pediatric Neurosurgery, The Laboratory for Oculo-Cerebrospinal Investigation, The Children's Memorial Medical Center and Northwestern University Medical School, Chicago, IL. Chiari II malformation is almost invariably associated with myelomeningocele and a progressive hydrocephalus. Associated anomalies include small posterior fossa, Luckenschadel of the skull, caudal displacement of pons, medulla, and basilar artery, and upward herniation of the superior cerebellum. Syringomyelia occurs in 50%, and aqueduct stenosis, polymicrogyria, cortical heterotopia, and agenesis of the corpus callosum occur occasionally. Previous theories include the follow: 1) Herniation of the posterior fossa contents resulting from supratentorial hydrocephalus with leakage of cerebrospinal fluid into the amnion and herniation of the hindbrain; 2) Traction theory suggesting that the caudal spinal cord may pull the cerebellum and medulla into the lower cervical canal because of tethering; 3) Dysgenesis of the hindbrain and developmental arrest; 4) Small posterior fossa due to mesodermal insufficiency and overgrowth of neuroepithelium causing a neural tube defect.

The unified theory proposed by the authors incorporates the previous observation of Padget that leakage of cerebrospinal fluid is one factor in the cause of a small posterior fossa and emphasizes the role of distention of the embryonic and fetal ventricular system in normal cerebral development. The neural tube defect and defective occlusion are the developmental factors that cause the Chiari II malformation and the interrelated cerebral and skull anomalies. Altered inductive pressure on the surrounding mesenchyme is the cause of the Chiari II malformation and Luckenschadel whereas the lack of distention of the developing telencephalic ventricles results in cerebral anomalies, e.g., dysgenesis of the corpus callosum, cortical heterotopia, and polymicrogyria. Chiari II malformation is the result of a series of interrelated time dependent defects in the development of the ventricular system leading to multiple anomalies in brain development, according to this theory. (McLone DG, Knepper PA. The cause of Chiari II malformation: A unified theory. *Pediatr Neurosci* 1989; *15*:1-12).

COMMENT. Chiari described three types of cerebellar malformation which he had found in cases of congenital hydrocephalus. In Type I the medulla was displaced downward into the spinal canal and was covered by peg-like processes arising from the cerebellar hemispheres, their lower ends opposite the origin of the third cervical roots. This anomaly was found in a girl of 17 in whom the malformation had caused no symptoms during life.

Type II was a similar malformation of the lower parts of the cerebellum associated with an elongation of the fourth ventricle which extended into the spinal canal in a six month old baby with hydrocephalus. There were heterotopic nodules of gray matter in the walls of the lateral ventricles, the cerebellum was small, the pons was elongated, the medulla was entirely in the spinal canal, and the lower cranial nerves were elongated. Hydromyelia and meningomyelocele were associated.

Chiari type III was a single case of cervical spina bifida in which there was herniation of the cerebellum through the bony defect, a form of occipital meningoencephalocele. Arnold's description of a case of meningomyelocele without hydrocephalus was less detailed than the earlier description by Chiari. Schwalbe and Gredig gave the name Arnold-Chiari malformation to type II which was always associated with meningomyelocele. For a full description of the historical and pathological aspects of Chiari malformations see *Greenfield's Neuropathology*, Baltimore, Williams and Wilkins Co. The section on malformations of the nervous system was written by Dr. R.M. Norman. - Editor. *Ped Neur Briefs* October 1989.

Arnold-Chiari Malformation
And Intermittent Hydrocephalus

Intermittent symptoms of obstructive hydrocephalus in a young woman with Chiari-I malformation are reported from the Neuroophthalmology Service, Wills Eye Hospital, Philadelphia, PA. A perviously healthy 26 year old woman experienced episodes of intermittent pressure headaches, dizziness, tingling in the right arm, and right anterior chest pressure for two months. These episodes lasted 5-15 minutes and occurred up to 15 times a day. They were followed by blurred vision with the appearance of a "green patch" inferiorly before the left eye. Bilateral optic disc elevation was identified with indirect ophthalmoscopy. Lumbar puncture showed an opening pressure of 190 mm H_2O. Intravenous fluorescein angiography demonstrated venous stasis, diffuse retinal hemorrhages, and disc edema interpreted as consistent with papillophlebitis. An MRI using multiple thin sagittal sections directed at the posterior fossa revealed the Chiari I malformation, and an intraventricular catheter confirmed that the malformation was causing an intermittent obstruction and increased intracranial pressure. In one attack in which the patient experienced several typical episodes of right hand and right chest paresthesias, headache, and blurred vision the simultaneous intracranial pressure readings were elevated to a maximum of 580 mm H_2O). The pressure was sustained for approximately 2 minutes; as it decreased the patient's symptoms abated. Following posterior fossa decompression and a C1 to C3 laminectomy the pressure was relieved and the patient was asymptomatic. (Vrabec TR et al. Intermittent obstruction hydrocephalus in the Arnold-Chiari malformation. (*Ann Neurol* Sept 1989; *26*:401-404).

COMMENT. Although this patient is outside the pediatric age group, Chiari I malformation becomes symptomatic in children and the transient nature of the signs and symptoms may prove misleading in diagnosis. Conventional CT and MRI may fail to reveal the malformation and posterior fossa directed MRI using multiple thin sagittal sections including the midline view may be necessary for diagnosis. - Editor. *Ped Neur Briefs* October 1989.

Ocular Signs Of Chiari Malformation

Twenty-eight patients (14 females and 14 males aged between four and 34 years) with myelomeningocele and Chiari malformations were examined neuro-ophthalmologically at the Karolinska Institute, Huddinge University Hospital, Huddinge, Sweden. The Chiari malformation, determined with MRI, was type I in three patients and type II in 25. All had hydrocephalus; mild in 12, moderate in 13, and marked in three. Shunt procedures had been performed in 20. Spontaneous or gaze related nystagmus and abnormal optokinetic nystagmus were the most common disturbances of ocular motility. Horizontal gaze paresis occurred in 14 patients and vertical gaze limitations in nine, all in upward gaze. Horizontal nystagmus occurred in 17 whereas vertical nystagmus was uncommon and downbeat nystagmus was not observed. Strabismus occurred in 11 patients and esotropia was more common than exotropia. No signs of optic atrophy or other changes in the visual pathways were found. (Lennerstrand G, Gallo JE. Neuro-ophthalmological evaluation of patients with myelomeningocele and Chiari malformations. *Dev Med Child Neur* May 1990; 32:415-422).

COMMENT. Downbeat nystagmus has been considered almost pathognomonic of the Chiari malformation but was absent in the cases in this study. A girl aged ten referred to me recently because of migraine headaches had downbeat nystagmus and a refractive error; the MRI was negative for Chiari malformation and brain stem auditory evoked responses were normal.

Lennerstrand G et al have used the MRI to determine the correlation between disturbances of ocular motility and the degree of hydrocephalus, tactile plate deformity, and dislocation of the cerebellum and medulla oblongata in 28 patients with myelomeningocele. (*Dev Med Child Neur* May 1990; *32*:423-431). All patients had Chiari malformations. Strabismus and spontaneous nystagmus were related to the degree of hydrocephalus and to the amount of lower brain stem deformities. Convergence defects correlated with upper brain stem deformities. - Editor. *Ped Neur Briefs* May 1990.

NEURAL TUBE DEFECTS

Overview Of Neural Tube Defects

In an overview of neural tube defects (NTDs), Dr. RJ Lemier of the Dept Pediatrics, Univ of Washington and Children's Hospital, Seattle, WA, divides them into 2 major groups: 1) *Neurulation* and 2) *postneurulation* defects.

Neurulation defects arising between the 17th and 30th day after fertilization are caused by nonclosure of the neural tube, leaving nervous tissue exposed, whereas postneurulation NTDs are covered by skin. Three general categories of neurulation defects are described: 1) craniorachischis (total dysraphism), 2) anencephaly, and 3) meningomyelocele. Environmental teratogenic factors implicated in neurulation defects include valproate sodium and nutritional and vitamin deficiencies. Prenatal diagnosis is made by screening for maternal serum a-fetoprotein (AFP) levels during the 16th-18th week of pregnancy with follow-up ultrasound and amniocentesis when AFP is elevated. Elevated amniotic fluid acetylcholinesterase levels are confirmatory of open NTD and eliminate possible false-positive results of AFP tests. The population incidence of open NTDs is about 2/1000 births but the chance of recurrence is 1/20.

Postneurulation or closed NTDs arising after the 30th day of fetal life include hydrocephalus, encephalocele, and lumbosacral lesions. The causes of hydrocephalus and associated abnormalities are listed as follows: Arnold-Chiari malformation with meningomyelocele, tumors and cysts, aqueductal stenosis, achondroplasia, tuberous sclerosis, Dandy-Walker syndrome, chromosome trisomy 13 and 18 anomalies, prenatal infection, and aneurysm of the vein of Galen. Comprehensive lists of lumbosacral NTDs and encephalocele syndromes are provided. Early resection of caudal NTDs is advised when practical. (Lemire RJ. Neural tube defects. *JAMA* Jan 22/29 1988; *259*:558-562).

> COMMENT. As an encouraging postscript to this depressing subject, the author notes a declining incidence of NTDs in several areas of the world, including the U.S., related in part to prenatal diagnosis, genetic counseling and nutritional supplementation. Folate treatment before and at the time of conception prevent recurrence of spina bifida. Exposure to spermicide contraceptives is not a risk factor. - Editor. *Ped Neur Briefs* February 1988.

Vitamins And Neural Tube Defects

The use of vitamin supplements by women around the time of conception was examined and compared in those having babies with neural tube defects, those with stillbirths or some other type of malformation, and in women who had normal babies. The study was performed at the National Institute of Child Health and Human Development, National Institutes of Health, Bethesda, Maryland; Northwestern University, Chicago; and the California Public Health Foundation, Berkley. The rate of periconceptional multivitamin use among mothers of infants with neural tube defects (15.8%) was not significantly different from the rate among mothers in either the abnormal or the normal control group (14.1% and 15.9%, respectively). There were no differences among the groups in the use of folate vitamin supplements. The authors conclude that the periconceptional use of multivitamins or folate-containing supplements did not decrease the risk of having an infant with a neural tube defect. (Mills JL et al. The absence of a relation between the periconceptional use of vitamins and neural-tube defects. *N Engl J Med* Aug 17, 1989; *321*:430-5).

COMMENT. Several studies have suggested that women who take multivitamins or supplements of folic acid around the time of conception may have a reduced risk of delivering an infant with a neural tube defect such as myelomeningocele or spina bifida. British studies have reported that folic acid in a dose of 4 mg/day or multivitamins can reduce the risk of recurrence in women who have already delivered an infant with such a defect. In a report published from the Atlanta Birth Defects Case Control Study, mothers of children with neural tube defects were significantly less likely to report vitamin use around the time of conception than were the mothers of infants with other malformations or normal control children. The results of the present study were strikingly different from those of the Atlanta Birth Defects case Control Study in which 7% of mothers with affected babies and 50% of controls reported using multivitamin supplements at least three times a week in the periconceptional period. It is possible that the use of vitamins was not itself protective but was a marker for other health conscious behavior that prevented the malformations. Other explanations for the difference in the results might include the variation in the years studied and geographic differences. It should be noted that the Vitamin A analog Isotretinoin is teratogenic and should be avoided during pregnancy. Further studies are obviously needed to confirm these results. In the meantime mothers might be advised to take vitamins in the recommended daily allowances but not to resort to megavitamin therapy with possible adverse effects. - Editor. *Ped Neur Briefs* August 1989.

Causes Of Neural Tube Defects

Investigators from the Greenwood Genetic Center, South Carolina and Department of Pediatrics, U. of North Carolina, Chapel Hill, studied 6 fetuses weighing < 1 kg with spinal defects detected through maternal serum-fetoprotein or ultrasound examination in the midtrimester. Infusion through the umbilical artery, using 5 ml or less of a mixture of barium and gelatin heated to 55°C, demonstrated abnormalities of the arterial supply to the region of the neural tube defects in all cases.

Since embryologically these arteries develop prior to closure of the neural tube, the authors propose that the vascular disturbances limit nutrition to the developing neural tissue and supporting structures, preventing neural tube closure. The vascular abnormalities are considered to be primary malformations that lead to neural tube defects rather than secondary morphologic disturbances resulting from neural tube defects. (Stephenson RE, Aylsworth AS et al. Vascular basis for neural tube defects: a hypothesis. *Pediatrics* 1987; *80*:102-106).

COMMENT. The authors comment that their hypothesis for the formation of spina bifida is in contrast to that of an overdistension and rupture of a previously closed neural tube, as suggested by Gardner and Breuer. Nutritional inadequacy is a proposed mechanism. Folate treatment before conception prevented recurrence of defects (Laurence KM et al. *Br Med J* 1981; *282*:1509), and periconceptional vitamin supplements containing folic acid, ascorbic acid, and riboflavin were also effective (Smithells RW et al. *Arch Dis Child* 1981; *56*:911). Among 397 given supplements only 3 had a second infant with a neural tube defect whereas of 493 mothers not receiving a vitamin supplement, 23 had recurrence of affected infants. Reports suggesting that the use of spermicides may increase the risk of neural tube defects (Huggins G et al. *Contraception* 1982; *25*:219) have not been supported by results of a study published by Louik C et al (*N Engl J Med* 1987;

317:474-8). The risks of five specific birth defects, including neural-tube defects and Down syndrome, were not increased by exposure to spermicide contraceptives in the first four months of pregnancy, at the time of conception, or at any time before conception. - Editor. *Ped Neur Briefs* August 1987.

Diabetes And Fetal CNS Malformations

Diabetic and healthy control pregnant women were followed in a multicenter collaborative study coordinated by the Epidemiological Branch, National Institute of Child Health and Human Development, Bethesda, MD. Major malformations, including anencephaly, arhinencephaly and holoprosencephaly, microcephaly, meningomyelocele and hydrocephalus, were detected in 4.9% of diabetic women who entered the study early compared to 9% in late-entry diabetic subjects (P=.032) and 2.1% in controls (P=.027). Mean blood glucose and glycosylated hemoglobin levels during organogenesis were not significantly higher in women whose infants were malformed, and hypoglycemia was not more common in the same group. Hyperglycemia during organogenesis was not correlated with malformation. The authors conclude that not all malformation can be prevented by good glycemic control but the lower incidence among women studied within 21 days of conception (early-entry group) as compared with the late-entry group justifies good metabolic control around time of conception. (Millis JL et al. Lack of relation to increased malformation rates in infants of diabetic mothers to glycemic control during organogenesis. *N Engl J Med* Mar 17 1988; *318*:671-6).

COMMENT. Previous studies have shown low malformation rates in diabetic women who achieved excellent periconceptional glycemic control. The present study suggests that poor glycemic control explains some but not all diabetes associated malformations. Metabolic factors other than glycemic control may be relevant according to animal studies. Genetic factors may also be involved and female offspring are more susceptible. Congenital optic nerve hypoplasia, not encountered in this study, has been reported in women whose mothers had diabetes mellitus. (Nelson M et al. *Arch Neurol* 1986; *43*:20). - Editor. *Ped Neur Briefs* March 1988.

Brain Anomalies And Heart Defects

The type, frequency, and clinical presentation of developmental brain anomalies in 41 infants with the hypoplastic left heart syndrome are reviewed from the Children's Hospital of Philadelophia, and the University of Pennsylvania School of Medicine, Philadelphia. A major or minor central nervous system abnormality occurred in 29% and included agenesis of the corpus callosum (3 cases), holoprosencephaly (1), micrencephaly (9), and cortical mantle malformation (8). Congenital brain anomalies were present in patients either with or without external dysmorphic features that involved the head, face and eyes, fingers, lung and kidney. In patients living only one day or less approximately 50% had recognizable malformations, microcephaly, and pulmonary anomalies. (Glauser TA et al. Congenital brain anomalies associated with the hypoplastic left heart syndrome. *Pediatrics* June 1990; *85*:984-990).

COMMENT. The authors recommend that infants with hypoplastic left heart syndrome deserve careful genetic, ophthalmologic and neurologic evaluations, including CT scan and long-term neurologic follow-up. In the same issue of *Pediatrics* the authors review their experience with acquired brain lesions associated with hypoplastic left heart syndrome, finding 45% with hypoxic, ischemic and hemorrhagic lesions secondary to CNS perfusion and glucose oxygen delivery. A duration of cardiopulmonary bypass with hypothermic total circulatory arrest longer than 40 minutes was associated with a higher incidence of acquired neuropathology. (Glauser TA et al. Acquired neuropathologic lesions associated with the hypoplastic left heart syndrome. *Pediatrics* June 1990; *85*:991-1000). - Editor. *Ped Neur Briefs* June 1990.

Incidence Of Neurologic Malformations

A 17-year survey of major congenital neurologic malformations among infants born in U.S. Army Hospitals worldwide
from January 1, 1971 through December 31, 1987 is presented
from the Neonatology Services, Walter Reed Army Medical
Center, Washington, DC and Travis Grant USAF Medical
Center, Travis Air Force Base, CA. From a population of 763
364 live-born and stillborn infants, 275 had anencephaly (0.36
per 1000 total births), 526 had spina bifida (0.69 per 1000),
112 had encephaloceles (0.15 per 1000), and 370 had hydrocephalus (0.48 per 1000 total births). The incidence of CNS
defects among stillborn infants was 24 times greater than among
live-born infants. There was a female preponderance of infants
with anencephaly, spina bifida and encephalocele and a male predominance for hydrocephalus. Black infants were less likely than
white infants to have spina bifida. Other congenital anomalies
were associated in 20% of infants with anencephaly, 40% with
encephaloceles, 37% with hydrocephalus, and 22% with spina
bifida. (Wiswell TE et al. Major congenital neurologic malformations. A 17-year survey. *AJDC* Jan 1990; *144*:61-67).

COMMENT. The racial background of the patient population in this study closely resembled that of the United
States as a whole and the results may reflect those of the
U.S. In the past 20 years, declines in the frequencies of
anencephaly and spina bifida have been noted in many
countries, particularly in the British Isles. In the present
study the incidence of neural tube defects decreased only
among white female infants and no etiological factor could
be implicated. - Editor. *Ped Neur Briefs* April 1990.

Management Of Neural Tube Defects:
Non-Closure V. Early Closure

Non-closure of open neural tube defects above L2 in 105
infants born between 1978 and 1985 resulted in a significantly
lower incidence (p<0.001) of hydrocephalus, shunt insertions,
and ventriculitis during the first few months of life, and mortali-

ty was not increased throughout the first year, in a study reported from the Royal Belfast Hospital for Sick Children, Belfast, Northern Ireland. This non-closure or deferred-closure group was compared with 109 infants born between 1964 and 1971 whose open neural tube defects were treated by early closure. Hydrocephalus correlated with the occurrence of ventriculitis (p < 0.001) during the first year of life in both non-closure and early-closure groups; 37 of 72 infants with hydrocephalus developed ventriculitis compared with 6 of 37 without hydrocephalus in those whose defect was not closed, and results were similar in those who received early closure. The authors conclude that non-closure of neural tube defects is associated with a better prognosis and a reduction in the number of shunt operations and revisions. (Deans GT, Boston VE. Is surgical closure of the back lesion in open neural tube defects necessary? *Br Med J* May 21 1988; *296*:1441-2).

COMMENT. A rate of infection of 20% or higher is reported with the operative treatment of hydrocephalus (see *Ped Neur Briefs* Sept 1987; 1(4):28), and patients with myelomeningocele are most susceptible. In those shunted at 1 week of age or earlier, the rate of infection was 48% but when shunt was performed at 2 weeks or later, the incidence of infection was lower. Since non-closure of myelomeningocele appears to be safe and reduces the necessity for shunt procedures, this method of management should be preferred. However, I am sure that other pediatric neurosurgeons have opposing opinions. - Editor. *Ped Neur Briefs* July 1988.

Prognosis Of Open Spina Bifida

The outcome of 117 consecutive cases of open spina bifida treated unselectively from birth between 1963 and 1970 and reviewed 16-20 years later is reported from the Department of Urology, Addenbrooke's Hospital, Cambridge, England. Forty-one percent died before their 16th birthday and most of the survivors were badly handicapped: 50% were wheelchair dependent,

30% were mentally retarded and 75% relied on an appliance or padding for incontinence. The majority had had a shunt inserted within hours of birth. 75% were incapable of employment and 50% were unable to live without help or supervision. The sensory level at birth provided a yardstick for predicting the range of handicap into adult life and was useful in counseling parents concerning the child's long-term prognosis. With a sensory level above T11 the disability would be severe, with no prospect of walking or of continence and with a 10% chance of independent living. A sensory level between T11 and L3 (from the umbilicus to the knees) should indicate a moderate disability in 60% and a capability of living independently in 45%. A sensory level below L3 should predict a survival rate of 75% and a normal intelligence in 80%; 90% would be ambulant as adults and 45% would be continent; and 85% would be totally independent with moderate or minimal disability. (Hunt GM. Open spina bifida: Outcome for a complete cohort treated unselectively and followed into adulthood. *Dev Med Child Neurol* Feb 1990; *32*:108-118).

> COMMENT. The impact of treatment on disability is far less than that on mortality. In groups of patients treated selectively, the mortality among the untreated cases is higher and those selected for treatment are born with a much lesser degree of disability. Thoracic scoliosis and horseshoe kidney that may be recognized during fetal life are associated with sensory levels in the thoracic region and are predictive of a poor prognosis. The author points out that the reliable discrimination between mild and severe cases of spina bifida in early pregnancy is not yet possible and parents should be informed of the likelihood of prolonged dependency into adulthood. - Editor. *Ped Neur Briefs* April 1990.

Tethered Spinal Cords

The diagnosis of tethered spinal cord by MRI in seven children with cutaneous lumbar hemangioma is reported from the

Children's Hospital of Pittsburg, University of Pittsburgh School of Medicine. The hemangiomas ranged in size from 4x6 cm to 8x20 cm and all overlapped the midline. All demonstrated tethered cords; four showed intraspinal lipomas, and two showed tight fila terminale. At surgery, all infants were found to have tethered cords and none had an intraspinal hemangioma. All patients were neurologically normal both pre- and postoperatively. (Albright AL et al. Lumbar cutaneous hemangiomas as indicators of tethered spinal cords. *Pediatrics* June 1989; *83*:977-980).

> COMMENT. The lumbar hemangiomas in these patients were large and the significance of small lesions is not known. Despite a normal neurological examination, infants or children with large lumbar cutaneous hemangiomas should be suspected of having tethered cords and magnetic resonance imaging should be obtained. If neurologic deficits are allowed to develop with increasing age, the likelihood of postoperative improvement is only 25-50%. Ultrasound may be used to diagnose tethered cords but magnetic resonance is usually required for better visualization. In addition to the association with cutaneous hemangioma, tethered cord occurs with subcutaneous lipoma, a hairy tuft, a prominent dimple, or a midline sinus tract or skin defect. - Editor. *Ped Neur Briefs* June 1988.

Anencephaly

A Medical Task Force on anencephaly presents a consensus statement limited to medical issues of organizations of physicians caring for fetuses and infants with anencephaly. The statement was approved by the AAP, AAN, ACOG, ANA, and CNS. Anencephaly is defined as a congenital absence of a major portion of the brain, skull, and scalp with its genesis in the first month of gestation. The primary abnormality is failure of cranial neurulation, the embryologic process that separates the precursors of the forebrain from amniotic fluid. Anencephaly does not mean the complete absence of the head or brain.

Craniofacial anomalies are associated and up to 1/3 have defects of the non-neural organs that could preclude their use for transplantation. The maternal serum a-fetoprotein level is elevated in 90% of cases, and elevated a-fetoprotein levels in amniotic fluid and the presence of acetylcholinesterase on electrophoresis occur in virtually all cases. Ultrasonography is also reliable in the prenatal diagnosis of anencephaly.

The postnatal diagnosis requires the following criteria: 1) Absence of a large portion of the skull, 2) absence of scalp over skull defect, 3) exposed hemorrhagic fibrotic tissue, 4) absence of recognizable cerebral hemispheres. The cause is usually not known and a polygenic or multifactorial etiology is suggested. Chromosome abnormalities and mechanical factors are recognized associations. Hyperthermia and deficiencies of folate, zinc and copper in the mother have been invoked. In recent years, 80-90% are aborted, 7-10% are stillborn, and 3-11% are live born. Most live born anencephalic infants have died within the first days after birth and survival beyond one week occurred in 0-9% in three series. Two months was the longest survival confirmed with accepted diagnostic criteria. The estimated incidence of anencephaly in the U.S. is 0.3-7/1000 births and the incidence of live born infants with anencephaly would be less than 100 per year. Anencephalic infants have no functioning cerebral cortex and are permanently unconscious. Brain stem functions are present in varying degrees and the diagnosis of brain stem death depends on the disappearance of previously existing brain stem functions, including loss over an observation period of at least 48 hours of measurable cranial nerve function and spontaneous movements, and a positive apnea test. Confounding factors such as drugs, hypothermia, or hypotension should be excluded. The use of organs from infants with anencephaly for transplantation is also discussed. (Stumpf DA et al. The infant with anencephaly. *N Engl J Med* March 8, 1990; *322*:669-674).

COMMENT. This comprehensive report on the infant with anencephaly provides medical information of importance in the analysis of social, legal, and ethical issues concerning transplantation of organs from anencephalic infants. - Editor. *Ped Neur Briefs* April 1990.

Optic Nerve Hypoplasia

The pathology, clinical features, and disorders associated with optic nerve hypoplasia in children are reviewed from the Tennent Institute of Ophthalmology, Weston Infirmary, Glasgow, Scotland. A total of 100 references is provided. Histologically a reduced number of optic nerve fibers can be demonstrated in a smaller than normal optic nerve. An overgrowth of retinal pigment epithelium surrounding the small optic disc gives rise to the "double ring sign". Failure of differentiation of the retinal ganglion cell layer between the 12 and 17 mm stages of embryonal development has been suggested as a cause of optic nerve hypoplasia (ONH). Other theories include axonal degeneration within the optic nerve or stretching of the optic nerve during the development of abnormal cerebral hemispheres. Factors predisposing to ONH include maternal diabetes mellitus, postmaturity, young maternal age, alcohol abuse during pregnancy, and maternal use of anticonvulsants, quinine, LSD, and phencyclidine.

Three clinical varieties are described: 1) Isolated abnormality in an otherwise normal eye; 2) In malformed eyes; 3) With other disorders involving the midline structures of the brain. Nystagmus, poor vision, and visual field defects occur. The differentiation from optic atrophy is important and may require examination with sedation and fundus photography. The electroretinogram is normal but the amplitude of the visual evoked response is reduced. ONH occurs with 25% of cases of agenesis of the septum pellucidum and 27% of patients with ONH have partial or complete absence of the septum pellucidum. The neurological features of this condition, known as *septo-optic dysplasia*, include mental retardation, spasticity, abnormalities of taste and impaired smell. The ability to learn tasks requiring spatial orientation may be impaired. A number of neurological conditions may be associated with ONH and these include porencephaly, cerebral atrophy, anencephaly, hydrocephaly, congenital suprasellar tumors, and Aicardi syndrome. The frequent association of endocrine problems with ONH should alert the physician to test for pituitary dysfunction early in infancy so that optimal replacement therapy can be given. Children with septo-optic dysplasia and a deficiency of growth hormone frequently have normal growth until their third or fourth year of life. Pituitary dysfunction with ONH may be manifested as diabetes insipidus, prolonged neonatal hyperbilirubinemia, hypotonia, infantile hypoglycemia, hypothyroidism, and growth retardation. All children with ONH should have a careful neuroendocrinology exam including a CT scan. (Zeki SM, Dutton GN. Optic nerve hypoplasia in children. *Br J Ophthalmol* May 1990, *74*:300-304).

> COMMENT. The early recognition of optic nerve hypoplasia and its differentiation from optic atrophy are important because of the frequent association with neurological and systemic abnormalities and particularly neuroendocrine disorders which may require early treatment. - Editor. *Ped Neur Briefs* May 1990.

Lissencephaly Syndromes

The diagnostic features and clinical signs of 21 patients with lissencephaly type I are reviewed from the Department of Neurology, Westeinde Hospital, The Hague, The Netherlands; the Departments of Child Neurology, Academic Medical Centre, Amsterdam, and Sophia Children's Hospital, Rotterdam. A multicenter study was conducted with the cooperation of all child neurology departments in The Netherlands. Lissencephaly was diagnosed at autopsy in two patients and by CT scan in 19. The criteria of Dobyns WB (1987) were used for the classification of Lissencephaly: *Type I* Isolated lissencephaly sequence (ILS), Miller-Dieker syndrome (MDS); *Type II*, Walker-Warburg syndrome, Fukuyama congenital muscular dystrophy; Rare forms, Neu-Laxova syndrome, Cerebro-cerebellar syndrome.

Lissencephaly type I is classified according to pathology and radiology as follows: Grade 1, complete agyria; Grade 2, agyria with some sulci; Grade 3, a mixture of about 50% agyria and 50% pachygyria; Grade 4, complete pachygyria. Of 21 patient with lissencephaly type I, 17 had isolated lissencephaly and 4 had the Miller-Dieker syndrome. More severe abnormalities in gross brain morphology occurred in MDS than in ILS. Facial dysmorphism was most frequent in MDS patients and microcephaly in combination with facial abnormalities increases the suspicion of MDS. All children with lissencephaly in this study were severely retarded, 86% developed epilepsy before the age of six months, and one-third had infantile spasms. The somatic signs of 19 patients with chromosome deletion 17p are described for the present series of patients and those in the literature: malformed fingers, congenital heart-defect, sacral dimple, cryptorchidism, and malformed kidneys. (De Rijk-van Andel JF et al. Diagnostic features and clinical signs of 21 patients with lissencephaly type I. *Dev Med Child Neurol* Aug 1990; *32*:707-717).

COMMENT. The diagnosis of lissencephaly is made by clinical and neuroradiological findings. Cases of isolated lissencephaly may be distinguished from the Miller-Dieker syndrome without the results of chromosome analysis in most cases. The CT signs of lissencephaly include smooth brain surface and no Sylvian fissure with figure 8 appearance, sharp demarcation between gray and white matter, and colpocephaly. Facial dysmorphism may show high forehead, bitemporal hollowing, and micrognathia. - Editor. *Ped Neur Briefs* September 1990.

Schizencephaly And Behavioral Correlates

The MRI appearance and neuropsychologic and speech/language evaluations in three patients with schizencephaly are described from the Department of Radiology,

Michigan State University, East Lansing, MI. All patients presented with a seizure disorder and they were left-handed without familial sinistrality in first degree relatives. The primary areas of cerebral involvement were the left parasylvian and pararolandic regions with varying degrees of secondary involvement of the right hemisphere. There was mild right-sided limb hypoplasia, and motor dexterity with the dominant left hand was better than with the right hand. Two patients showed significant impairment in finger localization and tactile form recognition particularly with the nondominant right hand.

The level of general intellectual functioning related to the amount of brain tissue involved, and neurobehavioral abilities reflected the location of the brain malformation and the prenatal onset of the disorder. The full scale IQ on the WAIS-R ranged from a low of 65 to a high of 87. Only one patient showed a higher verbal IQ than performance IQ and her visuospatial construction abilities and visual memory abilities were significantly impaired. There were varying degrees of linguistic deficit with relatively greater difficulties in syntactical speech than in semantic aspects. (Aniskiewicz AS et al. Magnetic resonance imaging and neurobehavioral correlates in schizencephaly. *Arch Neurol* August 1990; *47*:911-916).

COMMENT. Yakovlev and Wadsworth first described the schizencephalies as congenital defects in the cerebral mantle in 1946. The patients in the present study shared features in common with the *pathologic left handedness syndrome* of Orsini and Satz; predominantly left-sided cerebral lesion with onset before six years of age and involving speech/language areas of frontotemporal parietal cortex, atypical or right-sided hemispheric speech representation, impaired visuospatial abilities and preserved verbal cognitive abilities, right limb hypoplasia, right hand motor impairment, and absence of familial sinistrality. (Orsini DL, Satz P. A syndrome of pathological left-handedness: Correlates of early left hemisphere injury. *Arch Neurol* 1986; *43*:333-337). - Editor. *Ped Neur Briefs* September 1990.

Neural Maturational Delay In Sids

The pathological evidence for developmental delay in SIDS is reviewed from the Division of Neuropathology, The Hospital for Sick Children, University of Toronto, Toronto, Canada. Evidence of hypoxic ischemic insult to the brain includes astrogliosis and subcortical leukomalacia. Astrogliosis is most apparent in the region of the tegmentum in SIDS victims, a finding interpreted as hypoperfusion during episodes of bradycardia associated with apnea. Subcortical or periventricular leukomalacia was found in 21.6% of infants who died of SIDS. Term and prematurely born SIDS infants showed persistence of the reticular dendritic spines which suggests a delay of development to a mature, higher level of neuronal function. This delay may reflect a functional impairment of the higher levels of respiratory control in SIDS infants.

A number of reports suggest alterations in neurotransmitter levels of catecholamines, beta endorphin, met-enkephalin, and substance P in SIDS. Examination of 36 infants who had died of SIDS showed that the mean number of small myelinated vagal fibers was significantly decreased in the SIDS infants compared with controls, suggesting an abnormal or delayed development of the vagus nerve. This finding was similar to that reported in a two year old infant dying of persistent infantile sleep apnea (Ondine's curse). Elevated dopamine in the carotid bodies of SIDS victims suggests a role in pathogenesis: dopamine inhibits respiration by acting directly on the carotid bodies and the carotid body plays an important role in the development of respiratory maturation. The pineal gland influences diurnal rhythm and is significantly reduced in weight in SIDS patients compared to age matched controls; the significance of this reduction is unknown. Brains of SIDS victims born at term were significantly heavier than reference values matched for both age and body length. (Becker LE. Neural maturational delay as a link in the chain of events leading to SIDS. *Can J Neurol Sci* Nov 1990; *17*:361-671).

COMMENT. The authors emphasize a delay of neural maturation of both myelination and synapses in the etiology of SIDS. Other abnormalities such as brainstem astrogliosis may be secondary to hypoxic-ischemia. In Canada, the incidence of sudden infant death syndrome is 1.2 per 1000 live births. The peak age is 1-4 months. The highest incidence is in winter and more boys than girls are affected. A thorough autopsy ruled out SIDS in 10% of sudden unexpected deaths occurring under one year of age. The differential diagnoses included congenital heart disease, myocarditis, central nervous system trauma (child abuse), cardiomyopathy, encephalitis, meningitis, congenital diaphragmatic hernia, and medium chain acyl coenzyme deficiency. If an anatomical cause of death is found, the diagnosis is not SIDS. In SIDS the mechanism of death must be related to a central type of respiratory failure or cardiac dysrhythmia. - Editor. *Ped Neur Briefs* December 1990.

Acrocallosal Syndrome (Schinzel Syndrome)

The acrocallosal syndrome, first described by Schinzel (*Helv Paediatr Acta* 1979; *34*:141) and characterized by dysmorphic features, macrocephaly, polydactyly, mental retardation, and agenesis of the corpus callosum, is reported in two unrelated boys with consanguineous parents from the Centre de Genetique Medicale, Service de Pediatrie Generale and Radiologie, Hopital d'Enfants de la Timone, Marseille, France. An autosomal recessive mode of inheritance is suggested and echographic survey of further pregnancies is advised. Clinical manifestations included macrocephaly, bulging forehead, antimongoloid slant of eyes, broad short nose, posteriorly rotated ears, herniae, polydactyly, cardiac defect, mental retardation and corpus callosal agenesis. (Philip N et al. The acrocallosal syndrome. *Eur J Pediatr* Febr 1988; *147*:206-208).

COMMENT. Only 12 cases of the syndrome have been reported. Schinzel, who described the syndrome in 1979 and has at least 5 publications on the subject, deserves the eponym. - Editor. *Ped Neur Briefs* March 1988.

Congenital Callosal Defects

A lethal and previously undescribed syndrome in 3 siblings with hypoplasia of the corpus callosum is described from the Istituto Materno-Infantil de Pernambuco, and Laboratorio de Genetica, Universidade Federal de Pernambuco, Recife, PE, Brazil. The combination of anomalies, probably inherited as an autosomal recessive trait, included corpus callosum hypoplasia, microcephaly, severe mental retardation, preauricular skin tag, camptodactyly (fixed flexion of one or more fingers), growth retardation, and recurrent bronchopneumonia. The children lived for 10, 23 and 32 months. At autopsy in 2 patients, the brain weighed approximately 500 grams and showed marked hypoplasia of the corpus callosum, aqueductal stenosis, enlarged 3rd and 4th ventricles, widened cavum septi pellucidi, and diffuse degenerative changes with astrocytosis. The literature on anomalies associated with callosal defects is reviewed. (da-Silva EO. Callosal defect, microcephaly, severe mental retardation, and other anomalies in three sibs. *Am J Med Genet* April 1988; *29*:837-843).

> COMMENT. Congenital callosal defects occur alone or with other brain anomalies, e.g. septum pellucidum defect, hydrocephalus, porencephaly, polymicrogyria, and cerebellar hypoplasia. Mental retardation, seizures, and failure to thrive are commonly associated, but the callosal defect itself may be asymptomatic. At least 4 distinct syndromes include callosal agenesis as a major component: Aicardi (with infantile spasms, hypsarrhythmia, chorioretinal lacunae and coloboma), Schinzel acrocallosal syndrome (with macrocephaly, and polydactyly), Anderman's syndrome (with anterior horn cell disease), and Shapiro syndrome (with recurrent hypothermia). (See *Ped Neur Briefs* March 1988; *2*:17). - Editor. *Ped Neur Briefs* July 1988.

Agenesis Of The Corpus Callosum And Aicardi Syndrome

The postmortem findings in a two month old infant with the typical clinical features of Aicardi syndrome (i.e., infantile spasms, chorioretinal lacunae, and agenesis of the corpus callo-sum) are reported from the Division of Neurology, Saitama Children's Medical Center, Saitama, Japan. The rostrum of the corpus callosum was absent and the roof of the dilated third ven-tricle was covered with a thin leptomeningeal membrane. Cortical heterotropia were found adjacent to the anterior horn of the right lateral ventricle and consisted of small immature neurons. The article includes a review of five autopsied patients with this syndrome previously reported in the literature. (Hamano S et al. Aicardi syndrome: Postmortem findings. *Pediatr Neurol* July/Aug 1989; 5:259-61).

> COMMENT. In these cases, a high incidence of EEG lat-erality and an asymmetry of pathological lesions are of interest. Three of six patients had focal agenesis of the cor-pus callosum and three had papilloma of the choroid plexus. - Editor. *Ped Neur Briefs* October 1989.

Cerebellar Vermis Agenesis

The syndromes of vermal agenesis are reviewed from the Department of Pediatrics, Hopital des Enfants Malades, Paris, France. These include the *Dandy-Walker* syndrome and other complicated cases associated with multiple abnormalities. The Dandy-Walker syndrome consists of three abnormalities of development: 1) Partial or complete agenesis of the vermis of the cerebellum; 2) cystic formation in the posterior fossa com-municating with the fourth ventricle; and 3) hydrocephalus. Enlargement of the posterior fossa and elevation of the torcular and lateral sinuses are sometimes included among the diagnostic criteria. Associated abnormalities include agenesis of the corpus callosum (7-15% of patients), occipital encephalocele (18%), cleft lip and palate, cardiac malformations, urinary tract abnormali-ties, and minor facial dysmorphisms. The prognosis is guarded, 75% having borderline IQ or lower, and a mortality rate of 27% in some series. Various chromosomal abnormalities have been demonstrated in a few patients but their significance is unclear. There is a 1-2% chance of recurrence in the same family.

Syndromes of agenesis of the cerebellar vermis of genetic origin are distinguished from the Dandy-Walker malformation. These include Joubert syndrome, Walker-Warburg syndrome, Meckel-Gruber syndrome, and atypical Dandy-Walker with facial angioma. *Joubert* syndrome includes panting respirations, abnormal eye movements, facial asymmetry and ataxia, in addition to vermian agenesis. The MRI shows an umbrella shaped fourth ventricle. *Walker-Warburg* syndrome includes lissencephaly, retinal abnormalities and hydrocephalus. *Meckel-Gruber* syndrome is characterized by occipital encephalocele, polycystic kidneys, polydactyly and hydrocephalus. Some have congenital muscular dystrophy in addition. The inheritance pattern is autosomal recessive. An MRI with median sagittal cuts is usually required in the diagnosis of partial agenesis. No reliable metabolic marker has been determined but some cases of vermian agenesis are associated with abnormal urinary excretion of succinyl-purines and pipecolic acid. Shunting operations are required when hydrocephalus develops. Operations on the posterior fossa have a high rate of failure. Prognosis depends on the occurrence of other CNS abnormalities. (Bordarier C., Aicardi J. Dandy-Walker syndrome and agenesis of the cerebellar vermis: Diagnostic problems and genetic counselling. *Dev Med Child Neurol* April 1990; *32*:285-294).

COMMENT. In patients with agenesis of the cerebellar vermis a correct diagnosis is important in therapy, genetic counseling, and prognosis. Cases with complications which are usually autosomal recessive in inheritance and having a poor prognosis must be distinguished from the typical Dandy-Walker syndrome which is often amenable to surgical therapy. - Editor. *Ped Neur Briefs* April 1990.

Cerebellar Pathology And Autism

Magnetic resonance imaging scans (MRI) were obtained for 14 autistic patients, aged 4 to 19 yrs, diagnosed by DSM-III criteria at the Univ of Iowa Hospitals, Iowa City, and were compared to a control group. In coronal scans, the cerebellum of autistic patients was smaller and the IVth ventricles larger whereas axial scans showed no differences from controls. The authors refer to previous reports of postmortem evidence of cerebellar pathology in autism (Bauman M, Kemper TL. *Neurology* 1985; 35:866), and CT scans showing cerebellar atrophy (Damasio H et al. *Arch Neurol* 1980; *37*:504). The significance of cerebellar involvement in behavioral disorders is unknown. (Gaffney GR et al. Cerebellar structure in autism. *AJDC* 1987; *141*:1330-1322).

> COMMENT. The recognition of an organically based dysfunction of the brain as a major causative factor in infantile autism is gaining favor. It may be necessary to redefine the syndrome when the causal mechanisms are better understood and when primary and secondary symptoms have been distinguished. (Rutter M. *J Autism Child Schizophr* 1978; *8*:162). - Editor. *Ped Neur Briefs* December 1987.

Cerebellar Hypoplasia And Autism

The size of the cerebellar hemisphere and vermal lobules was measured in ten autistic and eight normal control subjects at the Neuropsychology Research Laboratory, Children's Hospital Research Center, and the Departments of Neurosciences and Radiology, School of Medicine, University of California at San Diego, LaJolla. On sagittal MRIs the cerebellar hemispheres of the autistic subjects showed hypoplasia and a near total absence of the cerebellar tonsils in one. In contrast, a comparison of the average cerebellar width measured on axial images revealed no significant differences between the autistic group and the normal control group. The mean area of the superior-posterior vermis in the autistic subject group was 20% smaller than in the normal control group, while there was no significant difference between the mean anterior vermis areas of the two groups. The results indicated that the decreased size of the cerebellar hemispheres and the vermal lobules VI through VII was associated with autism. (Murakami JW et al. Reduced cerebellar hemisphere size and its relationship to vermal hypoplasia in autism. *Arch Neurol* June 1989; *46*:689-694).

COMMENT. The results of this study confirm those of a previous study by the same authors that showed that hypoplasia of the superior-posterior vermis (lobules VI and VII) is frequently observed in autistic individuals. The nature of the link between cerebellar dysgenesis and autistic symptoms has not been determined. The authors refer to clinical and research observations indicating that the cerebellum also plays a role in a variety of cognitive functions, such as language, learning and memory, emotional behavior, and complex motivated behaviors. They believe that the hypoplasia of cerebellar hemispheres and vermis observed in many autistic individuals is linked with behavioral and cognitive symptoms. - Editor. *Ped Neur Briefs* May 1989.

Moebius Syndrome

Brain stem calcification on CT scan, suggesting prenatal brain stem ischemia, is reported in an infant with Moebius syndrome examined in the Department of Pediatrics and Neonatal Medicine, State University of Gent, Gent, Belgium. Attempts at oral feeding in the neonatal period resulted in cyanotic attacks and bradycardia. There were repetitive clonic flexion movements in the arms and tonic contractions of intercostal and diaphragmatic muscles leading to respiratory arrest. Anticonvulsant therapy including pyridoxine were without benefit. The face was mask-like, the tongue was small, the gag reflex weak, the voice low pitched, and there was inability to abduct either eye beyond the midline. When asleep, both eyes were incompletely closed. There was generalized hypotonia and areflexia. At six months of age head control with severe titubation was achieved but conjugate eye movements were absent. At 12 months of age she still could not sit independently and she was monitored at home because of an erratic bradycardia. EEGs were normal. Chromosome test was normal. The right facial nerve could not be stimulated and blink reflexes were absent bilaterally. Brain stem evoked response showed bilateral anomalies. CT scan of the posterior fossa showed pontomedullary calcification in the floor of the fourth ventricle and basal cisterns were large. The case provides in vivo support to a theory of disruption in the vascular territory of the subclavian artery in explanation of the Moebius syndrome. (Govaert P et al. Moebius sequence and prenatal brainstem ischemia. *Pediatrics* Sept 1989; *84*:570-573).

COMMENT. Congenital nonprogressive bilateral facial palsy and external ophthalmoplegia are the clinical features for the diagnosis of Moebius syndrome. (Moebius PJ. *Munch Med Wochenschr* 1888; *35*:91). Theories of etiology have included 1) primary brain stem nuclear hypoplasia, 2) secondary brain stem nuclear degeneration, and 3) brain stem atrophy secondary to muscular defect. The postmortem finding of focal brain stem mineral deposits in some patients with Moebius syndrome support prenatal ischemic necrosis as an alternative explanation. (Thakkar N et al. *Arch Neurol* 1977; *34*:124).

An infant with Moebius syndrome and MRI evidence of calcification in the medulla died recently at our institution and at autopsy was found to have atrophic lesions in the brain stem indicative of an ischemic pathology. (Clark HB. Personal communication). A case of a 13 year old boy with autosomal dominant congenital facial diplegia is reported from the Division of Neurology, Ramos Mejia Hospital, University of Buenos Aires, Argentina. Thirteen members of his family were affected over four generations. Electrophysiologic studies showed blink reflex abnormalities suggesting functional damage to the brain stem. (Garcia Etto MI et al. Familial congenital facial diplegia: Electrophysiologic and genetic studies. *Pediatr Neurol* July/Aug 1989; *5*:262-4). - Editor. *Ped Neur Briefs* October 1989.

MENTAL RETARDATION SYNDROMES

Causes Of Mental Retardation

The mechanisms of mental retardation with relative prevalence in a hospital referral experience are reported from the Developmental Evaluation Clinic, Children's Hospital, Boston, MA. Early alterations of embryonic development (including Down syndrome) account for 32%, unknown causes 30%, environmental problems (psychosocial deprivation, childhood psychosis) 18%, pregnancy and perinatal morbidity 11%, hereditary disorders 5%, and acquired childhood diseases 4%. This classification uses the timing of the putative noxious event. The patients with mental retardation were obtained from over 3000 children referred for general developmental assessment to a tertiary children's medical center. (Crocker AC. The causes of mental retardation. *Pediatr Ann* October 1989; *18*:623-636).

COMMENT. This issue of Pediatric Annals also includes articles concerning community services for children with mental retardation and special needs adoption agencies. - Editor. *Ped Neur Briefs* December 1989.

Life Expectancy Of Mentally Retarded

The life expectancy of profoundly handicapped people with mental retardation is reported from the Lanterman Developmental Center, Pomona, CA. Data were collected on mortality for 99,543 persons with developmental disabilities who received services from the California Department of Developmental Services between March 1984 and October 1987. Immobile subjects had a much shorter life expectancy than those who could move about. Those who required tube feeding had a very short life expectancy (4-5 additional years). Those who could eat if fed by others had a life expectancy of approximately 8 additional years. Those who were mobile though not ambulatory had a life expectancy of about 23 additional years. (Eyman RK, Grossman HJ et al. The life expectancy of profoundly handicapped people with mental retardation. *N Engl J Med* August 30, 1990; *323*:584-589).

COMMENT. The importance of mobility, toileting skills, and feeding skills to survival of the mentally retarded is confirmed by this study. Of all the variables examined, mobility was the best predictor of survival. - Editor. *Ped Neur Briefs* September 1990.

Williams And Down Syndromes

The neurological features of the Williams (WS) and Down (DS) syndromes were compared as part of a large multidisciplinary research center study and reported from the Departments of Neurosciences and Pediatrics, University of California School of Medicine, San Diego, CA. Eight patients with Williams syndrome and six with Down syndrome were matched for age (mean ages 16.7 and 18.8 years respectively) and WISC-R or WAIS scores revealed no significant differences between the two groups (WS: 53.8±7.3; DS: 52.5±8.8). DS patients demonstrated nonspecific features of global developmental delay but functioned fairly well for their developmental ages while those with WS demonstrated impaired oromotor skills, cerebellar dysfunction, difficulty with drawing, and higher verbal abilities than expected. WS patients also were small for gestational age and were more likely to have had early feeding problems and failure to thrive. One-half of the WS patients had epilepsy. The authors consider that neurologic distinctions between these two groups may reflect an underlying metabolic defect in Williams syndrome. (Trauner, DA et al. Neurologic features of Williams and Down syndromes. *Pediatr Neurol* May/June 1989; 5:166-8).

COMMENT. Williams syndrome is a disorder of unknown etiology characterized by distinctive elf-like facial features, mental retardation, cardiac defects and infantile hypercalcemia. A dissociation between language and cognitive skills described in patients with this disorder suggests a specific neuropsychologic profile. Seizures as a frequent manifestation of WS have not been reported previously. - Editor. *Ped Neur Briefs* August 1989.

Alzheimer Disease In Down Syndrome

A clinical prospective study of dementia of the Alzheimer type in 96 individuals with Down syndrome over age 35 years is reported from the Eunice Kennedy Shriver Center, Waltham, MA and the Massachusetts General Hospital and Harvard Medical School, Boston, MA. Approximately 50% had a clinical dementia and the average age at dementia onset was 54.2 years. The prevalence of dementia in institutionalized Down syndrome population in this study was 8% between 35 and 49 years, 55% between 50 and 59 years, and 75% of those over 60 years old. Seizures developed in 84% of demented individuals with Down syndrome and 20% had Parkinsonian features. Hypothyroidism had been treated in 59% of the demented patients. CT scans showed brain tissue loss most pronounced in the temporal lobes. Neuropathological examination of 12 autopsied demented cases of Down syndrome showed gyral and central atrophy especially of the temporal lobes, and large numbers of plaques and tangles distributed in the same locations (i.e. hippocampus, amygdala, neocortex) as in the non-Down syndrome cases of Alzheimer dementia. (Lai F, Williams RS. A prospective study of Alzheimer disease in Down syndrome. *Arch Neurol* Aug 1989; *46*:849-853).

COMMENT. The early age at onset of dementia in the Down syndrome population corresponds to the average age of onset (before age 52) in several large pedigrees of familial Alzheimer's disease. The gene for this form of autosomal dominant early onset Alzheimer disease has been mapped to the long arm of chromosome 21. An increased frequency of Down syndrome has been reported among relatives of early onset Alzheimer disease probands. The neuropathology and neurochemistry of Alzheimer's disease in aging individuals with Down syndrome and in the general population seem to be identical although the clinical expression of Alzheimer disease in Down syndrome shows some distinctive features, e.g. a high incidence of seizures. - Editor. *Ped Neur Briefs* August 1989.

Atlantoaxial Instability In Down Syndrome

Results of an investigation of 130 children with Down syndrome screened for atlantoaxial instability are reported from Our Lady's Hospital for Sick Children, Crumlin, Dublin, Ireland. Radiological screening at ages ranging from 1-16 years showed that seven (5.4%) had evidence of atlantoaxial instability. The incidence among children examined between one and five years of age was 5% whereas those x-rayed between six and ten years of age showed a higher incidence of 12.8%, which was close to that reported previously. The clinical history and complete neurological examinations were of no value in detecting the presence of atlantoaxial instability. The authors recommend that children with Down syndrome have a radiological screen between the ages of five and ten years and again at 15 years. (Cullen S et al. Atlantoaxial instability in Down's syndrome: clinical and radiological screening. *Irish Med J* June 1989; *82*:64-65).

COMMENT. The association between atlantoaxial instability and Down syndrome has been known for many years and the prevalence is reported between 10% and 30% with a preponderance of affected females. The detection of the instability is difficult since the majority of children affected had no symptoms or signs before major complications occur as the result of compression of the spinal cord. At the present time there is no evidence to suggest that repeated radiological screening is necessary in patients with Down syndrome. Children with Down syndrome who wish to participate in sports training and competitive activities should have cervical spine x-rays and those with a definite abnormality should be excluded from competitive sports. Recreational and play activities of a less strenuous nature are usually permitted. An x-ray taken before five years of age is less likely to detect the atlantoaxial instability than one performed in later childhood or adolescence. The Special Olympics Committee recommends that all children with Down syndrome should be examined for atlantoaxial instability before they participate in sports training and competitive physical activities which may result in hyperextension, flexion, or direct pressure on the neck or upper spine. Those found to have atlantoaxial instability should be excluded from participation in certain sports activities in the Special Olympics.

Atlantoaxial instability and odontoid hypoplasia are found in Morquio's syndrome (mucoplysaccharidosis Type IV), and other mucopolysaccharidoses, notably Hurler's (Type I), Hunter's (Type II), and Maroteaux-Lamy syndrome (Type VI). (Children's Memorial Medical Center Journal Club Newsletter, Ed. Stockman JA. August, 1989). - Editor. *Ped Neur Briefs* August 1989.

Laurence-Moon-Biedl Syndrome

Thirty-two patients with a form of Laurence-Moon-Biedl syndrome are reported from the Departments of Medicine, Ophthalmology, Radiology, and Community Medicine, Memorial University, St. John's, Newfoundland, Canada. The patients were located through the registry of the Canadian National Institute of the Blind, as a result of their attendance at an Ocular Genetics Clinic. Fourteen were male and 18 female with an age range of 12-54 (mean, 33 years). The estimated prevalence was 1 per 17500. The patients were distributed all over Newfoundland but were primarily in families of English West Country origin. Consanguinity was documented or presumed in six families. Mental retardation was present in 41% of patients. All patients had severe retinal dystrophy but only two had typical retinitis pigmentosa. Polydactyly occurred in 58%, 96% were overweight, and 48% were grossly obese. The majority were below the 50th percentile for height. Other abnormalities included small testes and genitalia, menstrual irregularities, low serum estrogen levels, diabetes mellitus, and renal abnormalities. (Green JS et al. The cardinal manifestations of Bardet-Biedl syndrome, a form of Laurence-Moon-Biedl syndrome. *N Engl J Med* October 12, 1989; *321*:1002-9).

COMMENT. The patients were classified as Bardet-Biedl syndrome rather than Laurence-Moon-Biedl syndrome. The authors conclude that the characteristic features of *Bardet-Biedl syndrome* are 1) severe retinal dystrophy, 2) dysmorphic extremities, 3) obesity, 4) renal abnormalities, and 5) hypogenitalism in male patients only. Mental retardation, polydactyly, and hypogonadism in female patients are not necessarily present.

The earliest reference to this condition appears in *II Samuel* 21:20, in which there is mention of "a man of great stature, that had on every hand six fingers, and on every foot six toes, four and twenty in number; and he also was born to the giant." (Millichap JG. *Proc Roy Soc Med* 1951; *44*:1063). This man was probably related to Goliath. Although the Hebrew word describing the stature is generally accepted to signify tall, the Aramaic translation uses a word "mashach", which means oily or fat. Pliny, in his Natural History, also refers to a baby with six fingers and six toes.

The cardinal signs of the syndrome described by Laurence and Moon (*Ophthal Rev* 1866; *2*:32), in order of their frequency, were obesity, retinitis pigmentosa, mental deficiency, genital dystrophy, familial incidence, and polydactyly. Spastic paraparesis mentioned in the present article was not included and was not present in my own case report. The early retinal changes do not usually conform with the classical picture of retinitis pigmentosa but these may appear in the later stages of the illness. Early retinal abnormalities are nonpigmented degeneration with loss of central vision, minimal peripheral pigmentation of the fundus, optic atrophy and fine retinal vessels. (Lyle DJ. *Amer J Ophthal* 1946; *29*:939). The need to separate patients in the present paper as examples of Bardet-Biedl syndrome seems questionable. Renal abnormalities have been reported in the Laurence-Moon syndrome and spastic paraparesis is not usually a dominant feature of that syndrome. As in most syndromes, individual expressions are variable and one or more of the cardinal features is often absent. - Editor. *Ped Neur Briefs* December 1989.

Prader-Willi Syndrome In Neonates

A retrospective study of 16 patients identifying physical features of neonates with Prader-Willi syndrome is reported from the Department of Pediatrics, Division of Genetics, William Beaumont Hospital, Royal Oak, MI and Section of Genetics, Department of Pediatrics, University of Arizona, Tucson. Medical records of 16 patients observed in the clinic at the University of Connecticut Health Center, Farmington, were reviewed for descriptions made during the newborn period. At the time of the chart review the patients ranged in age from eight months to 33 years. All initial examinations were performed at 22 days of age or earlier. Of 13 patients with high resolution chromosome analysis 12 showed the typical deletion of the long arm of chromosome 15.

Several of the characteristic features of Prader-Willi syndrome in early infancy were confirmed including hypotonia and genital hypoplasia. Features that have not previously been emphasized included an abnormal cry, disproportionately large head circumference and anterior fontanel, mild micrognathia, mild anomalies of gingivae or alveolar ridges, and changes in the appearance of the skin such as poor color, cyanosis, jaundice, ecchymoses, hirsutism, and foot edema. Hypoplasia of the scrotum was present with a normal appearing penis. Contrary to one previous report the hypotonia was associated with absence of deep tendon reflexes, and hyperreflexia was found in only one. (Aughton DJ, Cassidy SB. Physical features of Prader-Willi syndrome in neonates. *AJDC* Nov 1990; *144*:1251-1254).

COMMENT. Prader-Willi syndrome is a sporadic multisystem disorder characterized after infancy by obesity, acromicria, short stature, hypogonadism, and abnormal cognitive and behavioral functioning. Infants exhibit hypotonia, genital hypoplasia, and feeding problems with failure to thrive. The additional neonatal characteristics described in this paper may aid in early diagnosis and counseling of parents. - Editor. *Ped Neur Briefs* December 1990.

Floating-Harbor Syndrome

Six unrelated children with a unique association of short stature, dysmorphic features, and speech delay are reported from the Harbor/Univ of California at Los Angeles Med Center, the Kennedy Memorial Hospital, Boston, the Beilinson Med Center, the District General Hospital, Stanford, England, and the Cedars-Sinai Med Centr, Univ of California, LA. Two were French-Canadian, 2 British, 1 Iranian, and 1 Israeli ancestry. All had growth retardation during the first year, delayed bone age, severe speech delay, and normal or only mildly retarded intelligence. The strikingly similar facial features consisted of a large long nose, thick lips, broad mouth, deep-set eyes and long eyelashes. Growth hormone stimulation, somatomedin-C levels, thyroid, karyotype, and dermatoglyphics were normal. (Robinson P et al. A unique association of short stature, dysmorphic features, and speech impairment. (Floating-Harbor syndrome). *J Pediat* Oct 1988; *113*:703-706).

COMMENT. This unique syndrome was named after the hospitals where the first 2 patients were recognized (Pelletier and Feingold and Leisti et al. In: Bergsma D. ed. *Syndrome Identification*: Vol 1, No 1 and Vol 2, No 1. White Plains, NY:Nat Foundation-March of Dimes, 1973-74). The differential diagnosis includes the Rubinstein-Taybi syndrome, Russell-Silver syndrome, Williams and Noonan syndromes, and Dubowitz and Seckel syndromes. - Editor. *Ped Neur Briefs* October 1988.

Origins Of Cerebral Palsy

The causes of cerebral palsy were determined in a prospective study of 43,437 full term children from data collected in the

Collaborative Perinatal Study of the National Institute of Neurological and Communicative Disorders and Stroke, Bethesda, MD, and published from the Department of Pathology and Center for Biostatistics and Epidemiology, M.S. Hershey Medical Center, Pennsylvania State University College of Medicine, Hershey, PA. The diagnosis of cerebral palsy had been made by neurologic examination at seven years of age in 127 and at one year of age in 23 who then died before the seven year follow-up. The incidence of cerebral palsy in the group studied was 1 in 290 (0.34%).

Based on attributable risk estimates, congenital malformations explained over half (53%) of the cases of quadriplegic cerebral palsy. Only 14% of the cases of quadriplegic CP was attributable to birth asphyxia and 8% to CNS infections. Of 116 nonquadriplegic patients with cerebral palsy congenital disorders explained about one-third and CNS infections about 1 in 20; no cause could be identified for nearly 60% and birth asphyxia was not a significant antecedent. Characteristic consequences of birth asphyxia were more often the result of nonasphyxial disorders. These included meconium in the amniotic fluid, low 10 minute Apgar scores, neonatal apnea spells, seizures, persisting neurologic abnormalities, and slow head growth after birth. Congenital disorders explained nearly four times as many cases of quadriplegic CP then did birth asphyxia (attributable risks, 53% vs 14%, respectively). Congenital disorders were the only factor that explained a large number of the nonquadriplegic CP cases. Oxytocin, whose use was followed by an increased frequency of neonatal seizures, was not followed by a corresponding increase in the frequency of CP. (Naeye, RL et al. Origins of cerebral palsy. *AJDC* October 1989; *143*:1154-1161).

COMMENT. Many previous studies have labeled asphyxia as the cause of CP based on the occurrence of fetal distress and low Apgar scores. In the present study, low ten minute Apgar scores were more often associated with congenital disorders than with birth asphyxia in the CP cases.

Fetal distress and low Apgar scores cannot be used to distinguish CP of asphyxial origin from CP due to congenital malformation. Birth asphyxia or hypoxia that is severe enough to damage the fetal brain usually causes death before or soon after birth. The present authors underscore the importance of making accurate measurements and observations on neonates to avoid misattributing nonasphyxial CP to birth asphyxia. Carefully recorded observations of kidney, heart, and lung function can help to determine cause, because birth asphyxia that is severe enough to damage the brain usually damages the kidneys, lungs, and often the heart.

The purpose of the Collaborative Perinatal Study of the NINCDS was to determine the causes and methods of prevention of cerebral palsy. This present analysis of the data collected from the study shows that no cause could be identified for the majority of cases of cerebral palsy in term infants. Has the Collaborative Study failed in its designed purpose? In an editorial comment, Bedrick AD of the University of Arizona, Tucson, states that "prematurity and low birth weight are strong risk factors for CP. Prevention of preterm delivery would be a tremendous stride in preventing CP." This same comment was voiced by some of the committee members, myself included, 34 years ago in the early planning stages of the Collaborative NINCDS Study, Bethesda, 1955. The proposal of a prospective study restricted to the causes and prevention of prematurity in relation to CP which might have provided early answers was overruled in favor of the more general and involved study of all pregnancies. Much time and energy have been expended in the analysis of the data collected by this extensive study only to conclude that we probably do not know what causes most cases of cerebral palsy. - Editor. *Ped Neur Briefs* October 1989.

Corticospinal Tract In Newborns

The maturation and function of the corticospinal and corticobulbar tracts in the human newborn are reviewed from the Departments of Paediatrics, Pathology and Clinical Neurosciences, University of Calgary Faculty of Medicine, Calgary, Alberta, Canada. The myelination of these tracts begins in late gestation but is not complete until two years of age. Functions attributed to these descending pathways in the full term human newborn include the following: 1) Development of passive muscle tone and resting postures; 2) Enhancement of suck and swallow reflexes; 3) Relay of cortical epileptic discharges; and 4) Inhibition of complex stereotyped motor reflexes ("subtle seizures"). The antagonistic balance between flexors and extensors is controlled by the subcortical spinal and corticospinal pathways. If the corticospinal tract is impaired as with perinatal asphyxia the infant assumes distal flexion and proximal extension postures which reflect the influence of subcorticospinal pathways when corticospinal tract antagonism is lacking.

The "tonic seizures" of preterm infants with intraventricular hemorrhages are probably not true epileptic phenomena but rather episodes of decerebration. A weak suck, poor feed, and impaired coordination of swallowing are findings common to cerebral cortical disturbances in the newborn caused by hypoxia, meningitis, hemorrhage or hydrocephalus. Most human neonatal seizures are focal or multifocal and arise in the cerebral cortex and are relayed by the corticospinal tract to spinal motor neurons and to facial and hypoglossal nuclei by the corticobulbar tract. Some neonatal seizures are subcortical in origin. The corticospinal tract probably does not influence muscle maturation because muscle shows histochemical differentiation at 20-28 weeks gestation, long before myelination of the corticospinal tract begins. Cerebellar influence on muscle tone and coordination is mediated mainly by the corticospinal and corticobulbar tracts. Hypotonia is among the most constant clinical findings in infants with cerebellar hypoplasia. (Sarnat HB. Do the corticospinal and corticobulbar tracts mediate functions in the human newborn? *Can J Neurol Sci* 1989; *16*:157-160).

COMMENT. Dr. Sarnat's research concerning the development of the corticospinal tract in the newborn aids the clinician in his understanding of reflexes, seizures, and muscle tone and posture. In another recent study, acridine orange, a fluorochromic stain of nucleic acids, was used to study neural maturation in human brains during development. The increase in cytoplasmic RNA of neurons coincided with the onset of neurotransmitter synthesis, and the presence of orange fluorescence in heterotopic nerve cells served as a marker of the state of maturity and degree of migration. (Sarnat HB. *Rev Neurol* (Paris), 1989; *145*:127-133). - Editor. *Ped Neur Briefs* October 1989.

CHAPTER **8**

PRENATAL AND PERINATAL DISORDERS

Prenatal Asphyxia In Growth Retarded Fetuses

Members of the Department of Obstetrics at King's College Hospital, London SE5 have measured the umbilical venous oxygen and carbon dioxide tensions, pH, lactate and glucose concentrations, nucleated red cell (erythroblast) content, and haemoglobin concentration in 38 fetuses with intra-uterine growth retardation in which blood sampling was performed by cordocentesis. The oxygen tension was below the normal mean for gestational age in 33 cases (87%). The severity of fetal hypoxia correlated significantly with fetal hypercapnia, acidosis, hyperlacticaemia, hypoglycaemia, and erythroblastosis. The authors conclude that signs of asphyxia at birth are not necessarily due to the process of birth but may originate before birth. (Soothill PW, Nicolaides KH, Campbell S. Prenatal asphyxia, hyperlacticaemia, hypoglycaemia, and erythroblastosis in growth retarded fetuses. *Br Med J* 1987; *294*:1051).

COMMENT. Law courts often assume that any infant who develops cerebral palsy must have been damaged by obstetric mismanagement. This study demonstrates that what happens before delivery is sometimes more important than what happens during and after the birth process. Cordocentesis is attended by technical risks and cannot be used routinely. There is need for a non-invasive and repetitive test for the prenatal diagnosis of fetal hypoxia. (Symonds EM. *Br Med J* 1987; *294*:1046). - Editor. *Ped Neur Briefs* June 1987.

Intracranial Hemorrhage In Term Infants

The authors identified 12 cases of symptomatic intracranial hemorrhage (ICH) among 23,000 infants born at the Beth Israel and Brigham and Women's Hospitals in Boston, MA, in 1982 and 1983. The incidence of ICH was 5.2/10,000 live births or 5.9/10,000 term appropriate-for-gestation age infants (> 2,500 g and > 37 wks gestation). Delivery was spontaneous vaginal in 8, forceps in 3, and cesarean section in 1. Pitocin was used in 5 cases; the indications were induction for postdate in 3 and prolonged second state in 2. Mean Apgar scores at 1 and 5 mins were 5 (range 2-9) and 7 (1-10). Neonatal seizures were the most common presenting symptom, occurring in 7 (60%) infants. Most infants were symptomatic by the second day. Eleven survived the neonatal period. None developed hydrocephalus. The diagnosis of ICH was confirmed by CAT scan. In most cases the hemorrhage was in the subarachnoid space and the CSF obtained by lumbar puncture contained blood. Obstetrical risk factors were: 1) prolonged second stage of labor (> 2 hrs), 2) very rapid labor with rapid descent, and 3) Pitocin and forceps delivery. CAT scan or ultrasound were considered essential for diagnosis of ICH. (Sachs BP, Acker D et al. The incidence of symptomatic intracranial hemorrhage in term appropriate-for-gestation-age infants. *Clin Pediatrics* 1987; *26*:355).

COMMENT. Primary subarachnoid hemorrhage (SAH) was the most common form of hemorrhage in a previous study of 22 term newborn infants seen in a 5 year period with intracranial hemorrhage on CT examination (Fenichel GM et al. *Arch Neurol* 1984; *41*:30). All infants with diffuse SAH had seizures on the first day of life. Five of 10 infants with SAH were born after prolonged labors, traumatic deliveries, and intrauterine asphyxia; three had intrauterine asphyxia. Five of 8 infants with intraventricular hemorrhage (IVH) had difficult deliveries with trauma and asphyxia. In 3 infants with IVH and 3 with intracerebral hemorrhage (ICH) the cause was unexplained, i.e. in almost one-third of the total group. The occurrence of intracranial hemorrhage does not preclude a good outcome. Development was normal or near normal at follow-up in one-half the infants who suffered a SAH and in 3 of 7 with IVH. Seizures in the first week of life are an important sign of SAH, IVH and ICH, occurring in almost all cases. - Editor. *Ped Neur Briefs* August 1987.

Prognosis Of Neonatal Asphyxia

Of 86 asphyxiated full-term neonates with CNS complications admitted to the Intensive Care Unit at the Nagoya City University Hospital, Japan, during a 10 year period (1972-81), 63 (73%) survived the neonatal period. The CNS complications were hypoxic-ischemic encephalopathy (58), intracranial hemorrhage (27) and brain infarction (1). Of 54 survivors who were followed for 3-13 years, 8 (15%) had major handicaps such as cerebral palsy, epilepsy and mental retardation and 5 (9%) had minor CNS abnormalities. Factors predictive of long-term CNS sequelae were: 1) absent Moro-reflex over 6-days, and 2) abnormal neurological signs on discharge.

Each neonate had a 1 min Apgar score of 6 or less, neurological abnormalities including stupor or lethargy, hypotonia, abnormal respirations, jitteriness or seizures, and one or more abnormal findings on laboratory tests such as spinal tap, echoencephalography, cerebral angiography, EEG, and CAT scan. (Ogawa IT, Kanayama M, Wada Y. Long-term prognosis of asphyxiated full-term neonates with CNS complications. *Brain Dev* 1987; *9*:48-53).

> COMMENT. Another method of assessment of neurologic outcome in asphyxiated term infants is by use of serial CK-BB, or creatine kinase brain-type isoenzyme measurement (Walsh P. *J Pediat* 1982; *101*:988). Serum CK-BB activity, when measured in cord blood and at 6-12 hours of life, correlates with neurologic outcome after severe asphyxia, comparing favorably with CT scanning as a prognostic factor. The mean of elevations in CK-BB in the asphyxiated was 4-fold the values obtained in control infants. Normal CK-BB activity was a predictor of good neurologic outcome. - Editor. *Ped Neur Briefs* August 1987.

Serum CPK And
Hypoxic-Ischemic Encephalopathy (HIE)

The value of brain-typical creatine phosphokinase isoenzyme (CPK-BB) determinations in the assessment of brain damage due to neonatal asphyxia in 33 full-term infants has been assessed in the Services of Neonatology, Child Neurology and Radiology, Clinica Infantil, Cindad Sanitaria "La Paz", Madrid, Spain. Serum CPK activities measured at 4 hrs after birth were significantly higher in infants who died of HIE or developed neurological sequelae than in those asphyxiated infants who showed no neurological abnormalities during a 16 mo follow-up period or in a control group of 20 infants delivered normally. At 10 hrs afer birth, the enzyme levels in brain damaged infants had decreased markedly and overlapped with values obtained in infants without sequelae at follow-up. Compared to the neurological exams, EEGs, and CT scans obtained in the first or second week of life, the CPK assay was inferior as a predictor of neurological outcome. Normal CPK, CT and EEGs, and mild clinical encephalopathy were 96-100% predictive of a favorable outcome in asphyxiated full-term infants. (Fernandez F et al. Serum CPK-BB isoenzyme in the assessment of brain damage in asphyctic term infants. *Acta Paediatr Scan* Dec 1987; *76*:914-918).

> COMMENT. In this study, an elevated serum CPK measured within 4 hrs after birth was a sensitive indicator of brain damage in asphyxiated term infants but was of limited prognostic value in assessment of neurological outcome. These results contrast with those reported by Walsh P (*J Pediat* 1982; *101*:988), who found that serum CPK-BB activity measured in cord blood and at 6-12 hrs of life correlated with neurological outcome after severe asphyxia and compared favorably with CT scanning as a prognostic indicator. Normal CPK-BB activity was a predictor of good neurologic outcome in both studies. - Editor. *Ped Neur Briefs* February 1988.

Birth Complications And Risk Of Cerebral Palsy

Statisticians at the National Institutes of Health (NINCDS), Bethesda, MD have compared the follow-up neurologic status of full-term infants whose birth was complicated but who were free of signs of hypoxic-ischemic encephalopathy (HIE) in the nursery period with asymptomatic infants whose births were uncomplicated. The rate of CP was 2.3/1000 in asymptomatic infants with one or more birth complications and 2.4/1000 among asymptomatic infants whose births were uncomplicated. A total of 41,012 patients was evaluated at 7 years of age in the National Collaborative Perinatal Project (NCPP). The full-term infant whose birth was complicated but who was free from abnormal signs of HIE in the newborn period was not at increased risk of CP. The neonatal signs judged indicative of HIE were 1) decreased activity after the first day of life, 2) need for incubator care for three or more days, 3) feeding problems, 4) poor suck, 5) respiratory difficulty, and/or 6) neonatal seizures. (Nelson KB, Ellenberg JH. The asymptomatic newborn and risk of cerebral palsy. *AJDC* 1987; *141*:1333-1335).

COMMENT. Term infants whose brains have been injured during delivery show signs of damage in the neonatal period. Children with sustained neurologic abnormality in the newborn period are at a higher risk of CP than those with transient abnormalities. The risk increases directly with the number of abnormal signs. Neonatal seizures are the most reliable evidence of intrapartum asphyxia. The Apgar score is not the best indicator. In the NCPP, the proportion of CP attributable to asphyxia - as defined by a 5-min Apgar score of < 6 - was about 25%. Most children with CP do not have low Apgars at birth. Only about 12% of surviving children with Apgar scores of 0-3 developed CP (Nelson K, Ellenberg J. *Pediatrics* 1981; *68*:36). For babies over 2500 gm, irrespective of birth complication, most achieved 5-min Apgar scores of 7 or higher, and the risk of CP was not significantly higher than in children whose births were uncomplicated. The risk of CP attending low Apgars was conditioned on low birth weight, and 25% of CP cases are attributable to premature delivery (Freeman JM, Editor, Prenatal and perinatal factors associated with brain disorders. NIH Publication 1985; No 85-1149). - Editor. *Ped Neur Briefs* December 1987.

Brainstem Injury From Perinatal Asphyxia

The clinical, radiological and neuropathological features of selective hypoxic-ischemic injury of the brainstem with relative sparing of cortex and subcortical white matter in an asphyxiated term infant are described in a case reported from the Division of Neurology and Depts of Pediatrics, Pathology and Radiology, British Columbia's Children's Hospital, Vancouver, Canada. The infant was pale, flaccid and without respiratory effort at birth and seizures occurred during the first hour. The Apgar score was one at 1, 5 and 10 min. The signs of brainstem dysfunction included abnormal horizontal eye movements, facial diplegia and ptosis, tongue fasciculations, and abnormal auditory evoked potentials. CT showed increased attenuation in the basal ganglia at 2 wks, and dilation of the third ventricle at 1 mo.

Lateral ventricles and cortical sulci were normal, showing no atrophy.

The infant died of pneumonia at 4 mos of age. Neuropathological examination revealed scarring and pallor of the thalamus, basal ganglia and brainstem with neuronal loss and gliosis. (Roland EH et al. Selective brainstem injury in an asphyxiated newborn. *Ann Neurol* Jan 1988; *23*:89-92).

> COMMENT. In animal studies, selective brainstem damage occurs after acute total asphyxia whereas the cerebral cortex and subcortical white matter are predominantly affected by prolonged partial asphyxia. In the human infant, the localization of hypoxic-ischemic encephalopathy is generally more diffuse (Volpe JJ *Neurology of the Newborn* 2nd ed, Philadelphia, Saunders, 1987) and selective brainstem injury is rare and frequently fatal. - Editor. *Ped Neur Briefs* February 1988.

Cerebral Palsy

A professor of obstetrics at the Univ of California at Davis School of Med, Sacramento, reviewing the relationship of obstetric care and management of asphyxia to the subsequent development of cerebral palsy (CP), refers to his own previously published study at Oxford University (*Lancet* 1984; 2:827) and a similar study in progress at the Univ of Newcastle, England. Babies who were at risk for development of CP were compared with matched normal controls. The frequencies of substandard obstetric care were determined in the controls and in all cases of fetal death from asphyxia or trauma, those with severe asphyxia, convulsions in the first 48 hrs of life, and in children recognized to have CP at 18 months of age.

Quality of care during labor proved to be less important than prenatal care. Substandard care during labor was not related to severe asphyxia, neonatal convulsions, or CP. A delay in the initiation of treatment for diagnosed asphyxia was not observed in CP cases, was uncommon in the control group (1.4%), but was frequent in cases of fetal death (20%), convulsions (7.9%) and severe birth asphyxia (5.4%). Substandard intrapartum care and especially the lack or failure to react appropriately to electronic fetal monitoring was causally related to neonatal seizures but not to CP.

A possible causal relationship of perinatal asphyxia and CP should require the following: 1) severe newborn acidosis, 2) damage to other organs, 3) severe neurologic abnormalities in the first 24-72 hrs. (Niswander KR. Does substandard care cause cerebral palsy? *Contemporary Pediatrics* Jan 1988; 5(1):56-76).

COMMENT. This review and study tend to confirm the results and conclusions of the Neurological Collaborative Perinatal Project (NCPP) concerning prenatal and perinatal factors associated with brain disorders: only 25% of CP cases may be attributed to asphyxia at birth and CP is only very rarely preceded by potentially preventable perinatal asphyxia. (Freeman JM, Ed. NIH *Publications 85-1149*, April 1985). - Editor. *Ped Neur Briefs* February 1988.

Periventricular Leukomalacia And Bilirubin Toxicity
The role of bilirubin toxicity and other factors in the etiology of extensive periventricular leukomalacia of 5 preterm infants was investigated in the Department of Paediatrics, Tampere University Central Hospital, Tampere, Finland. Diagnosis was made by routine ultrasound screening, and the perinatal course and later development of affected infants was compared with 12 normal controls. Infants with leukomalacia were delivered more often by the vaginal route, their mean highest serum total bilirubin and blood pH were significantly higher than the controls. The authors speculate that bilirubin toxicity may play an important role in addition to ischemia in the severe cases of periventricular leukomalacia. (Ikonen RS et al. Possible etiological factors in extensive periventricular leukomalacia of preterm infants. *Acta Paediatr Scand* July 1988; 77:489-495).

COMMENT. The periventricular white matter in preterm infants is susceptible to ischemia and factors leading to hypotension can cause leukomalacia. Vaginal delivery and compression of the head of the preterm infant caused by uterine contractions during labor may lead to cerebral ischemia, but other causes include birth asphyxia, hypoxia, and hypocarbia. Although the basic cause of periventricular leukomalacia is ischemia, bilirubin toxicity may occur when the blood brain barrier is damaged by anoxia, permitting bilirubin to enter the brain even when bound to albumin. - Editor. *Ped Neur Briefs* August 1988.

Neuropathology Of Prenatal Brain Damage

Autopsy results of 89 infants who died at 7 days of age or less were analyzed in the Depts of Pathology and Pediatrics, University of California School of Medicine, Davis, CA. Twenty-two (25%) showed evidence of prenatal brain lesions; 10 (16%) were preterm and 12 (48%) were term infants. Term infants were affected more often than those born prematurely. The prenatal injuries in both premature and term infants were characterized by cerebral white matter necrosis and gliosis without hemorrhage. Hydramnios was the only maternal condition that predicted prenatal damage. Apgar scores were low, seizures were rare, and acute intracranial hemorrhage occurred equally often in infants with and without prenatal injury. The causes of death were primarily cardiorespiratory. The findings support growing evidence for the prenatal onset of brain injury in many infants who survive and later develop cerebral palsy. (Ellis WG et al. Neuropathological documentation of prenatal brain damage. *AJDC* Aug 1988; *142*:858-866).

COMMENT. Cordocentesis has been employed to detect prenatal hypoxia (see *Ped Neur Briefs* June 1987; 1:1) but the test is attended by technical risks and cannot be used routinely. As the authors comment, neonatal care will increase survival for prenatally damaged infants and the incidence of cerebral palsy may rise unless fetal/maternal abnormalities in late gestation are identified and corrected. There is need for a non-invasive and repetitive test for prenatal diagnosis of fetal hypoxia. - Editor. *Ped Neur Briefs* July 1988.

White Matter Necrosis In Neonates

The neuropathologic and ultrasonographic findings in 22 very low birth weight infants surviving at least 6 days are described from Michigan State University, East Lansing, MI., St. Luke's Roosevelt Medical Center and New York Hospital Cornell Medical Center, NY. White matter necrosis was found in 15 of the 22 subjects and affected hemispheric white matter in ten. The classic features of periventricular leukomalacia were absent from 7 of the 15 infants with necrosis. Intraventricular hemorrhage had occurred in 17. Increased parenchymal echogenicity and ventricular enlargement were present in 67% of infants with white matter necrosis. (Paneth N et al. White matter necrosis in very low birth weight infants; neuropathologic and ultrasonographic findings in infants surviving six days or longer. *J Pediatr* June 1990; *116*:975-984).

COMMENT. White matter necrosis need not be restricted to the periventricular regions and ultrasonographic scanning should include more peripheral areas of the brain. - Editor. *Ped Neur Briefs* August 1990.

Baer In High Risk Infants

Brainstem auditory responses (BAER) performed on 667 high risk infants from an infant special care unit were evaluated at the Department of Otolaryngology, University of Texas Medical Branch, Galveston, Texas. Infants who failed the test were classified into two groups; those who failed at 30 dB hearing level and those who failed at 45 dB hearing level. At follow-up examination in one, three, or six months, 8 (1.2%) had severe sensorineural hearing impairments (since only 50% returned for follow-up, 2.4% was a more accurate incidence). Conductive hearing loss was found in 15.7% (17/108) of those who passed

30 dB level and in 34.3% (12/34) of those who failed. The use of BAER testing at levels less than 45 dB permitted detection of middle ear disorders. All of the infants who failed at 45 dB hearing level and had abnormal results at the 3-4 month follow-up examination had severe sensorineural or moderate to severe mixed hearing losses. For the group that failed at 30 dB hearing level and were abnormal at follow-up, 80% had conductive hearing disorders and 20% had mild sensorineural hearing impairments. Infants enrolled in a parent-infant program for hearing impairment by 6 months of age were referred from the BAER program. (Kramer SJ et al. Auditory brainstem responses and clinical follow-up of high-risk infants. *Pediatrics* March 1989; *83*:385-392).

COMMENT. The brainstem auditory evoked response test (BAER) is effective in the early detection of hearing impairments in high risk neonates, and the degree and type of hearing loss may be predicted. However, the children who were referred to the BAER program represented only 31% of the total number of parent-infant program children with congenital hearing impairment and only 50% of the children with multiple handicaps. Some of the hearing impaired children entering the parent-infant program at this center during the period of the study were referred from sources other than the BAER program and were much older when enrolled. An infant hearing assessment program for only high risk infants would fail to identify approximately one-half of hearing impaired children. - Editor. *Ped Neur Briefs* May 1989.

Prognosis Of Very Low Birth-Weight Infants

The cognitive and motor abilities of 43 very low birth weight children (VLBW) and classroom controls are reported from the Greenwood Children's Centre, City Hospital, Nottingham, England. Children born in 1981 and weighing less than 1501 grams who had received treatment in the neonatal intensive care unit were followed up on entry to primary school at the age of 5 years. Those included in the study were apparently normal with no observed handicap or need for special educational services. The results on the McCarthy Scales of Children's Abilities were compared with those of matched class-mates. Significant differences were found between the two groups on all six scales and were most marked on the general cognitive index. The mean IQ score for the study children was 88 compared with 101 for the controls. No child in the control group scored below 74, whereas 8 of the study children scored below 70 and were in need of special education. (Abel Smith AE, Knight-Jones, EB. The abilities of very low birth weight children and their classroom controls. *Dev Med Child Neurol* July 1990; 32:592-601).

COMMENT. In addition to the immediate morbidity and mortality, the cognitive deficits of very low birth weight children are a concern. One third of the VLBW infants born in the Nottingham Centre died in the neonatal peri-od, but two-thirds appeared to be developing normally on the basis of early follow-up studies. Learning difficulties among the study group became increasingly apparent at higher educational levels, although in their first year of school none had been uncovered. - Editor. *Ped Neur Briefs* August 1990.

CHAPTER 9

CNS NEOPLASMS

Brain Tumors In Infants

The clinical manifestations, histological typing, location and results of surgical and oncological treatment in 76 children with intracranial tumors presenting during the first 2 years of life are reported from the Hopital Neurologique et Neurochirurgical Pierre Wertheimer, Service de Neurochirurgie Infantile, BP Lyon Montchat, Lyon, France. Patients were analyzed in groups according to age (29 under 1 yr and 47 between 1-2 yrs) and malignancy. A slight male preponderance was observed in children up to 1 year, while an equal sex distribution was found in the older group. Supratentorial tumors were most prevalent during the 1st year, and the posterior fossa location was most frequent after 1 year. Increased intracranial pressure and hydrocephalus were the chief clinical manifestations. Medulloblastoma and ependymoma were most frequent in the highly malignant group and astrocytoma in the low-malignant group.

The overall survival rate was 46% following operation; 22% recovered completely and have survived 8 mos to 14 yrs, and 13% have a mild neurological deficit. In those with medulloblastoma or ependymoma requiring radiotherapy, only 20% had favorable neuropsychological results. No patient with a highly malignant tumor operated on during the first year of life survived later. Brain irradiation in this age group leads to a severely handicapped child and chemotherapy is preferred for highly malignant tumors, especially when surgical excision is incomplete. Radical surgery is proposed as the ideal treatment. (Lapras C et al. Brain tumors in infants: a study of 76 patients operated upon. *Child's Nerv Syst* April 1988; *4*:100-103).

> COMMENT. In 17 children with intracranial neoplasms presenting within the first 2 months of life, alterations in behavior, anorexia, vomiting, irritability, or unusual quiet-ness were the most common symptoms and 10 had macro-crania and hydrocephalus (Jooma R et al. *Surg Neurol* 1984; *21*:165). The operative mortality was 40% and the total case mortality was 80%. These authors from the Hosp for Sick Children, Great Ormond St, London, felt that an aggressive approach to most of the cases in this age group was not warranted at present, and the radiation dose is lim-ited by the increased sensitivity of the immature brain.

> A first report of medulloblastoma in an 8-yr-old patient with *Coffin-Siris syndrome* (Rogers L et al. *Child's Nerv Syst* 1988; *4*:41) was diagnosed during an evaluation for neurogenic causes of apnea and feeding difficulties. This syndrome is a rare congenital disorder characterized by mental retardation, deficient postnatal growth, joint laxity, and brachydactyly of the 5th digit with absence of the nail bed. Several cases of Dandy Walker cysts and a case of brain stem heterotopia have been described previously as complications of the syndrome. - Editor. *Ped Neur Briefs* June 1988.

Neonatal Craniopharyngioma

A craniopharyngioma detected in utero using ultrasound is reported from the Depts of Neurosurgery, Neonatology,

Pathology, and Obstetrics and Gynecology, New York University Medical Center, New York, NY. The obstetric ultrasound study performed because of premature labor at 35 weeks showed poly-hydramnios and macrocephaly secondary to an intracranial, cal-cified lobulated mass. A CT scan performed at 2 hrs of life demonstrated a calcified intracranial mass extending to the base of the skull. The infant suffered cardiorespiratory arrest and died at the second day of life. At postmortem examination, the suprasellar mass was a granular tumor with multiple cysts filled with green mucoid material. Microscopically, the tumor showed branching cords and palisading of epithelial cells, focal calcifica-tions, and an inner zone of stellate cells, an appearance diagnos-tic of craniopharyngioma. The authors uncovered only four other reports of congenital intracranial neoplasm diagnosed pre-natally using ultrasound. Three were teratomas and one a dys-plastic mass. Calcifications have been observed in teratomas and meningiomas in utero and are not pathognomonic of cranio-pharyngioma. Low set ears and polydactyly are reported as associated congenital anomalies. Polyhydramnios occurred in all five cases of neonatal brain tumors diagnosed antenatally by ultrasound. Radical excision of the tumor in the neonatal period was not advised. (Freeman TB et al. Neonatal craniopharyn-gioma. *NY State J Med* Feb 1988; *88*:81-83).

COMMENT. Craniopharyngiomas comprise about 3% of all intracranial tumors at all ages and 9% in children. Only 10 cases of neonatal craniopharyngioma were culled from the literature. Radical excision for cases presenting in infancy is recommended by the following authors reporting their experiences with 50 cases in Paris. - Editor. *Ped Neur Briefs* May 1988.

Treatment Of Craniopharyngioma In Infancy

A retrospective analysis of the outcome of 50 cases of cran-iopharyngioma treated in infancy by radical or subtotal surgical excision and irradiation is reported from the services of Neurosurgery and Endocrinology, Hopital des Enfants Malades,

149, reu de Sevres, 75743 Paris Cedex 15, France. The authors concluded that 1) radical excision is the treatment of choice; 2) if radical excision is not possible, surgery should be followed by irradiation to lower risk of recurrence; and 3) radiotherapy should be delayed as long as possible because of hazards to growing brain and used only when tumor recurrence has been demonstrated. After radical excision, the rate of recurrence was lowest, with a 10 year recurrence-free survival rate of 88%. After subtotal removal, the recurrence-free survival rate, 10 yrs post-op, was 37%; this rate was significantly higher (72%) when subtotal removal was followed by irradiation, but deafness and severe neuropsychological and intellectual sequelae were frequent complications of irradiation. Post-operative mortality was low in pre-chiasmatic cases and high in retro-chiasmatic tumors. Surgical statistics may improve with newer techniques. (Pierre-Kahn A et al. Traitement des craniopharyngiomes de l'enfant. Analyse retrospective de 50 observations. *Arch Fr Pediatr* Mars 1988; *45*:163-167).

> COMMENT. The neuropsychological deficits ascribed to irradiation in this report may be explained in part by the location of the tumor. Cognitive defects have been correlated with frontal lobe abnormalities seen on MRI in 4 patients with craniopharyngioma (Stelling MW et al. *Am J Dis Child* 1986; *140*:710). - Editor. *Ped Neur Briefs* May 1988.

West Syndrome And Cerebral Tumors

Two infants, six and seven months of age, with West syndrome associated with cerebral tumors are reported from the Department of Neurology, Pediatric Hospital, Buenos Aires, Argentina. Initial neurologic examinations were normal and the diagnosis of the tumors was by ultrasound and CT. One infant had a Grade III glioma in the right thalamus and the other had an anaplastic ependymoma and cyst in the right hemisphere. EEGs revealed generalized hypsarrhythmia in both cases. Infantile spasms responded to ACTH 5 IU/kg/day. One patient died at 18 months of age and the other was seizure free after complete surgical resection of the ependymoma. (Ruggieri V et al. Intracranial tumors and West syndrome. *Pediatr Neurol* Sept/Oct 1989; *5*:327-9).

COMMENT. Other brain tumors associated with West syndrome have included choroid plexus papilloma, ganglioglioma, and optic nerve glioma. Infantile spasms and choroid plexus papilloma have also been described in Aicardi syndrome. - Editor. *Ped Neur Briefs* October 1989.

Chiasmatic/Hypothalamic Gliomas

Twenty-four children with progressive chiasmatic/ hypothalamic glioma (CHG) have been treated with actinomycin D and vincristine combination chemotherapy without radiotherapy and followed for a median of 4.3 yrs at the Children's Hospital of Philadelphia, PA. Diagnosis and treatment required a positive CT or MRI, histological confirmation in 15 without optic nerve involvement, and progressive neurological or visual deterioration. Fifteen (62.5%) are free of progression with normal IQs, 9 showing tumor regression, and 9 have radiographic or clinical progression of the tumor within 2-6 yrs after initiation of therapy. The authors allude to intellectual and endocrinological sequelae of radiotherapy for CHG in young children and conclude that chemotherapy may significantly delay the need for radiotherapy. (Packer RJ et al. Treatment of chiasmatic/hypothalamic gliomas of childhood with chemotherapy: an update. *Ann Neurol* Jan 1988; *23*:79-85).

COMMENT. Both radiotherapy and chemotherapy carry the risk of potentially serious adverse effects. Histological confirmation of the tumor type before initiation of therapy may now be possible since thin-needle biopsy with CT guidance is an accepted low risk procedure for neurosurgeons (Szeiniak et al. *Cancer* 1984; *54*:2385). - Editor. *Ped Neur Briefs* February 1988.

Optic Nerve Glioma

The clinical presentation, diagnosis, response to therapy, and visual outcome of 18 children with optic nerve glioma are reported from the Division of Neurology, Department of Pediatrics, University of British Columbia, Vancouver, Canada. Failing vision was the presenting symptom in 13 patients and 15 had an incorrect initial diagnosis which resulted in many years of treatment delay with consequent further visual impairment and reduced efficacy of treatment. In patients presenting with visual impairment, the time from presentation to diagnosis was 28 months whereas in five with increased intracranial pressure, the diagnosis was made within three months. Incorrect initial diagnoses included idiopathic nystagmus (3), congenital optic nerve atrophy (3), squint, diencephalic tumor, multiple sclerosis, and hysteria. Following radiotherapy, an improvement in vision was observed only in those children who presented with increased intracranial pressure and who were diagnosed early. Multiple cafe-au-lait spots were observed in five children. (Appleton RE, Jan JE. Delayed diagnosis of optic nerve glioma: A preventable cause of visual loss. *Pediatr Neurol* July/Aug 1989; 5:226-8).

COMMENT. In young children presenting with nystagmus, squint, optic atrophy, or visual impairment, the possibility of optic nerve glioma should be considered. The diagnosis is especially likely if signs of neurofibromatosis are associated. Early diagnosis may prevent visual loss and may influence the efficacy of radiotherapy. - Editor. *Ped Neur Briefs* October 1989.

Pineal Region Tumors Of Childhood

At the University Hospital, Hamburg, from 1980-85, 17 children had pineal region tumors among 102 children with CNS tumors. The authors conclude: 1) that the incidence in Germany is higher than assumed and at least equal to that in Japan, 2) radiation without histological confirmation is not justified, 3) surgical removal, successful in 20 cases, is reasonably safe, 4) cranio-spinal axis radiation, either post-operatively or alone, is indicated for germinomas that have a tendency for CSF ependymal proliferation and/or seeding, 5) all children treated successfully by both surgery and radiation have not relapsed. (Schulte FJ et al. *Eur J Pediatr* 1987; *146*:233-245).

COMMENT. Pineal tumors are of two main types: 1) germinomas of the pineal or suprasellar region, and 2) pineal parenchymatous tumors (pineoblastomas in younger children and pineocytomas in older children and adults). Spinal seeding, more common with germinomas, occurs in 2-15% of pineal tumors.

Parinaud's syndrome (impairments of upward gaze, convergence, and accommodation), is the classical presentation, usually with signs of increased intracranial pressure. Visual loss, diabetes insipidus, precocious puberty, and emaciation point to anterior hypothalamic involvement. Precocious puberty only occurs in males. Suprasellar teratomas present with visual loss, hypopituitarism, and diabetes insipidus.

Calcification occurs in 25-75% of pineal area tumors, rarely in children under 10 years of age, and especially in germinomas or embryonal carcinomas. CT scan demonstrates location but may not differentiate type of tumor. Oncofetal antigens (human chorionic gonadotrophin and alpha-fetoprotein) in serum and spinal fluid may help in diagnosis and response to therapy.

Operative mortality and morbidity in the past have been high. Shunt surgery and/or biopsy followed by radiotherapy has a 50-80% survival rate. The present authors make a point for surgical removal and postoperative radiation. (For further references see 1) Cohen ME, Duffner PK. *Brain Tumors in Children*, Raven Press, NY, 1984; 2) Sano K, Matsutani M. *Child's Brain* 1981; *8*:81-97; 3) Raimondi AJ, Tomita T. *Child's Brain* 1982; *9*:239-266). - Editor. *Ped Neur Briefs* July 1987.

Hypothalamic Hamartoma And Sexual Precocity

Four boys with hypothalamic hamartomas associated with sexual precocity are reported from the Departments of Pediatrics and Neurosurgery, University of Pittsburgh, and the Department of Pediatrics, Johns Hopkins University School of Medicine, Baltimore, MD. Two patients were treated surgically by resection using current microsurgical techniques and two received medical management. Precocious puberty caused by hamartomas occurs early in life with enlarged penis and muscular build noted in early infancy. Growth is accelerated and bone age is advanced. Deepening of the voice and the appearance of acne are common. Other clinical findings include mental retardation, behavioral disturbances, and seizures of gelastic, absence, and generalized tonic clonic patterns. In the two patients treated surgically, subsequent growth and development were normal and in two who were diagnosed late in childhood and treated medically, the adult height was not particularly compromised. The authors recommend surgical resection if the hamartoma is pedunculated or in cases where the patient is young and would require years of parenteral medical treatment. The nontreatment option exists because there is no evidence that the tumors will grow or subsequently cause other problems. (Starceski PJ et al. Hypothalamic hamartomas and sexual precocity. Evaluation of treatment options. *AJDC* Feb 1990; *144*:225-228).

COMMENT. The use of MRI with sagittal, coronal, and axial views enable better visualization of hamartomas and earlier diagnosis. Treatment to allow growth and pubertal development to occur at an age appropriate time may avoid considerable psychosocial stress and prevent premature skeletal maturation and a shorter adult stature. Medical treatment with long-acting gonadotrophin releasing hormone must be administered through childhood and surgery is sometimes preferred. - Editor. *Ped Neur Briefs* February 1990.

Meningiomas In Childhood

The clinical presentation and pathological characteristics of 18 meningiomas among 240 surgically verified intracranial space-occupying lesions in children are reported from the Depts of Neurosurgery and Pathology, National Inst of Mental Health, Bangalore and Nizam's Inst of Med Sciences, Panjagutta, Hyderabad, India. The tumor location was supratentorial in 15, infratentorial in 2, and intraorbital in 1 patient. The majority presented between 11-15 years of age and the sexes were equally affected. The most common presenting symptoms were headache in 11 and vomiting in 4 patients; hemiparesis, deteriorating vision and seizures were early manifestations in 3, 3 and 2 patients, respectively. The duration of symptoms before diagnosis was less than 1 month in 50% patients. The meningiomas were large, 4 showed sarcomatous change, 6 were cystic, and one recurred, requiring 3 operations. Two patients died postoperatively. (Kolluri VRS, Reddy DR et al. Meningiomas in childhood. *Child's Nerv Syst* 1987; *3*(5):271-273).

COMMENT. Meningioma is an uncommon intracranial tumor of childhood, accounting for less than 5% in previous reports and 7.5% in the above study. In some larger series, the incidence is quoted at 0.4-1.5%. Contrast CT is usually superior to MRI in radiologic diagnosis (Zimmerman RD et al. *AJNR* 1985; *6*:149). CT can distinguish orbital meningioma from optic nerve glioma in about 75% of cases. In the remainder, angiography shows a tumor blush with meningioma, a finding that is absent with optic nerve glioma (Jakobiec FA et al. *Ophthalmology* 1984; *91*:137).

Proptosis was an early presenting sign of orbital meningioma in the present study, leading to prompt diagnosis, whereas this manifestation was late in appearance in the following case-report of multiple meningiomas. - Editor. *Ped Neur Briefs* February 1988.

Multiple Meningiomas In A Child

The unusual case of a 4-yr, 5-mo-old boy with multiple meningiomas without neurofibromatosis is reported from the Children's Memorial Hospital and Northwestern University Medical School, Chicago, IL. The boy had presented with an external deviation, severe loss of vision and retinal "scar" in the right eye at 2 yrs of age and a history of progressive painless proptosis of the same eye for one year. At the time of diagnosis, a complete oculomotor nerve palsy with dilated pupil unreactive to direct and consensual light stimulation, ptosis, and a visual acuity of 20/300 were present on the right. Intracranial, intraorbital, and asymptomatic epidural cervical spine meningiomas were demonstrated by CT and MRI scans and by angiography. All tumors were surgically excised successfully. (Tomita T et al. Multiple meningiomas in a child. *Surg Neurol* Feb 1988; *29*:131-6).

> COMMENT. Proptosis was a late sign of the intraorbital meningioma in this case, preceded by external deviation of the eye and loss of vision for a period of 18 mos. Meningiomas may involve the nasal wall of the orbit and invade the olfactory groove as in the present case, or may originate at the sphenoidal ridge and cause the classical syndrome of unilateral anosmia, optic atrophy or papilledema, and exophthalmos. With extension of the tumor to the cribriform plate, the anosmia can be bilateral and more readily detected even in children.
>
> The young child is unlikely to react to an oil of wintergreen or toothpaste odor test. However, taste is partially perceived through the olfactory system, and the mother may have noticed a loss of appetite sufficient to excite an index of suspicion of involvement of the first cranial nerve, that often neglected part of the neurologic and eye examinations. Early diagnosis and treatment of meningiomas involving the orbit and presenting with loss of vision led to improved visual acuity in 9 of 10 patients with tumors less

than 3 cm in diameter and in 56% of a total of 85 patients followed postoperatively. (Kadis GN et al. *Surg Neurol* 1979; *12*:367). - Editor. *Ped Neur Briefs* February 1988.

Dysplastic Gangliocytoma And Partial Seizures

The clinical, radiologic and EEG features of three children with dysplastic gangliocytoma of the cerebral hemispheres and drug resistant partial seizures are described from the Comprehensive Epilepsy Center and Department of Neurology, Miami Children's Hospital, Miami, FL. A two year old girl had recurrent right-sided focal motor seizures that began within hours of birth; a 15 year old boy had habitual left-sided sensory seizures and infrequent grand mal attacks beginning at age three; and an eight month old boy was hospitalized following an episode of head trauma with unconsciousness and apnea followed by recurrent seizures consisting of staring, eye blinking and left versive head movement. None of the cases manifested a mass effect and the EEG findings lateralized to one hemisphere. Following cortical resection, two became seizure free and the third was almost seizure free. The authors consider that dysplastic gangliocytoma may be an important and surgically remedial cause of very early malignant partial seizures. (Duchowny M S et al. Dysplastic gangliocytoma and intractable partial seizures in childhood. *Neurology* April 1989; *39*:602-604).

COMMENT. Gangliocytomas are usually localized to the cerebellum and those originating in the cerebral hemispheres are much less common but may be epileptogenic. CT demonstrates hyperdense noncontrast enhancing regions and MRIs reveal medium intensity regions in the T-1 weighted and proton density images. The authors consider that subdural electrode recording can facilitate early surgical intervention by localizing epileptogenic regions and defining cortical regions of functional significance. The use of subdural electrodes to study the EEG features of simple partial seizures in seven patients is described in an additional article in this same issue of

Neurology. (Devinsky O et al. *Neurology* April 1989; 39;527-533). - Editor. *Ped Neur Briefs* April 1989.

Intracranial Lymphoma And Gradenigo Syndrome

A 13 year old black male patient with a T-cell lymphoma who presented with Gradenigo syndrome is reported from the Department of Pediatrics, Tulane University School of Medicine, New Orleans, LA. There was a seven day history of headache described as right-sided, throbbing pain, posterior to the eye and associated with right-sided facial numbness. After five days he developed double vision on right lateral gaze and marked decrease of pinprick sensation of the entire right face and loss of the right corneal reflex. Red glass testing confirmed diplopia from a weakness of the right lateral rectus muscle. CT revealed dural enhancement in the medial aspect of the right middle cranial fossa adjacent to the sella turcica. MRI showed the right internal carotid artery compressed and encased by the mass and the Meckel's cave segment of the trigeminal nerve was obliterated. A transphenoidal biopsy provided the diagnosis of T-cell lymphoma, Lennert type, and further evaluation revealed diffuse involvement of bone marrow, spleen, kidneys, and testes. Immunologic workup showed hypogammaglobulinemia. Chemotherapy and radiotherapy resulted in completed resolution of all symptoms and signs. (Norwood VF, Haller JS. Gradenigo syndrome as presenting sign of T-cell lymphoma. *Pediatr Neurol* Nov-Dec 1989; 5:377-380).

COMMENT. Gradenigo syndrome consists of cranial nerve VI palsy and abnormalities of the sensory component of ipsilateral cranial nerve V. Gradenigo described the symptom complex with middle ear infections and it has been reported as a result of tumors, most commonly neurofibroma. The primary neurologic presentation of lymphoma was unique and a new etiology for Gradenigo syndrome. - Editor. *Ped Neur Briefs* February 1990.

Epilepsy, Temporal Lobe Sclerosis And Tumors

Sixteen of 48 children undergoing temporal lobectomy for temporal lobe epilepsy at the Hospital for Sick children, Toronto, Ontario, were found to have tumors (12 patients), vascular malformations (3), and arachnoid cyst (1). Nine of these patients had concomitant mesial temporal sclerosis. In 11 of 18 operations (61%), it was necessary to extend the original cortical excision because of persistent epileptiform activity. The duration of seizures in the 16 patients varied from 1 and 13 years (average 6 years). Memory was impaired in 31% of patients, 39% had behavior problems, and 39% had deteriorating school performance.

Temporal lobectomy was performed on the right side in 8 cases and on the left side in 8. Four patients had an increased neurological deficit postoperatively and all had contralateral superior quadrantanopic defects. Of 15 patients followed for more than 1 year, 9 are seizure free (only 4 on medication), and 7 had more than 50% reduction in seizure frequency. (Drake J et al. *Neurosurgery* 1987; *21*:792-797).

COMMENT. The authors emphasize that simple excision of the tumor may not eradicate the seizures. The common occurrence of mesial temporal sclerosis in association with mass lesions requires extension of the resection to include removal of the hippocampus as well as the cortex adjacent to the tumor. It is suggested that hippocampal changes are secondary to repetitive seizure activity.

The late detection of cerebral gliomas as a cause of childhood epilepsy has been noted by other investigators. Diagnosis of supratentorial tumors was delayed for an average of 2 years after the initial seizure and 8 of 31 patients continued to have seizures for periods between 3 and 8 years before a tumor was demonstrated in a study of 291 cases at the Mayo Clinic. Seizures occurred in 17% of the total group — in 25% of patients with supratentorial tumors and in 12% of those with infratentorial tumors. They were the initial symptoms in 15% of patients with supratentorial tumors. Seizures were more common in patients with slowly growing astrocytomas, grades 1 and 2, than in those with more rapidly expanding astrocytomas, grades 3 or 4. (Backus RE, Millichap JG. *Pediatrics* 1962; *29*:978).

The MRI should permit earlier diagnosis of the temporal lobe glioma as a cause of childhood epilepsy. MRI is superior in defining the extent of gliomas grade I and II that may be poorly delineated by CT, and MRI should be a complementary examination in suspected tumor cases (Kormano M et al. *Acta Radiologica* 1987; *28*:369). The prompt surgical excision of the tumor before seizures become medically unresponsive may prevent the development of the mesial temporal sclerosis and dual pathology stressed in the present report. - Editor. *Ped Neur Briefs* January 1988.

Subarachnoid Hemorrhage From Brain Tumors

Six children with subarachnoid hemorrhage as the initial symptom of brain tumor are reported from the Depts of Neurosurgery, Univ of Occupational and Environmental Health, Kitakyushu, and Kumamoto Univ Med Sch, Kumamoto. They represented 3.6% of 167 new pediatric cases of brain tumor seen in 7-17 years at two centers in Japan. Two neonates presented with irritability, vomiting, cyanotic spells, and unilateral facial paresis. Four children, ages 4 to 15 years, developed sudden headache and vomiting with or without alteration of consciousness. The tumor locations were posterior fossa (2 medulloblastomas, one ependymoma, one hemangioma) and hypothalamus (one astrocytoma and one unverified). All were located close to the III or IV ventricles. The ultimate prognosis was poor. (Yokota A et al. *Child's Nerv Syst* 1987; *3*:65-69).

COMMENT. Medulloblastoma is more apt to bleed than other neuroectodermal tumors in pediatric patients. Compared to brain tumors in adults, those in children bleed more frequently and are more commonly located in the posterior fossa. Brain tumor should be considered as a possible etiology of subarachnoid hemorrhage in the neonate and child. - Editor. *Ped Neur Briefs* September 1987.

Intracranial Tuberculoma

In a report from the Dept of Pediatrics, All India Inst of Applied Sciences, New Delhi, India, intracranial tuberculoma was found in 20 (24%) of 83 patients with partial seizures complicated by increased intracranial pressure, systemic tuberculosis or focal neurologic deficit and in 12 (22%) of 55 patients with tuberculous meningitis. CT lesions consisting of ring enhancement, discs, and irregular coalescing masses with edema regressed within 12 weeks of starting medical therapy. Surgical excision was not required. Medical management was advocated, with surgery limited to drug treatment failures. (Bagga A et al. Intracranial tuberculoma. Evaluation and treatment. *Clin Pediat* Oct 1988; 27:487-490).

COMMENT. Tuberculoma mimics other space-occupying lesions and in India its reported prevalence has ranged from 4 to 40% of intracranial tumors. Effective chemotherapy and CT monitoring of treatment response have minimized the role of surgery. - Editor. *Ped Neur Briefs* October 1988.

Lipoma Of Corpus Callosoum

A lipoma of the corpus callosum diagnosed by CT at 7 mos and mistaken for hemorrhage in a premature infant is reported from the Medical College of Pennsylvania, Philadelphia, PA. The Apgar scores were 3 at one and five minutes, and the infant had hyaline membrane disease that progressed to bronchopulmonary dysplasia. Cranial ultrasound at 10 hrs demonstrated a subependymal hemorrhage with unchanged appearance at 17 days. Seizures associated with bilateral temporal polyspike and sharp-wave EEG activity were controlled with phenobarbital. His head circumference was at the 75th percentile and disproportionately large. A repeat ultrasound at 7 mos showed increased echogenicity in the midline with normal ventricles, interpreted as blood in the third ventricle with calcification. CT showed a large midline area of decreased density extending into the lateral ventricles, consistent with a lipoma of the corpus callosum and calcifications. At 18 mos the head is large and development is delayed at the 12 mo level. (Imaizumi SO et al. Lesion mistaken for hemorrhage in a premature infant: Lipoma of corpus callosum. *Pediatr Neurol* Oct 1988; 4:313-6).

COMMENT. Blood, fat, and calcium have similar echogenicity by cranial ultrasound, and all three media are hyperechoic when compared to the moderate echogenicity of cerebral white matter, low echogenicity of gray matter, and absent echogenicity of fluid-filled ventricles or cysts. Lipomas are characterized by hyperechoic densities on cranial sonograms. - Editor. *Ped Neur Briefs* November 1988.

Posterior Fossa Dermoids

Three children with dermoid cysts of the posterior fossa are reported from the Assaf Harofeh Medical Center, Zerifen, and Hadassa Medical center, Jerusalem, Israel. Two presented with acute meningitis at 1 and 2 yrs of age, and the third patient had hydrocephalus treated by ventriculoperitoneal shunt at 7 mos and complicated by meningitis and cerebellar abscess at 9 mos of age. CT scans with enhancement and bone window setting revealed the midline bony defect and low density lesion with ring enhancement in the posterior fossa. (Starinsky R et al. Dermoids of the posterior fossa. Case reports and review. *Clin Pediat* Dec 1988; 27:579-582).

COMMENT. Recurrent meningitis or brain abscess in an infant or young child should prompt a search for a sinus, fistula, and bone defect in the occipital area. Dermoid cysts of the cerebellum and posterior fossa account for 2% of intracranial tumors in children. Astrocytoma, medulloblastoma, brain stem glioma, and ependymoma of the IVth ventricle are the most frequently encountered IC tumors. - Editor. *Ped Neur Briefs* November 1988.

Epidermoid Tumors

Six patients with histologically proven epidermoid tumors are reported from the neurosurgical service, Brigham and Women's Hospital and Children's Hospital, Harvard Medical School, Boston, Mass. All patients were adults between 22 and 52 years of age at the time of diagnosis. Symptoms had been present for more than one to five years and the methods of presentation included seizures in two, ataxia (3), headaches (3), dysmetria (3), left-sided hearing loss (1), visual loss (1) and papilledema (1). The locations of the tumor were variable; cerebellar hemisphere in two, left temporal lobe (2), left cerebral hemisphere (1) and suprasellar cistern (1). Surgery was successful in all patients. None had symptoms related specifically to the tumor in childhood; one had been treated for bulimia for 17 years and another had meningitis at ten years of age. CT demonstrated a hypodense, smoothly contoured, extra axial paramedial mass with a lower density than cerebrospinal fluid. MRI showed an irregularly, but sharply marginated, mass with homogeneous density, variable enhancement with gadolinium, lack of edema in adjacent normal structures, extensive insinuation into cisternal and other cerebrospinal fluid spaces and a high signal intensity on proton-weighted images. Multiplanar magnetic resonance imaging was extremely helpful in showing the full extent of the lesion and its relation to other structures (Panagopoulos K P et al. Intracranial epidermoid tumors. A continuing diagnostic challenge. *Arch Neurol* July 1990; *47*:813-816).

COMMENT. Epidermoid, adamantinoma, cholesteatoma, and pearly tumor are terms used interchangeably to refer to this entity. Epidermoid tumors are congenital and arise from misplacement of ectoderm. They are usually benign and slow growing but malignant change may occur. The tumors may be very large at the time of diagnosis, with considerable mass effect but minimal edema. The MRI allows the distinction of an epidermoid from an arachnoid cyst. The MRI or CT is not diagnostic but the MRI is more likely to elucidate the extra axial-nature of the tumor and is preferred. Spinal epidermoid tumors may complicate a lumbar puncture performed 1 to 20 or more years previously. Symptoms are slowly progressive and manifested by back and leg pains progressing to gait difficulties. (Shaywitz BA. *J Pediatr* 1972; *80*:638). - Editor. *Ped Neur Briefs* July 1990.

Radiation-Induced Tumors

The relation between radiotherapy to the head and neck for tinea capitis childhood and the later development of tumors of the brain and nervous system have been investigated in 10,834 patients treated between 1948 and 1960 in Israel and the results evaluated at the Radiation Epidemiology Branch, National Cancer Institute, Bethesda, MD. Neural tumors developed in 73 patients, 60 in irradiated subjects, 8 among general population controls, and 5 among sibling controls. The increase in incidence among those irradiated was 7 times that of controls. The relative risk of all head and neck situated neural tumors among irradiated subjects was 8.4. Increased relative risks were greater for benign nerve-sheath tumors (18.8;n=25) than for meningiomas (9.5;n=19) and gliomas (2.6;n=7). A strong dose-response relation was shown, the risk approaching 20 after doses of 2.5 Gy. Radiation doses to the head and neck in childhood on the order of 1 to 2 Gy significantly increased the risk of neural tumors in those areas. (Ron E et al. Tumors of the brain and nervous system after radiotherapy in childhood. *N Engl J Med* Oct 20 1988; *319*:1033-9).

COMMENT. Radiation-induced tumors of the central nervous system are recognized as a consequence of combined treatments for leukemia chemotherapy and irradiation to the head. Therapeutic doses of radiation for childhood leukemia are higher than those used for the patients with tinea capitis in Israel and the relative risks are undetermined. - Editor. *Ped Neur Briefs* October 1988.

Chemotherapy For Medulloblastoma

The efficacy of adjuvant chemotherapy for patients with poor-risk medulloblastoma/primitive neuroectodermal tumors (MB/PNET) has been studied at the Children's Hospital of Philadelphia, University of Pennsylvania, PA. Chemotherapy consisted of vincristine during concomitant craniospinal radiation therapy and eight 6-week cycles of vincristine, cis-platinum, and cyclohexylnitrosourea. Twenty-five of 26 children (96%) treated remain alive and free of disease at a median of 24 months from diagnosis (range 6-50 mos). Actuarial disease-free survival was statistically significantly better than for control subjects who had received radiation therapy alone during an 8 year period prior to the use of adjuvant chemotherapy. The 2-year disease-free survival was 96% for patients on the protocol of adjuvant chemotherapy as compared to 59% for historical control patients treated with radiotherapy alone. (Packer RJ et al. Efficacy of adjuvant chemotherapy for patients with poor-risk medulloblastoma: a preliminary report. *Ann Neurol* Oct 1988; 24:503-508).

COMMENT. Surgical excision for the treatment of medulloblastoma has less than a 6 month survival rate, and postoperative radiation of the tumor bed alone has minimal benefit. Irradiation of the tumor bed and the entire neuraxis provides an overall chance of 30% to 50% for 5 year survival. Patients with clinical evidence of arachnoidal seeding or with gross evidence of seeding at surgery do poorly. Survival without evidence of recurrent tumor for a period exceeding the patients' age at diagnosis plus 9 months indicates a probable cure ("Collins' law"). Corticosteroids result in remarkable amelioration of root signs and symptoms and reduction of edema for a brief period. Experience with chemotherapy in the past 25 years has produced better survival rates, and used as an adjuvant these agents are indicated for the poor-risk patients, i.e. those less than 5 years of age at diagnosis or with disseminated tumors (Chang stages M1-M3). (Groover RV. In *The Practice of Pediatric Neurology*, Eds. Swaiman KF, Wright FS, CV Mosby, St. Louis, 1982). - Editor. *Ped Neur Briefs* November 1988.

Chemotherapy For Brain Tumors

The results of chemotherapy in the treatment of selected brain tumors in children are reviewed by the Division of Pediatric Hematology/Oncology, Children's Hospital and Health Center, San Diego. Chemotherapy was advocated in the following tumors: Malignant astrocytoma, glioblastoma multiforme, high risk medulloblastoma, malignant germ cell tumor, pinealoma, pinealoblastoma, and non-Hodgkin lymphoma. It was also considered of value in selected cases of optic glioma, brain stem glioma, ependymoma, and germinoma. The Children's Cancer Study Group and the Pediatric Oncology Group in the United States and the International Society of Pediatric Oncology in Europe have reported results favoring the addition of chemotherapy and a multimodal treatment of brain tumors.

In patients with cerebral hemisphere *astrocytoma*, the 5 year relapse free survival rate for those receiving chemotherapy (vincristine, lomustine, and prednisone for one year) was 45%, in contrast to 13% for those receiving neurosurgery and radiation therapy alone. There are reports of recurrent gliomas responding to chemotherapy for short periods. The authors favored chemotherapy for progressive *optic gliomas* to minimize the risk of adverse irradiation associated side effects in young children. In *brainstem gliomas*, chemotherapy is of unproved benefit but is being investigated because of the suboptimal current survival rate of approximately 20%.

In patients with *medulloblastoma* chemotherapy improved survival rates for children with subtotal tumor excision, children who were less than 2 years of age, and children with tumor extension into the brain stem. Those with small localized medulloblastomas may be given craniospinal irradiation after an attempt at surgical resection; those with extensive local or disseminated lesions may be best treated with neurosurgery, irradiation, and chemotherapy. Young children less than 3 years of age may receive chemotherapy in an attempt to delay radiotherapy, potentially reducing the risk of postirradiation side effects. In patients with large, invasive tumors plus CSF dissemination, the 5 year disease free survival rate with chemotherapy added was 45% versus 0% in patients not so treated. Children with large tumors without CSF spread of tumor also showed a trend that was less dramatic toward an increased disease free survival time with chemotherapy. Irrespective of the therapeutic regimen, children less than 4 years of age fared worse than older children. In *ependymomas,* some responses to chemotherapy have been noted in recurrent tumors but a consistently effective drug program has not been identified. *Malignant germ cell tumors* are often given combination chemotherapy plus irradiation. Recently, chemotherapy has also been used for *germinomas* to reduce subsequent irradiation dosage. Chemotherapy has also been used along with radiotherapy for the treatment of *pinealomas* and *pinealoma blastomas* which usually do not respond well to radiotherapy alone.

Acute leukemias (especially lymphoblastic leukemia, and non-Hodgkin lymphoma) may involve the central nervous system in children. Non-Hodgkin lymphoma of the brain is being reported with increasing frequency in patients with AIDS and is projected to be one of the most common neurologic neoplasms within several years. Treatment of *brain lymphoma* has traditionally involved systemic chemotherapy, intrathecal chemotherapy, and irradiation. Patients with AIDS have difficulty tolerating large doses of chemotherapy and may benefit from antiretroviral and immunomodulator drugs in future trials. The long-term adverse effects of therapy of brain tumors have assumed greater importance since increasing numbers of children survive treatment programs. Approximately one-half may manifest significant intellectual or behavioral retardation, particularly in those under 3 years of age. White matter abnormalities, calcifications, and brain atrophy may be demonstrated on CT scans and MRI. Histopathologic findings after cranial irradiation have included demyelinization and mineralizing microangiopathy. Short stature resulting from growth hormone secretory dysfunction occurs in brain tumor patients who received radiation therapy and hypothyroidism may occur after craniospinal irradiation. (Kadota R P et al. Brain tumors in children. *J Pediatr* April 1989; *114*:511-519).

> COMMENT. An estimated 1200-1500 new cases of brain tumors will be diagnosed annually in American children less than 15 years of age. Compared with other childhood cancers, brain tumors have not been intensively studied by pediatric oncologists. With the recent advances in chemotherapy and the concerns regarding adverse effects of radiotherapy, oncologists are playing a larger role in the treatment of brain tumors in children. Well designed controlled studies in multiple collaborative centers will be necessary to prove the effectiveness of this form of therapy. - Editor. *Ped Neur Briefs* April 1989.

Radiotherapy In Brainstem Gliomas

The results of a multiinstitutional phase I/phase II trial, using 100 cGy of radiation therapy twice daily to a total dose of 7,200 cGy in 31 children with high risk brainstem gliomas are reported from the Neuro-Oncology Program, The Children's Hospital of Philadelphia, the University of Pennsylvania, Philadelphia; New York University Medical Center; University of Minnesota; Children's Memorial Hospital, Chicago; and the Robert Wood Johnson Medical School, New Brunswick, NJ. Of the 35 patients evaluated, 24 (69%) had developed progressive disease and 11 (31%) remained in remission at the completion of the three year study period. Survival rate at 20 months was 32%. Patients relapsed at a median of eight months after diagnosis. Those in remission had been followed for a median of 18 months. No patient died as a result of treatment. Glucocorticoid therapy was tapered and discontinued during or soon after completion of treatment. In comparison to control patients and those treated in a previous trial using smaller doses of hyperfractionated radiotherapy, there was a statistically significant improvement in progression-free survival rate. Further studies seemed warranted. (Packer RJ et al. Hyperfractionated radiotherapy for children with brainstem gliomas: A pilot study using 7,200 cGy. *Ann Neurol* Feb 1990; *27*:167-173).

COMMENT. Brainstem gliomas account for approximately 10% of all childhood central nervous system tumors and are the most resistant to therapy. High risk patients with tumors involving the brain stem diffusely rarely survive after conventional doses of radiotherapy. Hyperfractionated radiation therapy offers greater potential benefit. - Editor. *Ped Neur Briefs* February 1990.

Papilledema In Children: Fluorescein Test

The use of oral fluorescein in the diagnosis of early papilledema in 23 children aged 1 mo to 10 yrs is reported from the Dr Rajendra Prasad Centre for Ophthalmic Sciences, All-India Inst of Med Sciences, Ansari Nagar, New Delhi, India. Of 15 children with suspected or early papilledema associated with hydrocephalus (10), seizures (3), possible tumor (1), and unilateral proptosis (1), late disc staining and retinal vascular fluorescence occurred in 12, the fluorescence at 60 min being significantly greater or of equal intensity to that at 30 min, denoting a positive test. All cases positive on oral fluorescein showed CT evidence of raised intracranial pressure, while those with negative fluorescein tests had normal CTs. In 8 children with pseudopapilledema examined after oral fluorescein, the retinal vascular fluorescence and slight disc head staining with sharp margins at 30 min declined markedly by 60 min, a negative result identical to that found in normal fundi. The authors caution that a negative result may occur with very early stages of papilledema manifested only by venous engorgement. (Ghose S, Nayak BK. Role of oral fluorescein in the diagnosis of early papilledema in children. *Brit J Ophthalmol* Dec 1987; *71*(12):910-915).

COMMENT. The necessity for conventional intravenous administration of fluorescein often precludes its use in small children with suspected papilledema. Oral fluorescein offers a more practical test that may gain acceptance if these results are confirmed. The funduscopic examination and diagnosis of early papilledema is often difficult, especially in small children, even for the experienced pediatric neurologist. Ophthalmologists may negate the neurologist's suspicions, but CT scan is nonetheless advisable if the clinical picture suggests a space-occupying lesion. - Editor. *Ped Neur Briefs* February 1988.

Spinal Cord Hemangioblastoma

A 6-month-old infant with a spinal cord hemangioblastoma located in the conus medullaris is reported from the University of Washington School of Medicine, Children's Hospital, Seattle, WA. At birth the physical examination was normal except for a lumbosacral dimple. By 1 month the dimple had deepened and a hemangioma developed at the site. CT and CT metrizamide myelography revealed a posterior filling defect at the level of the conus medullaris. At laminectomy, a congenital dermal sinus tract, cutaneous capillary hemangioma and cord hemangioblastoma were resected. There were no neurologic deficits either postoperatively or following removal of the tumor. (Michaud LJ et al. Hemangioblastoma of the conus medullaris associated with cutaneous hemangioma. *Pediatr Neurol* Oct 1988; *4*:309-12).

COMMENT. Spinal cord hemangioblastoma rarely presents in infancy and is usually manifest from the third to the fifth decades. It may be associated with a variety of cutaneous and other lesions, including von Hippel-Lindau and

Cobb syndromes. *Von Hippel-Lindau disease* is an autosomal dominant condition characterized by hemangioblastomas of the cerebellum, medulla and spinal cord; angiomas of the retina, liver, and kidney; pheochromocytomas, adenomas, or cysts of the kidney and epididymis; and pancreatic cysts. In *Cobb syndrome*, cutaneomeningospinal angiomatosis, spinal cord arteriovenous malformations are associated with cutaneous vascular lesions in corresponding dermatomes. These syndromes were not found in the above case report. - Editor. *Ped Neur Briefs* November 1988.

Medulloblastoma Prognostic Factors

The prognostic factors and outcome of treatment of 58 patients with posterior fossa medulloblastoma seen from March 1965 through December 1984 were reviewed in the Division of Radiation Oncology at the Mayo Clinic. The median age was 17 years and males were affected more frequently than females in a ratio of 1.5:1. The most common initial signs and symptoms were those associated with increased intracranial pressure and cerebellar dysfunction: nausea and vomiting 91%, headache 86%, ataxia 77%, papilledema 69%, nystagmus 67%. The overall 5- and 10-year survivals were 50% and 33% respectively; 5- and 10-year relapse-free survivals were 46% and 32%. Surgical and postoperative radiation therapy failed in 34 patients (59%). A significant improvement in ten year survival was associated with a posterior fossa radiation dose of 50 Gy or more, whole brain irradiation, and spinal axis irradiation. Total compared to subtotal resection correlated with better 10-year relapse-free survival but not overall survival. (Garton GR et al. Medulloblastoma - prognostic factors and outcome of treatment: Review of the Mayo Clinic experience. *Mayo Clin Proc* Aug 1990; 65:1077-1086).

COMMENT. The dose of irradiation to the posterior fossa was one of the most important determinants of overall survival and relapse-free survival in patients with medulloblastoma. Doses of 50 Gy or more are associated with improved survival and local control. Total removal of the tumor when possible and irradiation to the supratentorial area of the brain and spine in addition to the posterior fossa are recommended. Chemotherapy with or without additional irradiation was used for recurrent medulloblastoma. - Editor. *Ped Neur Briefs* September 1990.

Cerebellopontine Angle Lipoma

A cerebellopontine angle lipoma discovered incidentally in an asymptomatic 17 year old girl during evaluation for trauma is reported from the University of Alabama and Children's Hospital, Birmingham, AL. The CT had shown a low density nonenhancing 1.5 cm mass in the right cerebellopontine angle. The patient denied hearing loss, tinnitus, facial weakness or other neurologic symptoms. On examination she had a left-sided hearing loss, an audiogram showed left conductive hearing loss, and brainstem auditory evoked potentials were abnormal on the left. MRI was consistent with either an epidermoid or a lipoma. At surgical biopsy which confirmed the diagnosis the mass involved the 7th and 8th as well as portions of the 9th, 10th and 11th cranial nerves and was partially adherent to the brainstem. Surgical removal was not possible and postoperatively the patient made an uneventful recovery. (Ashkenasi A et al. Cerebellopontine angle lipoma in a teenager. *Pediatr Neurol* July/Aug 1990; 6:272-274).

COMMENT. The authors found only one other report of this tumor in a child and 17 in adults. They recommend that surgical removal should be avoided if possible because of postoperative cranial nerve injury. A mass with negative CT density and increased signal intensity on T1 and T2 weighted images on MRI should limit the differential diagnosis to lipomas, dermoids, or cholesterol granulomas, according to reports in the literature. - Editor. *Ped Neur Briefs* September 1990.

CHAPTER **10**

NEUROCUTANEOUS SYNDROMES

INTRODUCTION

The neurocutaneous syndromes (NCSs) or *phakomatoses* include tuberous sclerosis (TS), neurofibromatosis (NF-1), von Hippel-Lindau disease (VHL), ataxia telangiectasia (AT), and Sturge-Weber disease (SW). These five disorders affecting skin and the central nervous system are the major examples of more than 50 NCSs described. When classified according to genetics, TS, NF-1, and VHL are autosomal dominant, AT is autosomal recessive, and SW is non-hereditary.

Symposia in Europe and the US have addressed the distinguishing features of two types of neurofibromatosis, NF-1 and NF-2, and a joint meeting of the Royal Society of Medicine and the Tuberous Sclerosis Association of Great Britain has reviewed the recent advances in genetics, early diagnosis and prognosis of TS. Two excellent books authored and edited by Gomez MR

provide detailed descriptions of TS and NCSs, and the natural
history and pathogenesis of NF are outlined in a book by
Riccardi VM and Eichner JE.

This chapter includes reviews and comments of 9 articles
on neurofibromatosis, 2 on tuberous sclerosis, and 1 each on
hypomelanosis of Ito and leopard syndrome. The rare simultaneous occurrence of two NCSs in the same patient is reported.
Tuberous sclerosis is also covered in Chapter 1 in articles on
epilepsy, and particularly infantile spasms, and ataxia telangiectasia is reviewed in Chapter 16 under heredo-degenerative disorders and ataxia syndromes.

Tuberous Sclerosis And Renal Tumors

A 14-year-old girl with bilateral renal cell carcinoma
(hypernephroma) complicating a previously unrecognized tuberous sclerosis is reported from Cornell Univ Med College, NY,
and North Shore Univ Hosp, Manhasset NY, together with a
review of 6 similar cases culled from the literature. The patient
presented with a 6-month history of progressive weight loss and
anemia. She had an acne-like rash on her face and a nodule on
her tongue. Her father and paternal uncle were institutionalized
for convulsive and psychiatric disorders. Abdominal sonogram
and CAT scan showed a large mass arising from the right kidney
and a smaller mass in the left kidney. Areas of sclerosis and
periventricular calcifications were found in skull x-rays and CAT
scan of the head. Renal cell carcinoma and hamartomatous nodules were diagnosed at surgery. Epithelial-lined cysts of the kidney and adenoma sebaceum of the face were typical of tuberous
sclerosis. All abnormal hematological and chemistry values,
including hypercalcemia, anemia, thrombocytopenia, and
hypoalbuminemia returned to normal and the patient was
asymptomatic at 3 years after surgery. (Weinblatt ME et al.
Renal cell carcinoma in patients with tuberous sclerosis.
Pediatrics 1987; *80*:898-903).

COMMENT. Tumors occur more commonly in the kidney than in any other organ as a manifestation of tuberous sclerosis, their frequency being estimated at 80% (Critchley M, Earl CJC. *Brain* 1932; *55*:311). Hamartoma or multiple angiomyolipoma is the most frequent variety but hypernephroma, liposarcoma, adenosarcoma, myosarcoma, and perithelioma are also described (Wilson SAK. *Neurology* 1955, Williams and Wilkins, Baltimore). Mostly bilateral and often multiple, they sometimes undergo cystic degeneration. Of 29 cases of tuberous sclerosis reported by Fowler JS and Dickson WEC (*Quart J Med* 1910; *4*:43), 17 (58%) had renal tumors.

The present authors recommend that all patients with tuberous sclerosis should have periodic sonography of the kidney and frequent urinalysis, especially in adolescence and adult life when the incidence of renal masses begins to increase. Fortunately, most renal tumors associated with tuberous sclerosis are relatively benign and patients with renal cell carcinoma localized to the kidney have a 75% chance of recovery following surgery alone. - Editor. *Ped Neur Briefs* December 1987.

Tuberous Sclerosis: Prognosis And Early Diagnosis

A report of a joint meeting of the Forum on Mental Retardation of the Royal Society of Medicine and The Tuberous Sclerosis Association of Great Britain states that the prevalence of tuberous sclerosis (TS) for children under 15 years may be 1 in 10,300. Evidence for the assignment of the TS gene to chromosome 9 was reviewed, and high levels of carbohydrate specific to the glycoprotein-fibrinectin in the affected skin of TS patients noted. Infantile spasms associated with TS may have a better prognosis than in non-TS patients. Cognitive deterioration in TS is usually relative to underlying pathology rather than seizure frequency or severity. Of 88 children with TS followed until the age of 5 years, 81% of those who were walking showed severe psychiatric disorder, 59% were autistic, and 70% had hyperkinetic behavior disorders. Infantile spasms were associated with autism in 68%, 79% were severely mentally handicapped, and 47% were in special care units of schools. The detection of rhabdomyomata in echocardiography was a valuable diagnostic technique, positive in 47% of 60 children and adults with TS. A greater awareness and early diagnosis of TS is called for. (Corbett J, Hunt A. Recent research on tuberous sclerosis (TS), *JRSM* Aug 1988; *81*:481-482).

> COMMENT. Forehead plaques, smooth patches of slightly raised skin with a reddish or yellowish discoloration, can be one of the earliest skin manifestations of TS. Wood's light examination of the skin for hypopigmented maculae is important in all infants with myoclonic spasms and hypsarrhythmia. (See *Ped Neur Briefs* 1987; 1:3). MRI may help in predicting the eventual clinical severity of younger children with newly diagnosed TS, whereas the number of CT brain abnormalities does not correlate with prognosis. High-signal MRI lesions involving the cerebral cortex are characteristic of TS and correspond to hamartomas and gliotic areas seen pathologically. Periventricular calcification lesions are better visualized with CT than with MRI. (Roach et al. *Arch Neurol* 1987; *44*:301). - Editor. *Ped Neur Briefs* August 1988.

Neurofibromatosis Symposia And Classification

LINK (Let's Increase Neurofibromatosis Knowledge), the British Neurofibromatosis Association, organized a major European Symposium at Egham, Surrey, Feb 5-7, 1987, and clarified the distinguishing features of two syndromes with separate genetic markers: 1) von Recklinhausen's neurofibromatosis (VRNF), the so-called peripheral type, and 2) bilateral acoustic neurofibromatosis (BANF), the central variety.

VRNF with a prevalence of 1 in 3000 is inherited as an autosomal dominant condition with 100% penetrance and a high mutation rate. Serious complications, occurring in about 20%

include large plexiform neurofibromas, kyphoscoliosis, and optic nerve or chiasmal gliomas. Children should be examined twice a year to check for complications.

The gene responsible for VRNF, although not identified, was narrowed down to a few chromosomes by data that provided an "exclusion map" at this conference. The genetic analysis of BANF patients has shown deletions on chromosome 22, a step closer to the identification of the defective gene responsible for acoustic neuromas. (*Lancet* 1987; *i*:663-664).

> COMMENT. A similar conference on neurofibromatosis was scheduled July 13-15, 1987 in the U.S. and sponsored by the National Institutes of Health, Bethesda, MD. It was perhaps unfortunate that the European and U.S. sponsors could not have pooled their resources to make this an International Symposium. - Editor. *Ped Neur Briefs* June 1987.

Neurofibromatosis And Acoustic Neuromas

The criteria for diagnosis, treatment, family counseling and advances in genetics of neurofibromatosis are reviewed by a neurosurgeon and epidemiologist at the Massachusetts General Hospital, Boston, and the National Institute of Neurological Disorders, Bethesda, MD.

The neurofibromatoses consist of two distinct disorders, a peripheral and a central type, with genes located on separate chromosomes. The diagnosis of *neurofibromatosis 1* (NF1, von Recklinhausen's neurofibromatosis or VRNF in Europe) requires two or more of the following: 6 or more cafe-au-lait macules, 2 or more neurofibromas, axillary or inguinal skin freckles, optic glioma, Lisch iris nodules, osseous lesion and familial occurrence. *Neurofibromatosis 2* (NF2, bilateral acoustic neurofibromatosis or BANF in Europe) requires one of the following for diagnosis: a) bilateral eighth nerve tumors, or b) a positive family history plus a unilateral eighth nerve tumor or two of the following: neurofibroma, meningioma, glioma,

Schwannoma, or lenticular opacity. For patients with NF2 there is a 50% risk of transmission to any offspring, and close relatives should be screened for cafe-au-lait spots or neurofibromas, acoustic nerve tumors and lens opacities. Acoustic neuromas commonly become symptomatic during or soon after puberty and may be exacerbated in pregnancy, suggesting a hormone or growth factor important in tumor formation. The inherited gene for NF2 is on the long arm of chromosome 22. (Martuza RL, Eldridge R. Neurofibromatosis 2 (bilateral acoustic neurofibromatosis). *N Engl J Med* Mar 17 1988; *318*:684-8).

COMMENT. The British Neurofibromatosis Association - LINK, and two voluntary support organizations in the U.S. - The National Neurofibromatosis Foundation and the Acoustic Neuroma Association, organize medical symposia and provide valuable assistance to patients and their families. Newer diagnostic methods including brain stem auditory evoked potentials, CT and MRI and routine eye examination for subcapsular cataracts should afford earlier recognition.

Unidentified bright objects (UBOs), areas of increased signal on T1 or T2 weighted MRI, with concurrent negative contrast-enhanced CT are reported in 28 children with neurofibromatosis 1 and may possibly represent heterotopias. They were not correlated with the presence of learning disorders or retardation, and their significance is unclear. (Rubinstein AE et al and Dunn DW, Roos KL. *Neurology* Mar 1988; *38*(Suppl 1):282). I have a patient, a boy aged 12 yrs, with migraine headaches, macrocephaly, and cafe-au-lait patches, whose MRI shows UBOs. Although considered benign, such patients deserve careful long-term follow-up. - Editor. *Ped Neur Briefs* March 1988.

Von Recklinghausen
Neurofibromatosis: Clinical Features

A population-based study in southeast Wales and reported

Neurology, University of Wales College of Medicine, Cardiff, has identified 135 patients with neurofibromatosis type 1 (NF-1), a prevalence of approximately 1/5000. The major clinical features were multiple cafe-au-lait spots, dermal neurofibromas, Lisch nodules in the iris (93%), freckling in the axilla (67%) or groin (44%), macrocephaly (45%), and short stature (34%). Complications included plexiform neurofibromas in 40 (30%) patients, mental retardation in 13 (10%) severe in only 1, epilepsy 6 (4%), severe scoliosis 6, visceral and endocrine tumors 6, optic glioma 2, spinal neurofibroma 2, aqueductal stenosis 2, delayed puberty 2, and congenital glaucoma 1. No cases of acoustic neuroma were seen. The frequency of CNS and malignant tumors was 5%. The authors recommend regular biannual examinations during childhood, with particular attention to intellectual development and appropriate remedial education as necessary. In families of NF-1 patients, at-risk children who have not developed cafe-au-lait spots or Lisch nodules by 5 years of age are virtually certain to have escaped inheritance of the dominant gene. (Huson SM et al. Von Recklinghausen neurofibromatosis. A clinical and population study in Southeast Wales. *Brain* Dec 1988; *111*:1355-1381).

COMMENT. This article represents a major study and addition to the literature on neurofibromatosis type 1. Items of interest to the pediatric neurologist include the association of macrocephaly, mental retardation, and epilepsy. Hypsarrhythmia occurred more frequently than expected with NF-1 (2 cases) and this association has been noted previously (Riccardi VM, Eichner JE (1986) *Neurofibromatosis: Phenotype, Natural History, and Pathogenesis.* Baltimore, Johns Hopkins University Press). For correspondence, Dr. Huson's present address: Kennedy Galton Centre for Clinical Genetics, Northwick Park Hospital, Watford Road, Harrow, Middlesex HA1 3UJ, UK. - Editor. *Ped Neur Briefs* December 1988.

CNS Tumors And Neurofibromatosis

The association of CNS tumors and neurofibromatosis was studied in a population-based case control group of 338 patients, less than 15 years of age, diagnosed with a primary tumor of the central nervous system in a ten year period with 53 New York State counties and reported from the Cancer Etiology Unit, Division of Epidemiology, New York State Department of Health, Corning Tower, Albany, NY. The study included 676 controls and information on neurofibromatosis and congenital anomalies. The study confirmed the strong association of neurofibromatosis with the risk of CNS tumors.

Thirteen cases and no controls had neurofibromatosis. The types of CNS tumor were optic glioma in 9 patients, astrocytoma in 2, brain stem glioma in 1, and ependymoma in 1. Two fathers and three mothers of these cases had neurofibromatosis and five cases had siblings with neurofibromatosis. Seizures occurred in 37 (12% of 301) cases and in 18 (2.7% of 658) controls. The relative risk of seizures was 4.49 among patients with CNS tumors. There was no difference between cases and controls in the occurrence of congenital anomalies. (Baptiste M et al. Neurofibromatosis and other disorders among children with CNS tumors and their families. *Neurology* April 1989; *39*:487-492).

COMMENT. Neurofibromatosis carries an increased risk of CNS tumors including optic gliomas, other astrocytomas, acoustic neurinomas and meningiomas, also neuroblastoma, leukemia and other cancers. The coincidence of optic glioma and neurofibromatosis is especially frequent in children under 10 years of age and in this study the majority of the CNS tumor cases with neurofibromatosis were optic gliomas. Neurofibromatosis is due to an autosomal dominant genetic mutation with 100% penetrance. An important role for genetics in the etiology of some CNS tumors in children is supported by the strong association of neurofibromatosis with the occurrence of CNS tumors and the excess of neurofibromatosis in parents of CNS tumor cases.

Children with neurofibromatosis should be examined at regular intervals for possible optic glioma and those with optic glioma should be evaluated for manifestations of neurofibromatosis. - Editor. *Ped Neur Briefs* February 1989.

Learning Problems And Neurofibromatosis

A group of 32 children with von Recklinghausen's neurofibromatosis (VRNF) and school learning problems was compared to a matched sample of learning-disordered (LD) students without known genetic or medical disorders at the Division of Psychology, Department of Pediatrics, University of Iowa, Iowa City. VRNF children were found to differ from LD children on the frequency of WISC-R verbal-performance IQ discrepancies, perceptual organization, and on specific measures of visual-perceptual function. VRNF children were more likely to display nonverbal learning problems that may affect written language and organizational skills. Only 4% of the VRNF group showed pure language or memory deficits compared to 60% of LD children. Conversely, VRNF children were more likely to present with isolated visual perceptual deficits than LD children (56% versus 6%).

The VRNF population could be divided into distinct subgroups: 1) those with no cognitive disabilities; 2) those with mixed language and nonverbal dysfunctions (overlapping with LD children in the general population), and 3) those with nonverbal disabilities (visual perceptual deficits or more subtle organizational difficulties). The majority of VRNF children displayed impulsivity and social imperception, two behavioral features of visual perceptual disability. Eight children (25% of the group) with VRNF showed CNS complications and these children with CNS involvement had slightly lower IQ and cognitive measure scores than the uncomplicated VRNF children. The lower levels of performance may have been due to tumor variables or treatment variables (surgical intervention, cranial irradiation, or anticonvulsant medication). (Eliason MJ. Neuropsychological Patterns: Neurofibromatosis compared to developmental learning disorders. *Neurofibromatosis* Jan-Feb 1988; *1*:17-25).

COMMENT. The learning problems of children with VRNF have some similarities but some differences compared to children in the general population with learning disabilities. The similarities include a preponderance of affected males in both groups, average full scale IQ, and the presence of specific cognitive deficits. The differences include the high frequency of nonverbal dysfunctioning in the VRNF group, the less severe reading deficits in VRNF, and a greater reported frequency of behavior problems. The behavioral symptoms associate with visual perceptual disorder, speech impediments, and the cosmetic disfigurement among children with VRNF may all lead to a general impression of lower intelligence. Earlier studies of individuals with VRNF reported a high frequency of mental retardation and psychiatric disturbances, suggesting that 25-40% of individuals with VRNF were mentally deficient. More recent reports have included less severely affected individuals and the frequency of mental subnormality was closer to 8%. The rate of mental retardation was related to age: It was highest (17%) in the infant toddler group (based on the Bayley Scales), 22% in the preschool group (McCarthy Scales), 7% in the childhood adolescence group (WISC-R), and only 3% in the adult group (WAIS-R). - Editor. *Ped Neur Briefs* February 1989.

Neurofibromatosis And The MRI

The MRI was abnormal in seven of ten children with clinically proved neurofibromatosis reported from the Department of Radiology, the Oregon Health Sciences University, Portland, and the Departments of Neurology, Pediatrics and Radiology, University of Miami School of Medicine. Clinical diagnosis was based on six or more cafe-au-lait spots at least 1.5 cm in size. MRI was indicated because of mental retardation (5 patients), bilateral optic nerve tumors (1), shunt malfunction (1), learning disability (1), and possible brain tumor (2). The MRIs showed increased signal intensity on the T2-weighted images in the globus pallidus, brain stem, and cerebellum. The abnormalities most likely represented hamartomas. (Goldstein SM et al. A new sign of neurofibromatosis on magnetic resonance imaging of children. *Arch Neurol* November 1989; *46*:1222-1224).

COMMENT. The MRI in this study was more revealing than the CT scan which was normal in all except one of the patients studied. The neurologic and developmental examinations showed no correlation with the MRI findings. - Editor. *Ped Neur Briefs* December 1989.

Neurofibromatosis: Diagnostic Criteria

The diagnostic criteria, associated problems, genetics, pathogenesis, clinical evaluation and treatment of neurofibromatosis type I in childhood are reviewed from the Department of Pediatrics, Northwestern University Medical School and Children's Memorial Hospital, Chicago, Illinois. The National Institutes of Health Consensus Development Conference identified seven components of the syndrome, two or more required for the diagnosis: 1) six or more cafe au lait macules, 2) two or more neurofibromas or one plexiform neurofibroma, 3) freckling in axillary or inguinal region, 4) optic glioma, 5) two or more Lisch nodules, 6) osseous lesion such as sphenoid dysplasia or pseudoarthrosis and 7) a first degree relative with NF-1.

Other malignancies that occur in association with NF-1 include neurofibrosacroma, leukemia, xanthogranulomas, neuroblastoma, rhabdomyosarcoma and Wilms tumor. The full scale IQ is relatively low, but usually within the normal range. A visual perceptual disability occurs in 60 to 90% of the patients. The degree of intellectual deficit increases in direct proportion to the clinical severity. NF-1 and the Noonan syndrome may occur together. The localization of the NF-1 gene to chromosome 17 and the identification of linked markers has opened the door to prenatal and presymptomatic diagnosis of NF-1 and linkage analysis will soon be possible in families in which there are two or more affected members. Nearly 50% of persons with NF-1 do not have an affected parent and 50% are new mutations. Neurocristopathy, a generalized disorder of cells of neural crest origin, is the hypothesis for pathogenesis of NF-1. Histamine containing mast cells are found in high concentrations in peripheral neurofibromas and may be a factor in promotion of neurofibroma growth. Screening for optic gliomas by MRI is justified because of a high incidence (15%). Radiation therapy is the standard approach for optic glioma in children older than 5 years. Adverse effects include hypopituitarism, growth failure, cognitive deterioration, cataracts and secondary malignancies. Chemotherapy, if proven effective, would be preferable. Many optic gliomas are nonprogressive. Hormone treatment for precocious puberty associated with optic glioma may be efficacious.

Related neurofibromatosis syndromes include neurofibromatosis type 2, segmental neurofibromatosis and familial cafe-au-lait spots. Patients with multiple cafe-au-lait spots may not have any of the other stigmata of NF-1. The gene for neurofibromatosis type 2 with bilateral acoustic neurofibromatosis has been linked to chromosome 22. (Listernick R., Charrow J. Neurofibromatosis Type I in childhood. *J Pediatr* June 1990; *116*:845-853).

COMMENT. To this excellent review of NF-1 we may add a note concerning the simultaneous occurrence of neurocutaneous syndromes and a first report of a case of NF-2 and tuberous sclerosis in the same patient.

Neurofibromatosis I and tuberous sclerosis may occur simultaneously. This association is rare and the report by Schull and Crowe (*Neurology* 1953; 3:904-909) is the only case accepted by Gomez M (*Tuberous Sclerosis*, Raven Press, New York, 1988). Two patients reported by Vouge M et al (*Neuroradiology* 1980; 20:99-101) had clinical manifestations of neurofibromatosis I and also subependymal or intranuclear calcifications in the brain identical to the tubers of tuberous sclerosis.

I have recently evaluated a 14 year old girl with the simultaneous occurrence of neurofibromatosis type 2 and tuberous sclerosis. She presented with flaccid weakness and wasting of the left upper limb and electromyographic evidence of brachial plexopathy affecting primarily the upper and middle trunks. Examination of the skin showed a large depigmented patch over the right deltoid region, a small shagreen patch over the left lumbar region and a large pigmented area under the left axilla. The diagnosis of tuberous sclerosis was based on the skin lesions and typical calcifications shown in the CT scan of the head. The child had one seizure within 24 hours of a booster DPT immunization at 18 months. The diagnosis of neurofibromatosis type 2 was suggested by an MRI of the cervical spine showing enlargement of neural foramina C5-6 on the left side and was confirmed by a gadolinium MRI performed by Dr. Gomez at the Mayo Clinic. An asymptomatic right acoustic neuroma and a small meningioma at the level of C1 were also uncovered. The weakness and wasting of the left arm was explained by a plexiform neurofibroma. In addition the patient had a familial macular degeneration. She had inherited the neurofibromatosis from her father who had bilateral acoustic neuromas and other neurofibromata. No one in the family was known to suffer from tuberous sclerosis and examination of the mother was negative (Millichap JG, Gomez MR. Neurofibromatosis II and tuberous sclerosis: Simultaneous occurrence in a 14 year old girl. *Ped Neur Briefs* 1990; 4:50-51). - Editor. *Ped Neur Briefs* July 1990.

Hypomelanosis Of Ito: Neurologic Complications

The neurological complications in 34 Spanish children with hypomelanosis of Ito are described from the Paediatric Neurology Service, Hospital Infantil La Paz, and La Universidad Autonoma, Madrid, Spain. Most were referred because of mental retardation (65%) and seizures (53%), and the ages at time of the first visit were 2 months to 10 years. Skin lesions, observed within the first year of life in 70% of patients, consisted of hypomelanotic depigmented patches, cafe-au-lait spots, and angiomatous nevi; changes in hair color and alopecia also occurred. Noncutaneous abnormalities, observed in 94%, included macrocephaly, microcephaly, hemihypertrophy, kyphoscoliosis, coarse facial features, and hypertelorism. Autosomal dominant inheritance was demonstrated in some. (Pascual-Castroviejo I et al. Hypomelanosis of Ito. Neurological complications in 34 cases. *Can J Neurol Sci* May 1988; *15*:124-129).

COMMENT. The incidence of this disease was estimated at 1 per 1000 new patients consulting a pediatric neurology service, or 1 per 10,000 unselected patients in a children's hospital. It affects all races, but fair-skinned individuals may require a Woods lamp examination to detect the cutaneous lesions. - Editor. *Ped Neur Briefs* July 1988.

Leopard Syndrome And Gerstmann Syndrome

A 12 year old boy with multiple lentigines (Leopard) syndrome in association with Gerstmann syndrome and CT abnormalities is reported from the Department of Pediatrics and Pediatric Neurology, Beilinson Medical Center, Petah Tikva and Tel Aviv University, Sackler School of Medicine, Petah Tikva, Israel. Learning difficulties were first observed at five years of age. He had a single simple febrile convulsion at three years of age. Several hundred hyperpigmented skin lesions over the face, trunk, and extremities had appeared gradually after birth and had increased in number and size. Mild dysmorphic features included hypertelorism, epicanthal folds, cubitus valgus, and pterygium colli. A systolic cardiac murmur was indicative of pulmonic stenosis and was accompanied by EKG changes. The signs of *Gerstmann syndrome* included dyscalculia, left/right disorientation, finger agnosia, and dysgraphia. His IQ score was 86. Cranial CT showed dilatation of the left lateral ventricle especially in the occipital horn and mild atrophy of the left parietal lobe. (Garty B-Z et al. Gerstmann tetrad in Leopard syndrome. *Pediatr Neurol* Nov-Dec 1989; *5*:391-392).

COMMENT. The term Leopard is a mnemonic acronym for the features of the syndrome which may include: L - lentigines, E - EKG abnormalities, O - ocular hypertelorism, P - pulmonary stenosis, A - abnormal genitalia, R - retardation of growth, D - deafness. Mild mental retardation has been reported in patients with Leopard syndrome. Perhaps the "A" in the mnemonic should stand for acalculia in place of "abnormal genitalia". Some neuroradiologists would report the mild asymmetry of ventricles on the CT as a variant of normal and, in the absence of abnormalities of the white and gray matter, the diagnosis of parietal lobe atrophy may be questionable. As the author suggests, Gerstmann syndrome in children may be more common than indicated in the literature. In my experience this syndrome is not infrequent in children presenting with attention deficit disorders and normal CT scans are not unusual. It is possible that the MRI may be more revealing of associated cortical defects. - Editor. *Ped Neur Briefs* December 1989.

CHAPTER **11**

VASCULAR DISORDERS AND MALFORMATIONS

Arteriovenous Malformations: Surgical Indications

Twenty-three children with A-V malformations have been treated by neurosurgeons at the Children's Hospital of Eastern Ontario, Ottawa, Ontario. Fourteen were boys and 9 girls. The average age at presentation was 10 years. The majority (83%) presented with spontaneous hemorrhage and only one (4.3%) with seizures. Angiography was performed in 21 patients. The AVM could not be demonstrated in 5 (24%) who had an occult or cryptic AVM. Contrast-enhanced CT also failed to show abnormal vessels in 3 of the 5 occult AVMs.

Of 18 survivors, 15 were normal and 3 slightly disabled (2 with epilepsy). Aggressive surgical intervention resulted in improved survival and low morbidity. Overall mortality in the group was 22% while complete surgical excision carried a 7% mortality. The authors conclude that a spontaneous cerebral hemorrhage in a child is probably due to a vascular malformation, even when angiography and enhanced CT are negative.

CT contrast enhancement is not a reliable indicator of occult AVM and direct surgery is needed for diagnostic confirmation and prevention of further hemorrhages. Also, children presenting with symptoms other than hemorrhage (e.g. seizures) should undergo surgery to prevent bleeding, providing the lesion is accessible with low risk to healthy brain. (Ventureyra ECG, Herder S. *Child's Nerv Syst* 1987; *3*:12-18).

> COMEMNT. AVMs that bleed usually require neurosurgical management, and total excision seems the treatment preferred when feasible. Stereotaxic radiosurgery and the proton beam are available in some centers for cases not amenable to excision. The treatment of the AVM presenting with seizures or recurrent headache but without spontaneous hemorrhage is often a neurologist's responsibility. When should he involve his neurosurgical colleague? In the past, neurologists have sometimes chosen conservative management. The present study argues in favor of surgery for all AVMs in children diagnosed radiologically, given accessibility and low risk to surrounding brain tissue. Even the neonate with the AVM that involves the vein of Galen and presents with congestive heart failure has a better chance of survival with surgery. (See Hoffman et al. *J Neurosurg* 1982; *57*:316). - Editor. *Ped Neur Briefs* July 1987.

Arteriovenous Malformation: Rupture With Trauma

Three children, ages 5 to 9 years, with A-V malformations that ruptured after trivial head trauma, are reported from the Departments of Neurosurgery, University Medical School and Red Cross Hospital, Kumamoto City, Japan. They represented 12% of 25 consecutive patients with proven AVMs and 30% of 10 patients under 15 years of age. Two received blows on the forehead and one on the occipital region. Intracerebral hematomas were located in the subcortical area of the parietal or temporal lobe. Cerebral angiography revealed AVMs with feeding arteries from the anterior or middle cerebral arteries. At surgery there was no evidence of cortical contusion and excision of the AVMs was successful. (Nishi T et al. Ruptures of arteriovenous malformations in children associated with trivial head trauma. *Surg Neurol* 1987; *28*:451-7).

COMMENT. The authors found only 7 other case reports in the literature where hemorrhage from an AVM was associated with head trauma. All were in children. It is suggested that a larger shearing force can be produced in a child's brain than in an adult's, particularly during acceleration of the head in the AP or PA direction. - Editor. *Ped Neur Briefs* December 1987.

Intracranial Arterial Aneurysms In Early Childhood

Neurosurgeons from the Universita degli Studi di Roma "La Saspeinza", Rome, Italy, report a 4-year-old girl with a cerebral saccular aneurysm and analyze 71 cases under 5 years of age in the literature. The patient presented with headache, vomiting and immediate coma with opisthotonos and trismus. A CT scan revealed a round, hyperdense area near the midbrain, and an angiogram demonstrated an aneurysm on the left posterior cerebral artery. Recovery of consciousness and regression of nuchal rigidity took 3-4 days. At operation 12 days after the bleed, the artery was clipped above and below the aneurysm. A postoperative right facial-brachial paresis had resolved after 1 year but the hemianopia persisted.

Saccular aneurysms are rare in childhood, accounting for only 1-2% of cases. Most occur in the first year of life and affect the middle and anterior cerebral arteries in 40% and 12% of cases, respectively. Surgery appears to be tolerated better in early childhood than in adults, with operative mortalities after 1970 of 2.3% and 7.8% respectively. (Ferrante L et al. Intracranial arterial aneurysms in early childhood. *Surg Neurol* 1988; *29*:39-56).

COMMENT. Early versus delayed operation for ruptured intracranial aneurysm is controversial. An International

Comparative Study on Timing of Aneurysm Surgery in 3000 cases is expected to answer this question (Kassell NF, Torner JC. *Stroke* 1984; 15:566). The favorable outcome in this 4-year-old child would support a delay in operation until after recovery from the acute hemorrhage. The early age of presentation of the saccular aneurysm in children contrasts with an average age of 10 years for children with arteriovenous malformations (Ventureyra ECG, Herder S. *Child's Nerv Syst* 1987; 3:12). - Editor. *Ped Neur Briefs* January 1988.

Cerebral A-V Malformation In Neonate

A baby girl who developed congestive heart failure at 3 days of age and was shown to have an aneurysm of the vein of Galen is reported from the Dept Child Health, The Queen's Univ Belfast, Royal Maternity Hosp and Dept Radiology, Royal Victoria Hosp, Belfast. Treatment by embolization with helical stainless steel coils inserted along the straight sinus occluded the aneurysm. Postoperatively, recovery was rapid, the cranial bruit disappeared, and medical treatment for heart failure was discontinued. At 21 mos follow-up, the heart, head circumferences, and growth and development were normal. (McCord FB, Shield MD et al. Cerebral arteriovenous malformation in a neonate: treatment by embolization. *Arch Dis Child* Dec 1987; 62(12):1273-1275).

COMMENT. In this case nonsurgical treatment was successful. Ischemic brain lesions resulting from a steal phenomenon directing blood toward the aneurysm, as reported by Norman and Becker (*J Neurol Neurosurg Psychiat* 1974; 37:252), did not result. - Editor. *Ped Neur Briefs* February 1988.

Spinal A-V Malformation In A Neonate

A newborn male infant with flaccid paraplegia, without contractures, deformities or atrophy, caused by an arteriovenous malformation (AVM) of the dorsal spinal cord, is reported from the Depts Neurosurgery and Pediatrics, Hospital Infantil Nino Jesus and Dept Neuroradiology, Hospital Infantil La Paz, Madrid, Spain. Diagnosis was by lumbar puncture showing blood in the CSF, myelography demonstrating serpiginous filling defects and increased spinal cord diameter, and a spinal angiographic outline of the AVM with a large intraspinal aneurysmal sac. Following embolizations, clipping of feeding vessels, and surgical removal of the sac, the AVM was closed but the paraplegia had persisted at 10 mo follow-up. (Esparza J et al. Arteriovenous malformation of the spinal cord in the neonate. *Child's Nerv Syst* 1987; *3*(5):301-303).

COMMENT. Spinal cord A-V malformations may be dorsal extradural, compact intraspinal or diffuse intraspinal involving several vertebral segments. The latter presents in childhood or adolescence and carries a poor prognosis. Stereotaxic radiosurgery or proton beam therapy may offer better results than surgical intervention for large AVM's involving eloquent nervous tissue. (Kjellberg RN et al. *N Engl J Med* 1983; *309*:269). - Editor. *Ped Neur Briefs* February 1988.

Arteriovenous Malformation: Total Excision

The clinical characteristics and microsurgical approach to treatment of 39 children with AVMs are reviewed from the Neurosurgical Unit, Queen Elizabeth Hospital, Hong Kong. The pediatric cases represented 23% of 175 AVMs in all age groups. Age at diagnosis ranged from 1 month to 16 years, the majority between 11-16 years. Male to female ratio was 1.8:1. Hemorrhage in 87.5% was the most common presenting symptom. Total surgical excision was the treatment of choice, more than 80% leading a fully functional life. (Fong D. Chan S. Arteriovenous malformation in children. *Child's Nerv Syst* Aug 1988; *4*:199-203).

COMMENT. The reported mortality from the first hemorrhage in AVM is 10% and 12% from the second. AVM's in children are more apt to bleed than those in adults. Surgery is usually advised on operable lesions.

Cerebral cavernous malformations are discussed in a recent article (Rigamonti D et al. *N Engl J Med* Aug 11, 1988; *319*:343). In a study of 24 patients with histologically verified CCMs at the Barrow Neurological Institute, Phoenix, AZ, 13 were members of 6 unrelated Mexican-American families, and 11 had no evidence of a heritable trait. In the familial cases, 11% of relatives had seizures and 83% were asymptomatic. MRI revealed cavernous malformations in 14 of 16 studied, and 11 had multiple lesions. MRI was superior to CT and angiography in diagnosis of CCM. The authors conclude that CCMs are not rare, particularly in Mexican-Americans. There are 2 forms - sporadic and familial. The more prevalent familial form is transmitted as an autosomal dominant, and multiple lesions are common. - Editor. *Ped Neur Briefs* August 1988.

AV Malformations: Radiation Therapy

Clinical and radiologic follow-up of 86 patients with symptomatic, but surgically inaccessible, cerebral arteriovenous malformations treated with stereotactic heavy charged particle Bragg-peak radiation is reported from the Divisions of Neurosurgery and Neuradiology, Stanford University School of Medicine, California and the Lawrence Berkeley Laboratory, University of California. Ages at the time of treatment were from 9 to 69 years (mean, 33). Presenting symptoms were hemorrhage (60 patients), neurologic deficits (11), seizures (35), and headaches (40). Three years after radiation treatment the rate of complete obliteration of the lesions as detected angiographically was 100% for smaller lesions and 70% for those larger than 25 cm^3. Major neurologic complications occurred in ten patients (12%). Seizures and headaches were less severe in the patients who suffered from these initially. The authors concluded that heavy charged particle radiation is effective for symptomatic surgically inaccessible intracranial AV malformations.

Disadvantages of this therapy include the long delay in obliteration of the vascular lesion and a small risk of serious neurologic complications (Steinberg G K et al. *N Engl J Med* July 12, 1990; *323*:96-101).

> COMMENT. In an editorial comment by Heros R C and Korosue K of the University of Minnesota, Minneapolis, it is pointed out that the rate of serious morbidity from a hemorrhage from an arteriovenous malformation is about 30% and the mortality rate is about 10%. Not to treat is an unattractive choice for younger patients who will remain at risk for the rest of their lives. In considering the results of radiation therapy for AV malformations, the morbidity and mortality resulting from hemorrhage after treatment must be considered, particularly in comparing irradiation with surgical excision, a treatment method which eliminates the risk of hemorrhage. The delayed adverse effects of radiation on nervous tissue may limit this form of therapy in children. Only patients with previous hemorrhage, severe neurologic deficits, uncontrolled seizures, or disabling headaches were accepted in the authors' protocol which included mainly adults. - Editor. *Ped Neur Briefs* July 1990.

Surgical Treatment Of Childhood Moyamoya Disease

Neurosurgeons at the Hospital for Sick Children and Western Hospitals, Toronto, Canada, review their experiences during a 6 month to 15 year follow-up of 25 children with moyamoya disease 15 of whom underwent revascularization procedures. Five patients had superficial temporal artery-middle cerebral artery (STA-MCA) bypass procedures and 13 underwent encephalo-duro-arterio-synangiosis (EDAS), a procedure expected to induce collateral branches to sprout from the STA.

Of the untreated cases, 75% developed permanent neurological sequelae, including seizures, hemiparesis and mental retardation, and 2 died. Among the 13 treated cases, 10 were neurologically intact and the remainder were improved. The

STA-MCA was the procedure of choice in older children whereas EDAS, including opening of the arachnoid, a simpler technique, gave good results and was preferred in infants and young
children. The authors suggest that all pediatric patients be
offered the benefit of early surgical treatment before permanent
neurological deficits have developed. (Olds MV, Griebel RW,
Hoffman HJ et al. *J Neurosurg* 1987; *66*:675-680).

COMMENT. Moyamoya, a Japanese term meaning hazy
or misty like a "puff of smoke", describes the angiographic
appearance of the net-like collateral circulation that develops at the base of the brain as a result of stenosis of the distal internal carotid artery and its branches. Moyamoya disease has been classified in two forms: 2) a *primary* idiopathic nonprogressive form with alternating hemiplegia,
predominantly in girls of Japanese origin, often familial and
representing a hereditary malformation of the elastic lamina
of the cerebral vasculature, and 2) an *acquired* usually progressive form in both children ad adults with varying
underlying diseases. The diseases associated with moyamoya have included neurofibromatosis, basal meningitis,
hypertension, atherosclerosis, myopathy, sickle-cell anemia,
Fanconi's anemia, type 1 glycogenosis, congenital heart disease, Down syndrome, and conditions requiring radiation
therapy. The postradiation pathogenesis was reported by
Drs. Rajakulasingam, Cerullo, and Raimondi at
Northwestern UMS (*Child's Brain* 1979; *5*:467), one case
occurred in the present series, and a patient of mine, a girl
aged 16, developed the syndrome following irradiation of
the neck for Hodgkin's disease.

The present authors point out that the early concepts
of moyamoya disease as a relatively benign disorder in
Japanese girls have been modified in recent reports. The
sexes were equally affected and the majority of patients
were Caucasian in their series. The clinical course depends
on the rapidity and extent of vascular occlusion and the

ability to develop a collateral circulation. The progressive nature and serious sequelae of cases left untreated are stressed. - Editor. *Ped Neur Briefs* July 1987.

Moyamoya Disease Involving Posterior Cerebral Arteries

Sixteen children with moyamoya disease and involvement of the posterior cerebral artery are reported from the Departments of Neurophysiology, Neurosurgery, and Radiology, faculty of Medicine, Kyushu University, Fukuoka, Japan. Eight patients had complete occlusion of posterior cerebral arteries and the other eight had nonocclusive disease. All patients showed patent ophthalmic arteries bilaterally. Pattern-reversal visual-evoked potentials showed abnormalities in 75% of the posterior cerebral artery occlusive group and no abnormalities in the nonocclusive group. Abnormalities were also found in positron emission tomography, computed tomography, and the clinical examination of the visual fields. The authors concluded that the pattern-reversal visual-evoked potentials was the most practical means to explore posterior cerebral artery occlusion in the course of moyamoya disease. (Tashima-Kurita S et al. Moyamoya disease. Posterior cerebral artery occlusion and pattern-reversal visual-evoked potential. *Arch Neurol* May 1989; *46*:550-553).

> COMMENT. Moyamoya disease is characterized by progressive occlusion of cerebral arteries and predominantly the anterior and middle cerebral arteries. The incidence of posterior cerebral artery involvement and visual disturbances is approximately 25% and the clinical manifestations include decreased visual acuity, homonymous hemianopsia, constriction of the visual fields, and scintillating scotoma. - Editor. *Ped Neur Briefs* May 1989.

Neonatal Stroke: Left Middle Cerebral Preponderance

The prevalence of left middle cerebral artery involvement in 15 patients with neonatal stroke has been investigated at the

Department of Neurology and Pediatrics, Strich School of Medicine, Loyola University of Chicago, Maywood, IL. Of 15 patients reviewed retrospectively, 12 had left middle cerebral artery infarction, and this preponderance was the same as that observed in 36 previously reported cases. Transcranial Doppler measurement of mean blood flow velocity in the right and left middle cerebral arteries of 20 normal newborns demonstrated no significant difference between the 2 sides. The authors postulate that the turbulent flow of blood from the ductus arteriosus in the perinatal period favors the passage of an embolus traveling up the arch of the aorta into the left common carotid artery. (Coker SB et al. Neonatal stroke: Description of patients and investigation into pathogenesis. *Pediatr Neurol* July-August 1988; 4:219-223).

> COMMENT. Neonatal seizures were reported in 12 of the 15 infants with stroke, and the birth was complicated in 13. Cesarean section was performed in 8 (53%). Subsequent examination at 1-4 years of age showed hemiparesis in 10, near normal function of the involved extremity in 8, and persistent epilepsy requiring anticonvulsant treatment in 4 patients. Neonatal stroke is not usually correlated with birth asphyxia, birth trauma, and type of delivery, and an embolic etiology is more likely. - Editor. *Ped Neur Briefs* August 1988.

Neonatal Stroke Outcome

The clinical outcome of 17 children, 1 to 11 years of age, who experienced cerebral artery infarctions as neonates has been studied in the Depts of Pediatrics and Neurology, Univ of Kentucky Med Center, Lexington, KY. The left middle cerebral artery (MCA) was involved in 9 (53%) and the right MCA in 5 (30%). Fourteen (82%) who developed neonatal seizures became seizure free and neurologically normal within the first year and anticonvulsants were discontinued. Three patients had recurrence of seizures after 1 to 8 years and anticonvulsants were renewed. Eleven patients (65%) have normal neurologic development but one of 2 attending school has cognitive deficits. (Stan SK, Baumann, RJ. Outcome of neonatal strokes. *AJDC* Oct 1988; *142*:1086-1088).

> COMMENT. The authors conclude that infants with a unilateral arterial stroke generally have a favorable prognosis initially but require long-term follow-up for possible recurrence of seizures and development of learning disabilities. Comparing these results with a previous report on neonatal stroke (*Ped Neur Briefs* Aug 1989; *2*:63-64), the increased prevalence of left middle cerebral artery infarction and the frequent complication of neonatal seizures are in agreement, but the recovery of neurologic function within 1 year is in contrast to a persistent hemiparesis in 66% of patients examined at 1-4 years of age. - Editor. *Ped Neur Briefs* September 1988.

Ischemic Stroke In Childhood: Causes And Symptoms

Juvenile ischemic cerebral vascular disease was studied over a 15 year period in 34 patients in the Department of Neurosurgery, Neurological Institute, Tokyo Women's Medical College, Tokyo, Japan. Intracranial occlusions were attributed to cerebral thrombosis or embolism in 23, and to Moya Moya disease in 11. An embolism based on congenital heart disease was found in 8, with trauma in 3, and with infection in 1. Cerebral angiography confirmed stenoses or occlusions in 17 of 21 patients tested. The initial symptoms of juvenile ischemic cerebral disease were hemiparesis in 22 (47.8%), convulsion in 9 (19.6%) and speech impairment in 7 (15.2%). The prognosis in patients with an unknown etiology for the occlusion had good outcomes whereas those with congenital heart disease had a relatively poor prognosis. Three patients had abscesses after their ischemic lesions. (Wanifuchi H et al. Ischemic stroke in infancy, childhood and adolescence. *Child's Nerv Syst* Dec 1988; *4*:361-364).

COMMENT. Cerebral arterial occlusion in children is uncommon and only 3% of cerebral infarctions occur in patients under the age of 40. A thorough diagnostic search to prevent recurrences is of importance in the young stroke victim. Despite a lengthy differential diagnosis of cerebral infarction several predominant etiologies account for the majority of cases. The category of uncertain etiology includes 35% of patients in whom the cerebral infarction was associated with mitral valve prolapse, migraine and oral contraceptive use. Each of these conditions is frequent enough in healthy young adults that causality cannot be assumed until other causes have been eliminated (Hart, Miller. *Stroke* 1983; *14*:110).

The causes of infarction in 100 young adults were listed as cerebral vascular atherosclerosis (18), cerebral embolism (31), cerebral vasculopathy (10), coagulopathy and systemic inflammation (9), peripartum (5), and uncertain etiology (27). Ergot preparations and oral contraceptives were contraindicated in patients with migraine headaches and cerebral infarction. Platelet antiaggregates were advised in migraine patients with cerebral infarction and in the idiopathic cases. In the present paper from Tokyo, some of the patients with arterial occlusion of unknown etiology had had frequent episodes of inflammation such as measles or tonsillitis in their past history and the occlusion and inflammation were thought to be indicative of arteritis. Patients with occlusion of the internal carotid artery often show pathological findings consistent with the early stages of Moya Moya disease in childhood (Suzuki J Takaku A. *Arch Neurol* 1969; *20*:288). - Editor. *Ped Neur Briefs* April 1989.

Neonatal Transverse Sinus Thrombosis

Four full-term newborns with transverse sinus thrombosis (TST) and a benign outcome are described from the Children's Hospital of Los Angeles and USCSM, and the University of

Texas Medical School, Houston, TX. The infants presented with irritability, jitteriness, and mild hypertonia. One had seizures and 3 had abnormal EEGs with temporal or central sharp waves. The CSF was xanthochromic and contained excess red blood cells. IN 2 of 4 followed up, the neurological exam was normal. MRI scans which permit diagnosis of TST shows a hyperintense signal of the sinus thrombosis in T1- and T2- weighted images and subdural and subarachnoid hemorrhages. Partial thrombosis can be seen as a ring of central hyperintense signal surrounded by a halo of signal void that corresponds to flowing blood. The authors suggest that TST may be relatively common, with a wide spectrum of severity. (Baram TZ et al. Transverse sinus thrombosis in newborns: clinical and magnetic resonance imaging findings. *Ann Neurol* Dec 1988; *24*:792-794).

COMMENT. Sinus thromboses in newborns are most commonly associated with birth trauma and intracranial hemorrhage. A mild tentorial laceration was considered likely in the cases reported. An inherited protein C deficiency may be manifested by massive venous thromboses in the newborn (Seligsohn U et al. *N Engl J Med* 1984; *310*:559), an etiology to be considered in the absence of a history of brain trauma. - Editor. *Ped Neur Briefs* December 1988.

Transposition Of Great Vessels And Mobius Syndrome

The vascular theory of embryopathogenesis for Mobius syndrome is proposed in a case report of a 3-month-old boy from the University of New Mexico School of Medicine, Albuquerque, NM. At birth, he had bilateral facial and abducens palsies, left acheiria (congenital absence of the hand), and transposition of the aorta and pulmonary artery. He was lethargic, cyanotic, and in respiratory distress, and he expired after an arterial switch procedure with closure of a septal defect. The authors cite 2 reports of Mobius syndrome with cardiac anomalies, both presenting with dextrocardia and the Poland anomaly (unilateral hypoplasia or absence of pectoral muscles, nipple, and upper limb). An intrapartum insult during the fourth to seventh week of gestation is consistent with the vascular theory of embryopathogenesis. (Raroque HG, Hershewe GL, Snyder RD. Mobius syndrome and transposition of the great vessels. *Neurology* Dec 1988; *38*:1894-5).

COMMENT. Congenital facial diplegia and abducens palsy, *Mobius syndrome*, has been explained as either a primary hypoplasia of cranial nerve nuclei or a primary deficiency of the muscles derived from the first two branchial arches. A dysgenesis of both neural and muscular tissue has been proposed in some cases. In the above case report, the concomitant occurrence of the vascular anomaly supports the theory of impaired cranial nerve nuclear development due to interruption of vascular supply at or around the sixth intrauterine week. - Editor. *Ped Neur Briefs* December 1988.

Cerebral Vasculitis And Diet Pills

A 17 year old girl who developed cerebral vasculitis and hemorrhage following the ingestion of an overdose of phenylpropanolamine diet-aid pills is reported from the Schneider Children's Hospital, Long Island Jewish Medical Center, New Hyde Park, NY. She developed headache and vomiting five hours after taking five diet-aid pills, equivalent to a total dose of 375 mg of phenylpropanolamine. Neurological examination showed early papilledema and minimal nuchal rigidity. A CT scan revealed a large right parietooccipital hemorrhage with deviation of the midline to the left and deformation of the right lateral ventricle. Angiography showed beading of the branches of the right carotid, basilar, and both posterior cerebral arteries, compatible with bilateral cerebral vasculitis. Following craniotomy for the removal of the clot and treatment with dexamethasone, the patient recovered rapidly and neurological examination revealed only a left homonymous hemianopsia. (Forman HP et al. Cerebral vasculitis and hemorrhage in an adolescent taking diet pills containing phenylpropanolamine: Case report and review of the literature. *Pediatrics* May 1989; *83*:737-741).

COMMENT. This case report was the eleventh documented example of phenylpropanolamine associated intracerebral hemorrhage with vasculitis. Necrotizing angiitis has been described with abuse of drugs such as amphetamine, methamphetamine, and ephedrine. Intracerebral hemorrhage may also occur as a complication of over-the-counter diet pills even with recommended doses. The authors comment that this report should alert pediatricians to the potential use of nonprescription medications containing phenylpropanolamine, whenever unexplained acute cerebral symptoms are present. - Editor. *Ped Neur Briefs* May 1989.

BLOOD DISORDERS

Iron Deficiency Anemia And Neurologic Deficits

A 14 year old black female adolescent with focal neurological abnormalities complicating severe iron deficiency anemia is reported from Duke University Medical Center, Durham, North Carolina. The anemia was caused by bleeding from generalized intestinal polyposis and hereditary hemorrhagic telangiectasia complicated by nasal and gingival bleeding. Neurologic symptoms and signs began with occipital headache and neck pain, intermittent diplopia, transient right-sided numbness and weakness, and a brief syncopal episode. On admission the patient was somnolent and the neurological examination revealed bilateral VI nerve palsies, facial palsies, papilledema, and generalized muscle weakness with normal reflexes. After transfusion with packed erythrocytes and treatment with ferrous sulfate orally the facial palsy resolved within 12 hours and the VI nerve palsy and somnolence resolved by the fifth day. A normal hemoglobin was maintained by iron supplementation and the neurologic exam remained normal despite continued gingival and nasal bleeding from telangiectases. (Bruggers CS et al. Reversible focal neurologic deficits in severe iron deficiency anemia. *J Pediatr* Sept 1990; *117*:430-432).

COMMENT. An iron deficiency anemia is reported in 23% of cases of *breath-holding spells* in infants and young children. (Holowach J, Thurston DL. *N Eng J Med* 1963; *268*:21). The neurologic abnormalities with iron deficiency anemia may result from tissue hypoxia, increased capillary permeability, cerebral edema, and abnormal cytochrome enzyme function involved in oxygen metabolism. - Editor. *Ped Neur Briefs* October 1990.

Factor XIII Deficiency And Intracranial Hemorrhage

A 38 month old boy with excessive bleeding following circumcision as a newborn and two episodes of intracranial hemorrhage at four months and at 8-1/2 months of age is reported from the Scott and White Clinic, Temple, TX. The diagnosis of Factor XIII deficiency was made in infancy and the bleeding was stopped with cryoprecipitate. Since 11 months of age he was treated with Fibrogammin at four week intervals and no further hemorrhages had occurred. MRI at three years demonstrated a left temporoparietal encephalomalacia and no vascular malformations. (Larsen PD et al. Factor XIII deficiency and intracranial hemorrhages in infancy. *Pediatr Neurol* July-August 1990; *6*:277-278).

COMMENT. Repeated intracranial hemorrhage can occur spontaneously and without evidence of trauma in infants with Factor XIII deficiency. Routine coagulation studies do not detect this factor deficiency and examination for Factor XIII may avoid a misdiagnosis of child abuse. Replacement therapy should be maintained throughout life. - Editor. *Ped Neur Briefs* October 1990.

CHAPTER **12**

CNS TRAUMA

Ice Hockey Injuries

The school of Public Health Institute for Athletic Medicine, and Departments of Orthopedic Surgery and Biomechanical Engineering, University of Minnesota, Minneapolis, MN, conducted an epidemiological study of ice hockey injuries among 12 high school varsity teams in the 1982-83 season. A major finding was a high incidence of concussion (9%), accounting for 12% of the total injuries. In addition, dizziness in 34%, headaches in 30%, blurred vision in 12%, and tinnitus in 11%, followed a blow to head or neck. Residual symptoms, including neck pain, back pain, reduced strength in upper extremities, were reported in 28% of players with a blow to head, neck or back. The older, taller, heavier player was injured most frequently, except that the risk to the 14-year old player was equal to that for 18-year olds. Injured players had greater playing experience, and defense and wings accounted for the highest percentage of injuries.

Injuries occurred primarily during competition (82%) and breakout plays accounted for 23% of head injuries. Colliding with another player (35%) and hitting the boards (20%) were the major mechanisms of injury. Playing hockey to allay tension and aggressions resulted in a risk of concussion four times that of alternative motivations such as enjoyment of the game, a scholarship for college, or peer relations. The use of the face mask may have promoted a more aggressive style of play and also increased risk of concussions and other injuries. The authors advocate elimination of body checking, the cushioning of boards, and the use of breakaway goal posts. (Gerberich SG, Finke R et al. *Child's Nerv Syst* 1987; *3*:59-64).

> COMMENT. These statistics are alarming. Other studies have shown that one-third of all hockey related injuries have occurred in children aged 5 to 14 years. Epidemiological studies are needed in the younger age groups and Little Leagues. Coaches should be aware that the development of vertebrae and adjoining cartilage is incomplete in children and susceptibility to neck injury is greater than in adults. Coaches, players and parents should be better educated regarding potential risks of serious injuries associated with collision forces to the head and neck in young hockey enthusiasts and aggressive behavior should not be condoned.

Other sports-related CNS injuries in children and adolescents reviewed by Lehman LB (*Postgrad Med* Sept 15 1987; *82*:141) include closed head and cervical spine injuries associated with boxing, wrestling, judo, karate, gymnastics, football, soccer, and rugby. The most important step in reducing cervical spine injury has been the elimination of "spearing", which involves the use of the helmeted skull as a battering ram. Episodes of mild cerebral concussion, a frequent occurrence in competitive sports, are deleterious. Recently, the cheerleaders "pyramid" formation has been implicated in a number of neurological injuries and even deaths. - Editor. *Ped Neur Briefs* September 1987.

Head Injury In Infants And Children

Of 738 children with head injuries (0-16 yrs) admitted to the Children's Memorial Hospital, Chicago, IL during a 5-year period from 1981-85, 318 (43%) were less than 3 years of age and almost half of the younger group were under 1 year. A fall was the most common mechanism of injury in children under 3 years, followed by a motor vehicle accident. Posttraumatic seizures developed more commonly in children under 2 yrs (16%) than in older children (9%, entire group). The most reliable indicators of poor outcome were absent or impaired oculovestibular reflex and bilateral fixed dilated pupils. Intracranial pressure greater than 40 torr with coma scores of 3, 4 or 5 spelled fatality. The mortality of the entire group with severe head injury was 22%. (Hahn YS et al. Head injuries in children under 36 months of age. Demography and outcome. *Child's Nerv Syst* Feb 1988; 4:34-40).

COMMENT. A modified Glasgow Coma Scale - *Children's Coma Scale* - was developed as an objective neurological assessment and prognostic indicator for the children under 3 yrs of age in this study. Points for eye-opening responses (4-1) were the same but those for best motor response and best verbal response were different for infants. Smiling, orientation to sound or verbal stimulus, or following objects were given a subscore of "5" (oriented); consolable crying but inappropriate interaction "4"; inconsistent consolable crying and moaning "3"; inconsolable crying and irritable, restless interaction "2"; no response "1". One-third of the younger group showed a sequence of labile symptoms following the initial loss of consciousness, becoming agitated and irritable, followed by vomiting, sleep, and waking and playful within 24 hrs in the majority. When children were comatose longer than 6 hrs, 75% (12/16) had a poor outcome with a 50% (8/16) mortality. - Editor. *Ped Neur Briefs* May 1988.

Conscious Level Assessment In Infants

Neurosurgeons at the Adelaide Children's Hospital, King William Street, North Adelaide, SA 50067, Australia have used a paediatric version of the *Glasgow Coma Scale* since 1977 for assessing conscious level in infants and young children. For the best verbal response, during the first 6 months the normally conscious infant is expected to cry or grunt spontaneously or when disturbed and the expected normal score is 2. Between 6 and 12 months, the normal infant babbles and begins to vocalize and scores 3. After 12 months, words are expected with a score of 4. Orientation by 5 years of age gives a score of 5. The normal aggregate scores at different ages are as follows: birth-6 months: 9; 6-12 months: 11; 12-24 months: 12; 2-5 years: 13; over 5 years: 14. A disadvantage of the scale is the reduced sensitivity, especially in the neonate. (Reilly PL et al. Assessing the conscious level in infants and young children: a paediatric version of the Glasgow Coma Scale. *Child's Nerv Syst* 1988; *4*:30-33).

> COMMENT. In an editorial comment, Dr AJ Raimondi corroborates the need for children's and infant's coma scales as substitutes for the well known Glasgow scale suitable mainly for adults. He favors an 11-point sale for infants, which incorporates ocular responses (ranging from normal pursuit to fixed pupils), verbal responses (ranging from crying to apnea), and motor responses (from flexion/extension to flaccidity). A uniformly tested and accepted coma scale for infants and children would be advantageous. Coma scores as low as 3-4 carry the same prediction of poor outcome at any age; coma scores of 5-8 may carry a less serious significance in young children than in adults. - Editor. *Ped Neur Briefs* May 1988.

Alpha Coma In The Electroencephalogram

Recorded EEG rhythms within the alpha-frequency band, paradoxically resembling waking patterns but in apparently comatose patients, a pattern termed alpha coma, have been reviewed over a 10 year period in the Division of Electroencephalography, University of Washington School of Medicine, Seattle, WA. Of 50 patients with records showing the alpha-pattern coma, 49 were admitted with cardiopulmonary arrest and one had developed alpha coma with hyperglycemic, hyperosmolar coma. In addition to the alpha activity, arrhythmic delta waves were present diffusely in 25% and theta waves in 23%. The outcomes of patients with or without alpha coma after cardiac arrest did not differ significantly, the majority not regaining consciousness and dying in hospital. The single patient with hyperglycemic coma regained consciousness and was discharged but did not fully recover cognitive function. A review of the literature did not preclude neurological recovery following alpha coma. (Austin EJ et al. Etiology and prognosis of alpha coma. *Neurology* May 1988; *38*:773-777).

COMMENT. Alpha coma usually follows cardiac arrest and can be identified in 25% of patients. It also follows brain stem lesions, sedative drug overdose, respiratory arrest, and severe disturbance of glucose metabolism. Where alpha coma follows a condition other than cardiac arrest or a brain stem lesion the outcome is usually good. The prognosis is especially favorable after drug overdose. - Editor. *Ped Neur Briefs* May 1988.

Severe Head Injuries: Clinical Predictors

The clinical predictors of severe head trauma in 55 children, 1 to 15 years of age, were compared with CT scan findings at the Dept of Pediatrics, Medical College of Wisconsin and Children's Hospital of Wisconsin, Milwaukee, WI. Severity of head trauma was determined according to the presence or absence of clinical variables, including altered mental states, duration of loss of consciousness greater than 5 min, vomiting, headache, focal neurologic deficit, seizures, and soft-tissue injury. Injury was considered severe if one or more of the following variables were present: altered mental status, increased intracranial pressure, and seizure or focal neurologic deficit. Thirty-seven (84%) of 44 patients with severe head trauma had a positive CT scan. Six (13%) with a Glasgow coma Scale (GCS) score of 12 or greater had abnormal CT scans. All patients with mild or moderate head trauma had normal CT scans. Historical information and clinical examination were the most accurate predictors for abnormal CT scans regardless of GCS scores. (Hennes H et al. Clinical predictors of severe head trauma in children. *AJDC* Oct 1988; *142*:1045-1047).

COMMENT. THE GCS may have limited application in the evaluation of acute head trauma in the pediatric population. A classification based on clinical findings more accurately identifies the severity of head trauma and the need for CT scans.   A further clinical objective evaluation of children with acute head injury includes tests of neuropsychological function. Investigators from the Dept Pediatrics, Univ of Maryland, Baltimore, report cognitive deficits immediately after closed head injury in adolescents that may interfere with school, home and peer activities (*AJDC* Oct 1988; *142*:1048). - Editor. *Ped Neur Briefs* September 1988.

Brain Injury And Shaking

The mechanism of brain injury in 24 infants with a diagnosis of *shaken baby syndrome* was investigated at the University of Iowa Hospitals and Clinics, Iowa City, IA. Half of the patients demonstrated signs of external head trauma. Intracranial injuries were indistinguishable in infants with and without evidence of external trauma. The mortality rate was the same in both groups. These findings indicated that shaking by itself is sufficient to cause severe or fatal intracranial injury and child abuse injuries associated with shaking may include direct trauma or only shaking. (Alexander R et al. Incidence of impact trauma with cranial injuries ascribed to shaking. *AJDC* June 1990; *144*:724-726).

COMMENT. From an anatomical standpoint one might expect that shaking would cause damage to the brain in the distribution of the vertebral arteries. Brain stem and occipital hemorrhage or ischemia was not documented in this report however. Apparently, shaking may cause hemorrhage from various sites including the retina and the intracranial bridging veins and the subdural space. The data in this study suggests that shaking alone is sufficient to cause serious intracranial injury or death.

Brain injuries among infants, children, adolescents, and young adults are reviewed from the Department of Epidemiology School of Public Health, UCLA, Los Angeles, CA. (Kraus JF et al. *AJDC* June 1990; *144*:684-691). The distribution of injuries by external cause varied with age. For infants, more than two-thirds of all brain injuries were from falls but only 8% were severe in nature. For preschool children, falls and motor vehicle accidents accounted for 51% and 22%, respectively. For school aged children five to nine years old, injuries were equally divided among motor vehicles, falls, and sports and recreation-related activities (31%, 31%, and 32%, respectively). Among adolescents aged 10-14 years, sports and recreation-related activities accounted for 43% of all brain injuries but only 7% were serious. Among young adults, 55% of injuries involved motor vehicles and one-third were serious. - Editor. *Ped Neur Briefs* June 1990.

Brain Injury And Drowning

The epidemiology and clinical course of immersion brain injury of childhood drowning cases are reviewed from the University of California, Davis, Sacramento. In 1986 there were 2,122 childhood drownings in the United States. Children 0-4 years of age accounted for 36% of all deaths and most of these occurred in residential pools. Children with a seizure disorder are at increased risk for drowning with rates several times higher than expected. Alcohol use is a contributing factor among adolescents in 40-50% of males. The outcome of drowning is largely determined by events occurring in the first ten minutes after the incident. Consciousness is lost after two minutes of anoxia, and irreversible brain damage occurs after four to six minutes. Survival is unusual after immersions of longer than five minutes.

Prompt resuscitation is vital; almost all subjects who ultimately survive are making a spontaneous respiratory effort within five minutes after extraction from the water and most do so within two minutes. Children who still require CPR in the emergency department have a poor prognosis: 35-60% die, and 60-100% of the survivors are severely brain damaged. Resuscitative measures may achieve somatic survival of the heart and other vital organs but brain function remains severely impaired. The patient in the permanent vegetative state breathes spontaneously and may exhibit random movements but has no purposeful activity or thought. Life expectancy of these children is estimated to average 18 months in institutions and longer in home care. Failure to provide timely resuscitation and lack of knowledge of CPR techniques among pool owners is associated with a poor outcome in drowning and near-drowning incidents. Pentobarbital therapy, at one time thought to be a promising addition to standard therapy for near drowning, has recently been shown to be ineffective. (Wintemute GJ. Childhood drowning and near-drowning in the United States. *AJDC* June 1990; *144*:663-669).

COMMENT. Since the outcome of an immersion event is determined within a few minutes of the onset of the incident, the emphasis is on primary prevention. Mandatory pool fencing and training in cardiopulmonary resuscitation for pool owners should be stressed. Children with epilepsy are often permitted to swim in pools but not in lakes with poor underwater visibility. Strict supervision must be observed since the risks of drowning are several times higher than for the average child. - Editor. *Ped Neur Briefs* June 1990.

Hyperglycemia And Cerebral Blood Flow In Drowning

Serial blood glucose levels and cerebral blood flow within 48 hours of admission were correlated with the clinical courses of 20 children with severe near-drowning in the Division of Child Neurology, the Department of Pediatrics, and Section of Neuroradiology, Loma Linda University School of Medicine, Loma Linda, CA. Seven children died, nine were in the persistent vegetative state, and four were normal. Ages ranged from nine month to ten years. Blood glucose levels on admission in the patients who died (511 ± 110 mg%) or who survived in a persistent vegetative state (465 ± 104 mg%) were significantly elevated compared with children who were normal at follow-up (238 ± 170 mg%). The blood glucose values returned to normal by day three of hospitalization.

Cerebral blood flow measured by stable xenon computed tomography was significantly decreased in patients who died compared with those who were normal or in a persistent vegetative state. An increase in intracranial pressure was correlated with decreased cerebral blood flow but not with the elevated blood glucose. An elevated initial blood glucose on admission was highly predictive of patients who died or those with vegetative survival. Cerebral blood flow measurements were predictive of eventual death but did not differentiate patients who survived in a vegetative state from those who became normal. Combining blood glucose and cerebral blood flow values improved predictability of outcome in near-drowning. (Ashwal S et al. Prognostic implications of hyperglycemia and reduced cerebral blood flow in childhood near-drowning. *Neurology* May 1990; *40*:820-823).

COMMENT. Cerebral blood flow and blood glucose determinations on admission are useful predictors of the outcome of children with near-drowning and like the Glasgow Coma Scale, they are objective measurements of prognosis. - Editor. *Ped Neur Briefs* June 1990.

Cognitive Sequelae Of Mild Head Injury

The sequelae of mild head injury one to five years after injury, assessed in a longitudinal study of 13,000 British children born in one week in 1970, are reported from the Albert Einstein College of Medicine, Bronx, NY and Bristol Polytechnic and University of Bristol, England. Parental reports of mild head injury in 114 children treated with ambulatory care or admission to hospital for one night were compared with those of 601 children with limb fractures, 605 with lacerations, 136 with burns, and 1726 without injury. When the children were five and ten years of age the parents completed the Rutter Child Behavior Questionnaire. At age ten teachers also answered questions from both the Rutter and Conners' questionnaires. The picture vocabulary test was used to assess overall intelligence at age five and subtests of the British Abilities Scale were used at age ten.

Children with head injuries were statistically indistinguishable from uninjured children on all tests except the teachers' report of hyperactivity which was 4/10 of a standard deviation higher. The authors concluded that mild head injury in school aged children does not have an adverse effect on global measures of cognition, achievement, and behavior one to five years after injury. (Bijur PE et al. Cognitive and behavioral sequelae of mild head injury in children. *Pediatrics* Sept 1990; *86*:337-344).

COMMENT. Head injuries reported as concussion and which result in ambulatory care or hospitalization of one night do not have an effect on general intelligence, achievement, and aggression measured one to five years after the injury. The increase in hyperactive behavior was considered of doubtful significance. The teachers reports of hyperactivity were not likely to be biased but hyperactivity unrecognized by the parents before the injury may have resulted in greater vulnerability to head injury. Evaluated as a group, the occurrence of hyperactivity may not be remarkable but in those children who lost consciousness and required admission to hospital, the sequel of hyperactivity might be significant and worthy of careful follow-up and management. - Editor. *Ped Neur Briefs* November 1990.

CHAPTER **13**

INFECTIOUS DISEASES

Acquired Immune Deficiency Syndrome (AIDS)

Central nervous system involvement is reported in 61 of 68 infants and children with asymptomatic AIDS (13 with ARC-AIDS-related complex) followed for 1 to 48 months (average, 18 mos) in the Depts of Neurology and Pediatrics at SUNY, Stony Brook, NY. Acquired microcephaly in 34 patients (55%), cognitive deficits in 38 patients (62%), and spastic paresis in 52 patients (85%) were the most frequent CNS complications. Seizures in only 6 patients, ataxia in 6, extrapyramidal rigidity or dystonia in 5, and tremor in 3 were uncommon manifestations of CNS dysfunction. Lymphoma of the CNS, cerebrovascular accidents, and CNS infection occurred in 10 children (15%) who showed a rapidly progressive encephalopathy. Neurological deterioration was subacute but progressive in 11, and began with a plateau in 31 patients. A static course with cognitive deficits was noted in 17 children. CT scans performed on children with a subacute or plateau course frequently showed cerebral atrophy, white matter attenuation and bilateral symmetric calcification of the basal ganglia. Neuropathological findings in

16 of 34 children who died during the study period included an inflammatory response, reactive astrocytosis, foamy macrophages, multinucleated cells, and pyramidal tract degeneration. Calcification of the basal ganglia was present in all cases. (Belman AL et al. Pediatric acquired immunodeficiency syndrome. Neurologic syndromes. *AJDC* 1988; *142*:29-35).

COMMENT. This longitudinal study of neurological complications of AIDS in children is the largest yet reported and is a valuable informative article for the pediatric neurologist called as a consultant on these cases. The neurological complications of AIDS in children differ from those in adults (Snider WD et al. *Ann Neurol* 1983; *14*:403). The incidence of CNS involvement is higher in children but unlike adult patients, CNS opportunistic infections appear to be uncommon, occurring in only 8% of the children in this study. A progressive dementing encephalitis (AIDS dementia complex) accompanied by regional cerebral metabolic alterations is the chief neurological complication of AIDS in adult cases (Rottenberg DA et al. *Ann Neurol* 1987; *22*:700). Peripheral neuropathy with painful dysesthesias and retinopathy with cotton-wool spots reported in 16% and 20%, respectively, of adult cases were not recognized in the pediatric group. The static encephalopathy diagnosed in 17 (28%) children was cause for optimism but this was tempered by a later progressive course in 5 similar cases. The incidence of potential AIDS cases in children may be higher than expected: a recent survey showed that 1 in 61 babies born in NY City carried antibodies to AIDS virus, indicating that their mothers were infected. About 40% of infants showing antibodies are estimated to be infected and may develop AIDS. - Editor. *Ped Neur Briefs* January 1988.

Treatment Of Aids Encephalopathy

A 3-year old boy who had acquired HIV infection transplacentally and developed AIDS encephalopathy is reported from the Depts of Paediatrics and Immunology, Newcastle General Hospital, Newcastle upon Tyne, England. During Hemophilus influenza pneumonia at 26 months his speech regressed to expressive aphasia and he developed spastic diplegia with inability to walk. CT scan showed cerebral atrophy. CSF showed no cells and normal glucose and protein; IgG antibiotics to HIV were increased. Treatment with intravenous gamma globulin 300 mg/kg and oral zidovudine (Retrovir-Wellcome) 100 mg/m² 4x daily every 4 weeks for 8 months led to considerable clinical improvement and an almost normal CT. Spasticity regressed allowing him to run unaided and his speech in single words became articulate. (Matthew J et al. AIDS encephalopathy with response to treatment. *Arch Dis Child* May 1988; 63:545-547).

COMMENT. AIDS encephalopathy may be acute and rapidly progressive (15%), subacute but progressive (18%), and static with cognitive deficits (28%). A plateau course is apparent in many. The reported case was subacute in onset and without treatment further progression might have been expected. - Editor. *Ped Neur Briefs* May 1988.

Stroke And Aids

The occurrence and causes of stroke in children with acquired immunodeficiency syndrome are reported from the Albert Einstein College of Medicine, Bronx, and the State University of New York at Stony Brook, NY. The report includes seven children with HIV infection who had clinical evidence, pathological evidence or both of stroke. An estimate of the clinical incidence of stroke based on four of 68 cases followed in a longitudinal study for 4-1/2 years was 1.3% per year. Of the seven children with stroke, four had hemorrhage in the CNS and six had non-hemorrhagic infarcts. The prevalence of cerebrovascular disease in a consecutive autopsy series was higher than the clinical incidence and was documented in six (24%) of 25 children with HIV infection, including those children who had clinical evidence of stroke. In four children with immune thrombocytopenia, hemorrhage was catastrophic in one and clinically silent in three. Arteriopathy of meningocerebral arteries and aneurysmal dilatation of the circle of Willis were found in two patients, and two had co-existing cardiomyopathy and subacute necrotizing encephalomyopathy. (Park YD et al. Stroke in pediatric acquired immunodeficiency syndrome. *Ann Neurol* Sept 1990; *28*:303-311).

> COMMENT. In children with AIDS who develop focal neurological signs, cerebrovascular disease and stroke are likely explanations. The most frequent CNS complications of HIV-1 infection in children are developmental delays, cognitive impairment, acquired microcephaly, and bilateral corticospinal tract signs. Movement disorders and cerebellar signs are less frequent and seizures are uncommon. (Belman AL. *Am J Dis Child* 1988; *142*:29-35; *Neurologic Clinics*, W.B. Saunders, Philadelphia, August 1990; *8*:571-603). - Editor. *Ped Neur Briefs* October 1990.

New England Lyme Disease In England

A 6 year old boy seen this month after recovery from severe neurological complications of Lyme disease prompts this report to alert pediatricians and neurologists to the increase in incidence of this seasonal infectious disease, especially among campers in the United States, Europe, and Australia.

The patient whose case was reported from St. Helier Hospital, Carshalton, Surrey, presented 6 months ago with headache, drowsiness, vomiting, photophobia, and neck stiffness. He was afebrile and had papilledema and Babinski signs. The CT was normal and the CSF was compatible with viral meningoencephalitis. His condition rapidly deteriorated and bulbar, 6th and 7th nerve palsies, and spastic paralysis developed. *Borrelia burgdorferi* serology was positive and IgG and IgM titers were elevated in the serum but not in the CSF. Benzylpenicillin IV in high doses for 14 days resulted in slow but complete recovery. (Bendig JWA, Ogilvie D. *Lancet* 1987; *1*:681-2).

COMMENT. This patient lacked the history of tick bite, fever, arthralgia, and characteristic rash, erythema chronica migrans. He had been camping in France 4 months before and had been close to deer in Richmond Park 5 months before the onset of symptoms. About 15% of patients with Lyme disease develop neurological problems. A triad of meningoencephalitis, cranial neuritis, and radiculoneuritis is described. Early treatment with penicillin in children aborts the progress of the disease.

One case recently reported (Broderick JP et al. *Mayo Clin Proc* 1987; *62*:313), a girl from Wisconsin who had classic untreated Lyme disease at 13 years of age, developed severe focal inflammatory encephalitis with positive serologic tests 6 years later. She presented with headaches, global aphasia, and apraxia of her right upper extremity. The EEG showed slow-wave activity over the entire left hemisphere. Treatment with penicillin G 20 mill units daily for 2 weeks was followed initially by clinical deterioration but later by gradual and steady improvement. The early diagnosis of Lyme disease is important because of the serious neurological complications that accompany delay in treatment. - Editor. *Ped Neur Briefs* July 1987.

Lyme Disease And CNS Complications

Four adult patients with chronic meningoencephalitis caused by tick-transmitted Borrelia burgdorferi infection are reported from the Depts of Neurology, University of Freiburg, Freiburg, and University of Koln, Koln, Federal Republic of Germany. All patients lived in wooded areas in which the transmitting tick (Ixodes ricinus) was widely distributed. IgG antibody titers were higher in CSF than in serum, indicating a specific intrathecal immune response against the B burgdorferi antigen and suggesting *neuroborreliosis (Bannwarth's syndrome)*, although the characteristic painful meningopolyneuritis was absent.

MRI showed either multiple lesions of high signal density in the white matter suggestive of MS or evidence of vascular involvement, as in other spirochetal infections, such as meningovascular syphilis. The authors consider the clinical spectrum of neuroborreliosis to be comparable to the different forms of neurosyphilis. Only one patient had a complete clinical remission after intravenous penicillin therapy, in 2 there was no further progression, and one showed no improvement. (Kohler J et al. Chronic central nervous system involvement in Lyme borreliosis. *Neurology* June 1988; *38*:863-867).

COMMENT. The manifestations of Lyme disease are in 3 stages: *Stage I*, erythema chronicum migrans, in 80-95% cases, minor flu-like symptoms with headache, fatigue, fever, myalgias, and other signs of disseminated disease such as arthralgias; *Stage II*, neurological complications in 15% cases, onset at 2-11 wks, with meningitis, Bell's palsy, and peripheral radiculoneuropathy; carditis (8%); and *Stage III*, arthritis (60%) and chronic neurological syndromes as described above. The most common neurological complication is aseptic meningitis which presents with headache and stiff neck and associated encephalitic symptoms including somnolence, emotional lability, memory loss, poor concentration and behavioral changes. Seventh nerve palsy is seen in 50% patients with meningitis or it occurs alone. Peripheral neuropathies are motor or sensory or mixed. Less common neurological complications include mononeuritis multiplex, transverse myelitis, Guillain-Barre syndrome, chorea, cerebellar ataxia, and pseudotumor cerebri. Maternal-fetal transmission has been described, although no definite link to fetal anomalies has been documented.

Treatment recommended in the literature varies with the age: for children over 8 yrs and adults, oral tetracycline; for children under 8 yrs, phenoxymethyl penicillin. (For details, see Hurwitz S. *Contemporary Pediatrics* June

1988; 74-82; Stechenberg BW. *Pediatr Infec Dis J* June 1988; *7*:402-409). Preventative methods include: 1) avoidance of wooded, grassy areas; 2) use of tick repellants such as Deet and permathrins on clothes; 3) removal of ticks by pulling straight out with tweezers. - Editor. *Ped Neur Briefs* June 1988.

Lyme Disease: CNS Manifestations

Six patients with central nervous system manifestations of Lyme disease are reported from the Department of Neurology, Georgetown University School of Medicine, Washington, DC. Behavioral changes, ataxia, and/or weakness in bulbar or peripheral muscles developed weeks to years after the initial infection. Four patients had lymphocytic pleocytosis in the CSF and two had MRI evidence of demyelination. All patients had elevated antibody titers to B burgdorferi in serum and all were treated with high-dose intravenous penicillin. Four had recovered completely within one to three months. One patient had persistent brief episodes of vestibular neuronitis and optic neuritis 15 months after antibiotic therapy for myelitis. One patient in whom antibiotic therapy had been delayed for two years after the onset of CSF abnormalities failed to respond to repeated course of IV penicillin and showed a progressive neurologic involvement with bilateral peripheral facial weakness, double vision, weakness of triceps, wrist and finger flexors and loss of sensation in hands and arms. (Pachner AR et al. Central nervous system manifestations of Lyme disease. *Arch Neurol* July 1989; *46*:790-795).

COMMENT. A case of latent Lyme neuroborreliosis is reported in a 17 year old boy from the University of Munich, Germany (Pfister H-W et al. *Neurology* August 1989; *39*:1118). Borrelia burgdorferi was isolated from the CSF, serum IgG antibody titers were elevated, but concurrent inflammatory signs of CSF as well as intrathecal antibody production were absent. Bilateral tinnitus was the only clinical symptom and this could not definitely be attributed to the Borrelial infection.

Lyme disease is the subject of Medical Progress (Steere AC. *N Engl J Med* Aug 31, 1989; *321*:386). Lyme disease commonly begins in summer with a characteristic skin lesion, erythema migrans, accompanied by flu-like or meningitis-like symptoms. Weeks or months later the patient may have neurologic or cardiac abnormalities, migratory musculoskeletal pain or arthritis. After the first several weeks of infection almost all patients have a positive antibody response to the spirochete and serologic determinations are currently considered the most practical laboratory aid in diagnosis. The author concludes that appropriate antibiotics are usually curative but longer courses of therapy are often needed later in the illness and some patients may not respond. The fetus may be at risk in mothers treated for the disease; a pregnant woman in Europe whose erythema migrans was treated with oral antibiotics gave birth to an infant who died of Lyme encephalitis. (Weber K et al. *Pediatr Infect Dis J* 1988; *7*:286). - Editor. *Ped Neur Briefs* August 1989.

Chronic Neurologic Manifestations Of Lyme Disease

The chronic neurologic symptoms and signs in 27 patients with previous signs of Lyme disease and current evidence of immunity to Borrelia burgdorferi are reported from the Departments of Neurology and Medicine, Tufts University School of Medicine, New England Medical Center, Boston, MA. The median age was 49 years with a range of 25-72 years. Signs and symptoms of chronic neurologic abnormalities included encephalopathy in 89% with memory loss, depression, sleep disturbance, irritability, and difficulty finding words; polyneuropathy in 70% with spinal or radicular pain, distal paresthesia, and sensory loss; leukoencephalitis in 4%; and miscellaneous symptoms including fatigue (74%), headache (48%), hearing loss (15%), fibromyalgia (15%), and tinnitus (7%). Seventeen patients (63%) had abnormalities of both the central and peripheral nervous systems, seven (26%) had encephalopathy alone, two (7%) had polyneuropathy alone, and the remaining patient (4%) had leukoencephalitis.

At the time of examination chronic neurologic abnormalities had been present from three months to 14 years, usually with little progression. Six months after a two week course of intravenous Ceftriaxine (2 g daily), 17 patients (63%) had improved, 6 (22%) had improved and then relapsed, and 4 (15%) had no change in their condition. The early signs of infection were erythema migrans (85%), and headache and neck stiffness in 41%. The most common early neurologic abnormality was a facial palsy in 30%. Arthritis had occurred in 70% before the chronic neurologic symptoms developed and it was still present in ten patients (37%) when the chronic neurologic abnormalities were noted. (Logigian EL et al. Chronic neurologic manifestations of Lyme disease). *N Engl J Med* Nov 22, 1990; *323*: 1438-44).

COMMENT. The criteria for case inclusion in this study were previous signs of Lyme disease, neurologic symptoms lasting at least three months that could not be attributed to another cause, and current evidence of humoral or cellular immunity to B. burgdorferi, as shown by elevated serum IgG or IgM antibody titer of at least 1:400, five or more IgG antibody bands to spirochetal polypeptides, or a stimulation index of 10 or more in response to Borrelia antigens. The chronic neurologic abnormalities began months to years after the onset of infection, sometimes after long periods of latency and similar to the course of neurosyphilis. The most common form of chronic CNS involvement was subacute encephalopathy affecting memory, mood, and sleep sometimes with subtle disturbances in language. Diagnosis could be difficult because of the nonspecific nature of the symptoms. Although this report concerns adults, the findings might be pertinent to Lyme disease contracted during childhood. - Editor. *Ped Neur Briefs* December 1990.

Congenital Syphilis

Seven infants with congenital syphilis who became symptomatic between 3 and 14 weeks of age are reported from the Bronx Municipal Hospital Center and Albert Einstein College of Medicine, Bronx, NY. At delivery four infants and their mothers had negative rapid-plasma- reagin tests for syphilis. The other three mothers had been seronegative and were not tested at delivery; two of their infants were seronegative at birth and one was not tested. When the infants became symptomatic all seven and the five mothers available for testing were seropositive for syphilis. A characteristic diffuse rash was the presenting symptom in four and three presented with fever and aseptic meningitis. All infants had multisystem disease evidenced by hepatosplenomegaly, increased aminotransferase and alkaline phosphatase levels, anemia, and monocytosis. All responded to parenteral penicillin. Radiological evidence of bone involvement was seen in three of six patients tested. Renal disease occurred in the youngest child, a three week old boy who had severe nephrosis. A Jarisch-Herxheimer reaction, consisting of a sudden elevation of temperature, occurred in all children within two to six hours after they received the first dose of antibiotics. (Corfman DH, Glaser JH. Congenital syphilis presenting in infants after the newborn period. *N Engl J Med* Nov 8, 1990; *323*:1299-1302).

> COMMENT. At least in areas where the disease is prevalent, serologic tests for syphilis should be included in the evaluation of all febrile infants and especially if associated with aseptic meningitis, hepatomegaly, or hematologic abnormalities, even if previous tests for syphilis have been negative at birth. The incidence of syphilis has reached epidemic proportions in some areas. In New York the rate of primary or secondary syphilis in women rose only marginally between 1983 and 1986 but it increased almost four-fold between 1986 and 1988. In the same two year period the number of reported cases of congenital syphilis rose from 57 to 357. The pediatrician's suspicion of congenital syphilis

must remain high to avoid misdiagnosis. (McIntosh K. Congenital syphilis - breaking through the safety net. Editorial. *N Engl J Med* Nov 8, 1990; *323*:1339-1341). - Editor. *Ped Neur Briefs* November 1990.

Acute Viral Encephalitis

In a retrospective study of children with viral encephalitis admitted to the University Paediatric Unit, Queen Mary Hospital, Hong Kong, during the past 10 years, 57 satisfied the diagnostic criteria. The presumed viral etiology was determined in 15 (26%) patients of whom 9 had post-infectious encephalitis (mumps - 4, measles - 1, rubella - 1, influenza A - 2, influenza B - 1). The viruses isolated were: influenza (3 cases), Coxsackie (2), adenovirus (2), mixed adenovirus and cytomegalovirus (1), and herpes simplex (1).

Presenting neurologic features included focal signs (33%), convulsion (30%), headache (25%), drowsiness (18%), nuchal rigidity (10%), and coma (9%). Seven (12%) who developed status epilepticus within 24 hrs of admission died subsequently. A total of 16 (28%) died, and 5 were less than 1 year old. Indicators of a poor outcome were an onset in infancy and rapid deterioration in the level of consciousness.

Recovery was complete in 76% of 41 survivors; focal neurological deficits remained in 29% and epilepsy in 4% of 31 with sequelae. Eight children with suspected herpes simplex encephalitis on admission were treated with Acyclovir and none died; one in whom the diagnosis was confirmed developed spastic quadriplegia, mental retardation, and infantile spasms. (Wong V, Yeung CY. Acute viral encephalitis in children. *Aust Paediatr J* 1987; *23*:339-342).

COMMENT. Unlike previous reports from the USA and Scandinavia which have emphasized herpes simplex virus (HSE) as a major cause of acute sporadic viral encephalitis, only 1 case was identified in this study and none of the 16 patients who died had histological evidence of herpes simplex infection. Brain biopsy, a controversial diagnostic test, was not performed.

A consensus panel of the Jrnl of Pediatric Infectious Disease has recommended early brain biopsy as a prerequisite for diagnosis and treatment of HSE. This view is supported by Hanley et al, Johns Hopkins Hospital, but is considered invalid by Fishman RA, Univ of California, San Francisco (*Arch Neurol* 1987; *44*:1289-1292). Brett EM, at the Hospital for Sick Children, Great Ormond Street, London, has spoken against routine diagnostic brain biopsy for suspected HSE in children (*Br Med J* 1986; *293*:1388). Noninvasive magnetic resonance imaging (MRI) may provide early diagnosis without the immediate risks of biopsy and its later complications (Schroth G et al. *Neurology* 1987; *37*:179). - Editor. *Ped Neur Briefs* January 1988.

Subacute Sclerosing Panencephalitis (SSPE)

In England and Wales, unlike the United States, SSPE is a persisting problem. The number of new notifications of SSPE in a 6 year period (1980-86) was 60 (10 cases per year). There were 62 deaths from SSPE in the same period! Immunization against measles increased from 50 to 68% between 1980 and 1986. Of those children who developed SSPE, less than 5% had been immunized (Drs Miller and Barnes, personal communications). - Editor. *Ped Neur Briefs* June 1987.

Subacute Sclerosing Panencephalitis

A 20-year old Nicaraguan boy with SSPE was treated with intraventricular biosynthetic alpha 2b interferon (Schering, Intron A), 1 million units twice weekly for 5-1/2 months, at the Children's Hospital of Los Angeles, Neurology Division, Los Angeles, CA. Measles history was unknown; CSF and serum measles titers were greater than 1:64 and 1:256,000, respectively. Fever developed for several hours and dystonic posturing worsened after each dose. The child remained in a vegetative state and neither clinical nor CSF indices improved with treatment. The authors question whether the choice of a biosynthetic form instead of the natural alpha interferon, used successfully in 3 patients previously (Panitch HS et al. *Neurology* 1986; *36*:562), might account for the lack of response in their patient. (Mitchell WF, Crawford TO. Intraventricular alpha 2b interferon for SSPE. *Neurology* 1987; *37*:1884).

COMMENT. The National SSPE Registry, now located at the Dept Neurology, Univ South Alabama College of Medicine, Mobile, Alabama, has recently begun to track results of treatment of SSPE (Dyken PR. *Neurology* 1987; *37*:1883). The use of the standard neurological disability scale as employed in the present study helps to eliminate bias in the evaluation of new therapies. The course of the disease is variable and the results of treatment in only a few cases are probably unreliable.

While on sabbatical at the Hospital for Sick Children, Great Ormond Street, London, 1986-87, I observed 6 cases of SSPE treated by intraventricular interferon, part of a large scale study with long-term results not yet evaluated. The treatment appeared to be arduous and poorly tolerated, sometimes interrupted by secondary infections, and stressful to the child, family, nurses, social workers as well as physicians involved. The EEGs were often worse after the initiation of therapy. Preliminary observations suggested that interferon might prolong the course of the disease but seemed to have no specific curative effect. An international collaborative study with standardized treatment protocol should be considered together with more effective WHO measles immunization programs to prevent this distressing disease. - Editor. *Ped Neur Briefs* December 1987.

Herpes Simplex Encephalitis

The successful outcome of a case of herpes simplex encephalitis (HSE) in a pregnant woman at 29 weeks gestation is reported from the Depts of Neurology and Gynecology and Obstetrics, Royal Perth Hospital and the State Health Lab Services, Perth, Western Australia. The diagnosis was suspected from the clinical presentation with fever, headache, stupor, generalized convulsion, a focal EEG, and a hypodense area in the right temporal lobe on CT. It was confirmed retrospectively from evidence of specific antibody production in the CSF. Acyclovir 800 mg/d IV every 8 hours and in a reducing regime was continued for 22 days. She recovered after 2 months and delivered a normal unaffected baby. Mother has led a normal life except for right sided focal motor and grand mal seizures controlled with anticonvulsants for 3-1/2 years and secondary to post-encephalitic temporal lobe atrophy. The child, aged 3-1/2 years, is well. Infection with HSV in this patient was not disseminated and did not cross the placenta. Acyclovir was non-toxic to mother and fetus when used in the 3rd trimester of pregnancy. (Hankey, GJ, Bucens MR, Chambers JSW. Herpes simplex encephalitis in third trimester of pregnancy: successful outcome for mother and child. *Neurology* 1987; *37*:1534-1537).

COMMENT. This case of HSE is the sixth to be reported in pregnancy and the second to survive. Only one previous fetus has survived a pregnancy complicated by HSE and the mother, treated with idoxuridine, died 5 days postpartum. Acyclovir reduces mortality of neonatal HSE and is well tolerated but morbidity in surviving infants is high especially if treatment is delayed. Early diagnosis is facilitated by MRI. (Scroth G et al. *Neurology* 1987; *37*:179). For a review of the natural history of HSV infection of mother and newborn and therapy of neonatal HSV infection, see Whitley RJ et al. and Infectious Disease Collaboration Antiviral Study Group. *Pediatrics* 1980; *66*:489-501). - Editor. *Ped Neur Briefs* October 1987.

Neonatal Herpes Simplex Encephalitis: EEG In Diagnosis

The sequential EEGs of 15 neonates with herpes simplex virus meningoencephalitis were correlated with clinical and laboratory findings at the Children's Hospital, Harvard Medical School, and Massachusetts General Hospital, Boston, MA. EEGs were abnormal in seven (88%) of eight neonates examined during days one to four of the illness and three (38%) showed a multifocal periodic pattern. In three patients with an early abnormal EEG the CT and ultrasound were normal. All patients examined during days five to 11 of the illness had abnormal EEGs and three had multifocal periodic patterns. Nine patients with severe neurologic sequelae and vegetative state examined after day 11 of the illness showed markedly abnormal EEGs with very low voltage or electrocerebral silence. The authors concluded that the EEG is a sensitive test that may be superior to radiologic procedures in the early diagnosis of neonatal herpes simplex encephalitis. The multifocal periodic pattern in the presence of CSF pleocytosis is highly suggestive of the diagnosis. (Mikati MA et al. Neonatal herpes simplex meningoencephalitis: EEG investigations and clinical correlates. *Neurology* Sept 1990; *40*:1433-1437). - Editor. *Ped Neur Briefs* October 1990.

COMMENT. The cranial CT and ultrasound studies may be normal when the EEG is abnormal during the first few days of neonatal herpes encephalitis. An MRI with T2 weighted images may be more revealing than the CT and will show multiple small disseminated lesions. - Editor. *Ped Neur Briefs* October 1990.

Herpes Zoster Ophthalmicus

A 17-month-old boy with HZO and delayed contralateral hemiparesis following intrauterine varicella exposure is reported from the Dept of Neurology, Univ Texas Med Sch, Houston, TX. He presented with ataxia and a progressive right-sided weakness. His mother had chickenpox at 8 months of gestation but he appeared normal at birth. A vesicular rash developed four weeks before examination in the distribution of the ophthalmic and mandibular divisions of the left trigeminal nerve. CSF showed mononuclear pleocytosis, CT demonstrated multiple areas of hypodensity in the left basal ganglia, and angiography revealed occlusion of the left lenticulostriate arteries. Treatment with Acyclovir for 10 days was followed by recovery except for minimal right hemiparesis. (Leis AA, Butler LJ. Infantile herpes zoster ophthalmicus and acute hemiparesis following intrauterine chickenpox. *Neurology* 1987; *37*:1537-1538).

COMMENT. The authors cited only one similar previous case in a child, a 7-year-old boy. Delayed focal cerebral angiitis and infarction may occur after an interval of days to months between HZO and neurologic complications in adults. Passive immunization of exposed susceptible women reduces risks of maternal and fetal varicella. (McGregor JA et al. *Am J Obstet Gynec* 1987; *157*:281). - Editor. *Ped Neur Briefs* October 1987.

Ocular Signs Of Congenital Varicella

Ocular abnormalities associated with congenital varicella are described in 3 children examined at the Hospital for Sick Children, Great Ormond Street, London, England. The syndrome followed a maternal varicella infection during the second trimester of pregnancy. Ocular findings included chorioretinitis, atrophy and hypoplasia of optic discs, cataract, and Horner's syndrome. Neurological abnormalities included bulbar palsy, hemiparesis, learning difficulties, and psychomotor retardation. The authors stress that the ocular lesions may be subtle and routine ophthalmological evaluation in infants with the congenital varicella syndrome is advisable. (Lambert SR, Taylor D et al. Ocular manifestations of the congenital varicella syndrome. *Arch Ophthalmol* Jan 1989; *107*:52-56).

COMMENT. Chorioretinal scarring occurs after intrauterine rubella, toxoplasmosis, syphilis, and less frequently with intrauterine herpes simplex and cytomegalovirus infections. Varicella chorioretinitis should be included in the differential diagnosis of congenital chorioretinal scarring. Optic nerve hypoplasia has not previously been reported in association with congenital varicella syndrome. - Editor. *Ped Neur Briefs* January 1989.

Varicella With Delayed Hemiplegia

Acute hemiplegia developed seven weeks to four months after varicella infection in four children reported from the Division of Child Neurology, Institute of Neurological Sciences, Tottori University School of Medicine, Yonago, Japan. Carotid angiography demonstrated segmental narrowing and occlusion of the middle cerebral artery in two patients, findings that were similar to those associated with hemiplegia after herpes zoster ophthalmicus. Cerebral angiitis was cited as the cause. A survey of infectious diseases in the San-in District of Japan showed 26,000 varicella patients and a frequency of varicella with delayed hemiplegia of 1:6500. (Ichiyama T et al. Varicella with delayed hemiplegia. *Pediatr Neurol* July-August 1990; *6*:279-281).

COMMENT. The neurological complications of varicella may be caused by viremia with encephalitis, post exanthematous encephalitis or cerebral angiitis. Cerebellar ataxia is the most frequent neurologic complication and hemiparesis is unusual. Of the four children reported with delayed hemiparesis, two recovered completely and two had residual weakness, clumsiness, or dystonia. - Editor. *Ped Neur Briefs* October 1990.

Congenital Rubella And CNS Defects

The University Department of Pediatrics and Child Health, Leeds, and the Department of Microbiology, Hospital for Sick Children, London, collaborated in a study of the time relations between maternal rubella infection in pregnancy and the presence and types of defects in 422 children with confirmed congenital rubella registered in the National Congenital Rubella Surveillance Program at their institutions.

In 106 cases with maternal rubella confirmed by a 4-fold rise in hemagglutination inhibition (HI) titer and/or detection of rubella-specific IgM, 66 (62%) had defects; 44 (67%) were exposed to rubella during the 3rd and 12th weeks of pregnancy and the remaining 22 (33%) between the 13th and 17th weeks. Multiple defects involving the CNS, heart, eye, and hearing were recorded only in children exposed early and up to the 12th week, deafness was also found in some exposed up to the 17th week, and no defects occurred in 20 children exposed after this time. Deafness was the most common defect, reported in 62 (58%) of 106 children; it was sensorineural in 55 (89% of the 62) and mixed conductive and nerve deafness in 7 (11%). Of 9 children with CNS defects, 6 had microcephaly, 2 cerebral palsy, and 1 mental retardation.

Among 316 cases with confirmed congenital rubella but without laboratory confirmation of maternal infection, 265 (84%) had defects. Deafness occurred in 75%, eye disorders in 30%, CNS defects in 25% and the heart was affected in 20%.

School placements for 148 affected children were as follows: 62 (42%) schools for the deaf, 33 (22%) partial hearing units in normal schools, 3 educationally subnormal, 3 blind, and 40 (27%) attend normal schools. Three-quarters of children with confirmed congenital rubella attend special schools. (Munro ND, Jones G et al. Temporal relations between maternal rubella and congenital defects. *Lancet* 1987; 2:201-204).

COMMENT. These data demonstrate that the risk of fetal damage from maternal rubella is very small with exposure later than the 16th week of pregnancy. Before that time the risk of congenital defects is high. The incidence of defects in this study (62%) is considerably higher than that reported previously (20%) by Miller E et al. (*Lancet* 1982; 2:781). The increased incidence is explained by the high proportion (65%) of infants exposed up to the 16th week of pregnancy as contrasted by 38% in the earlier study. A small head circumference (< 10th percentile) occurring in 18% of 102 affected infants was an additional abnormality in the Miller study but was not included among the reported rubella defects. - Editor. *Ped Neur Briefs* August 1987.

Immunizations And Seizures

The Committee on Infectious Diseases of the American Academy of Pediatrics issue 2 reports in the current issue of Pediatrics recommending immunization of children against measles and pertussis despite a positive family history for seizures. The recommendations were in response to data from the Centers for Disease Control that suggested an increased risk of convulsions following these immunizations among children with a family history of seizures. A positive family history was obtained in 17.3% and 16.7% of children who had febrile and nonfebrile convulsions, respectively, following DPT vaccine c.f. 4.8% without neurologic complications. (*Pediatrics* 1987; *80*:741-743).

COMMENT. The authors wisely add a footnote, albeit in small print, to these reports that their recommendations do not indicate an exclusive course of treatment or procedure to be followed and that variations, taking into account individual circumstances, may be appropriate. The dangers of measles encephalitis and its sequelae in unimmunized children far outweigh the risks of vaccine-induced seizures, and the committee recommendation for measles vaccine is sound. Children suffering from epilepsy should be examined by a neurologist before immunization as a precaution and anticonvulsant drug levels should be adjusted to optimal therapeutic amounts when necessary.

Regarding pertussis immunization, the statement that "there is no reason to treat children with a family history of convulsive disorder or of "neurologic disease" any differently from children without such a history" may be misleading without qualification. Again, a pediatrician may be well advised to consult the neurologist caring for a sibling or parent with epilepsy to determine the etiology of the seizures and the degree of familial susceptibility before proceeding with DPT immunization in an infant at increased risk.

The debate concerning DPT vaccine-induced encephalopathy continues in the courts (*Br Med J* 1987; *295*:1053) with experts quoted as favoring and others opposing a causal relation. In my experience of 14 cases of DPT-related seizure disorders evaluated in the past three years, 6 had infantile spasms with onset temporally related to the immunization. (*ACTA Paedtr Jpn* 1987; *29*:54-60). - Editor. *Ped Neur Briefs* November 1987.

Pertussis Immunization And Convulsions

A follow-up study of 18 infants and children who suffered convulsions (9 cases) or "hypotonic-hyporesponsive" episodes (9 cases) within 48 hours following DTP immunization was conducted in the Depts of Pediatrics, UCLA Hospital and Clinics, and the Kaiser Permanente Medical Group, Los Angeles, CA. After an interval of 6 to 7 years, of 16 children contacted and considered normal by the parents, 2 had delayed language or a speech problem, 1 was a grade behind in school, 1 was hyperactive and required Dexedrine, 4 (31%) of 13 tested had minor neurological abnormalities, 6 (46%) had full-scale IQ scores below 90, and 7 (54%) had below average verbal IQ scores that the authors explained by the proportion of Hispanic and bilingual children in the sample. It was concluded that none of the 16 children suffered any serious neurologic damage as a result of either convulsions or "hypotonic-hyporesponsive" episodes related to prior DTP immunizations. (Baraff LJ et al. Infants and children with convulsions and hypotonic-hyporesponsive episodes following diphtheria-tetanus-pertussis immunization: Follow-up evaluation. *Pediatrics* June 1988; *81*:789-794).

COMMENT. A previous study quoted in the article failed to demonstrate IQ deficits following febrile seizures (Ellenberg JH, Nelson KB. *Arch Neurol* 1978; *35*:17). The low IQ scores recorded at follow-up in approximately 50% of the children with seizures related to DTP immunization might suggest a febrile seizure of the complex type with residual brain pathology. This possibility was discounted because the present study population included 7 (44%) Hispanic and 3 (19%) bilingual children, although all spoke English at school. - Editor. *Ped Neur Briefs* June 1988.

Hypoxaemia In Pertussis

Breathing movements, airflow and arterial oxygen saturation were recorded in 6 infants aged 3 weeks to 7 months with apneic and cyanotic episodes associated with pertussis and compared with 12 healthy controls at the Dept of Paediatrics, Cardiothoracic Institute, Brompton Hospital, and Communicable Disease Unit, St. George's Hospital Medical School, London. Infants with pertussis had a greater frequency of apneic pauses, episodes of hypoxemia, and dips in oxygen saturation even during continued breathing movements. Apnea accompanied by mismatch between ventilation and perfusion of the lungs may produce the rapid onset of severe hypoxemia in infants with pertussis. Electroencephalographic recordings during prolonged pauses in inspiratory efforts with hypoxemia in one patient did not show a seizure discharge, but convulsions occurred in association with apnea and cyanosis in 4 patients. The twin sister of one patient, with an identical history of pertussis, died during a cyanotic convulsion while the infants were being brought to the hospital. That the convulsions are secondary to severe cerebral hypoxemia is suggested by these recordings and findings. (Southall DP et al. Severe hypoxaemia in pertussis. *Arch Dis Child* June 1988; *63*:598-605).

COMMENT. This excellent study and method of investigation offers advantages over epidemiological research in demonstrating the potential hazards of pertussis in small infants and the need for early immunization and less toxic pertussis vaccines. In my practice, I have encountered no cases of convulsions as a result of pertussis in the USA, a reflection of the excellent compliance with immunization programs perhaps, while children with convulsive disorders related temporally to pertussis immunization have been referred to me often for neurologic evaluation and treatment. DPT vaccine was listed as one of 7 drugs most commonly implicated in hospital admissions prompted by adverse reactions (Mitchell AA et al. *Pediatrics* July 1988; *82*:24). - Editor. *Ped Neur Briefs* June 1988.

CNS Effects Of Coughing In Cystic Fibrosis

Neurological symptoms complicating the paroxysmal coughing associated with cystic fibrosis were studied in 273 patients, aged 10 to 44 years, attending the Cystic Fibrosis Research Center, Divisions of Pediatric Pulmonology and Neurology, Case Western Reserve University School of Medicine and Rainbow and Children's Hospital, Cleveland, OH. Lightheadedness in 47% and headache in 50% of those with paroxysms were the most common neurological symptoms. Confusion, visual loss or dimming, paresthesias, speech disturbance, tremors, paralyses of extremities and face, and syncope were less frequent, transient abnormalities. The pathophysiology of these symptoms was explained by high intrathoracic pressure, as in cough syncope, that is transmitted to the cerebrospinal fluid, compressing cranial vessels and resulting in a "bloodless brain" or transient cerebral ischemia. In some patients with headache, marked hypoxemia and hypercapnia accompanied the coughing paroxysm and aggravated the symptom, but in most this mechanism was unlikely, and irreversible sequelae were not observed. (Stern RC et al. Neurological symptoms during coughing paroxysms in cystic fibrosis. *J Pediatr* June 1988; *112*:909-912).

COMMENT. Unlike pertussis, in which paroxysmal coughing, episodic apnea and cyanosis, or disturbed ventilatory perfusion may result in severe hypoxemia and neurological dysfunction, the coughing in cystic fibrosis is rarely accompanied by significant hypoxemia and serious neurological sequelae. A direct effect of B pertussis toxins on surfactant function leading to alveolar atelectasis has been invoked as the cause of hypoxemia in pertussis. - Editor. *Ped Neur Briefs* June 1988.

Mumps, Measles And
Rubella Vaccination And Encephalitis

A case of encephalitis in a 14 month old girl occurring 27 days after immunization with MMR vaccine is reported from the Department of Child Health, Charing Cross Hospital, London, England. She was admitted with a 24 hour history of fever and vomiting and a generalized convulsion. Shortly after admission she went into status epilepticus and the seizures continued for a further two hours despite heavy sedation. She required artificial ventilation for four days. She had received mumps, measles and rubella vaccine 27 days before admission. There was a fourfold rise in the S antibody titer to mumps virus by complement fixation. The family history was negative for epilepsy or febrile convulsions. Recovery was slow and when discharged 28 days after admission she had odd behavior and visual impairment. Recovery was complete after four months. (Crowley S et al. Mumps, measles, and rubella vaccination and encephalitis. *BMJ* Sept 9, 1989; *299*:660).

COMMENT. The authors found one case of mumps meningitis as a post immunization complication in a report from Canada but none in the United States. There were three unpublished reports of mumps meningoencephalitis associated with mumps, measles and rubella vaccine in the United Kingdom. It is suggested that at least 30 days follow-up is needed to exclude a possible neurological complication of the mumps vaccination. The failure to follow patients for a sufficiently long interval after immunizations might explain the lack of neurological complications reported with other vaccines. - Editor. *Ped Neur Briefs* September 1989.

Guillain-Barre Syndrome And Oral Polio Virus Vaccine

An unexpected rise in the number of patients hospitalized with Guillain-Barre syndrome (GBS) was concomitant with a nationwide oral polio virus vaccine (OPV) campaign in Finland in 1985 and is reported from Clinical Neurosciences Institute of Occupational Health; Department of Neurology, University of Helsinki; Department of Virology, National Public Health Institute; and National Board of Health, Helsinki, Finland. The analysis was based on hospital records covering the population of 1.7 million. Seventy-one patients with GBS were recognized during the six year period and ten developed GBS within ten weeks after OPV vaccination. The mean onset occurred after 31 days. Meningeal signs and fever were absent and the electroneuromyography was not compatible with poliomyelitis. An increase in CSF protein was seen in all patients but one and the CSF white count varied from 0-15 (mean 3). The study suggests that live attenuated polio virus may sometimes trigger the GBS (Kinnunen E et al. Incidence of Guillain-Barre syndrome during a nationwide oral poliovirus vaccine campaign. *Neurology* Aug 1989; *39*:1034-36).

COMMENT. The authors comment that there are no previous reports of the possible triggering role of oral polio vaccine for Guillain-Barre syndrome. The mean age in the OPV-associated GBS cases did not differ from that in the other cases (43.5 years, range 4-74 years). The report indicated that OPV should not increase the risk of GBS in children.

GBS is an immunopathologic reaction usually preceded and probably triggered by nonspecific infections of the respiratory or gastrointestinal tract, by cytomegalovirus, or Epstein-Barr virus. An increase of GBS was reported in the United States in 1976-77 within ten weeks after a massive A/New Jersey influenza vaccination campaign. Lyme disease is another infection that sometimes causes a Guillain-Barre syndrome in children and adults. - Editor. *Ped Neur Briefs* September 1989.

Bacterial Meningitis: Presenting Complaints

The presenting complaints and their relation to age were investigated in 110 cases of childhood bacterial meningitis diagnosed at the Depts of Pediatrics, Universities of Oulu, Helsinki, and Turku, Finland. Fever and vomiting were the most frequent reasons for consulting a physician (60% and 31% respectively). Despite the frequency of irritability (85% of infants 1-5 mos), impaired consciousness (79% of infants 6-11 mos), and neck rigidity (78% of children 12 mos or older), these symptoms and signs prompted consultation infrequently (6%, 22%, and 3%, respectively). A short duration of symptoms correlated with absence of neck stiffness even in children older than 12 mos. The age-specific frequency of convulsions in 11-14% cases resembled that of simple febrile convulsions. Respiratory symptoms, a long duration of pre-diagnostic symptoms, and pre-diagnostic prescription of antimicrobial therapy were more frequent in patients with H. influenzae meningitis than in those with meningococcal disease. Earlier consultation and better prognosis might follow the better education of parents in the recognition of irritability and lethargy in addition to fever and vomiting as important suspect signs of meningitis in infants and children. (Valmari P et al. Childhood bacterial meningitis: initial symptoms and signs related to age, and reasons for consulting a physician. *Eur J Pediatr* 1987; *146*:515-518).

COMMENT. In a busy ER the missed diagnosis of meningitis is not a rare occurrence, unfortunately. Physicians as well as parents might be reminded of the importance of irritability and lethargy as early signs of meningitis in the febrile child and the absence or late appearance of neck rigidity, especially in the infant.

The decision to perform *lumbar puncture in febrile children*, even in those with an accompanying seizure, remains controversial. Of 241 children aged 6 mos to 6 yrs who came to the ER at Sinai Hospital or Johns Hopkins Hospital, Baltimore, with a first seizure and fever and who received a lumbar puncture, 94.6% did not have meningitis. Items in the history and examination predictive of meningitis were: 1) a visit to a physician in the prior 48 hours, 2) seizure in ER, 3) focal seizure, 4) petechiae, cyanosis, grunting respiration, and 5) abnormal neurologic signs. Item (5) was the most sensitive factor in diagnosis and the use of items (1) or (5) or both in the selection of children for LP would have identified all those with meningitis (5.4%) and would have spared 144 the need for LP. The authors concluded that routine LP is not warranted if these risk factors are absent and provided that immediate follow-up is available. (Joffe A et al. *Am J Dis Child* 1983; *137*:1153). This analysis approach may be useful for house staff but each child is an individual and the intuitive judgment of the experienced pediatrician is perhaps the best predictor of the need for LP. - Editor. *Ped Neur Briefs* November 1987.

Bacteremia and Febrile Seizures

The frequency of occult bacteremia among children treated as outpatients for simple febrile seizures has been investigated in the Dept of Pediatrics, Univ of Maryland School of Medicine and St. Agnes Hospital, Baltimore, MD. Patients seen with fever but without a history of febrile seizures had blood cultures performed more frequently than those with a history of seizures. Of 115 patients with febrile seizures, 93 had blood cultures of which 5 (5.4%) were positive, all for Streptococcus pneumoniae. Follow-up blood cultures on return to the ER were negative. Three of the five had been treated with amoxicillin suspension for otitis media and two had not received antibiotics. There was no significant difference in the occurrence of positive blood cultures in those with and without a history of febrile convulsions.

The leukocyte count was the most valuable predictor of bacteremia. A temperature less than 39°C and leukocyte count less than 15x10⁹/L were predictive of a negative blood culture. Of those with a positive culture, the mean leukocyte count was 20.9x10⁹/L and the mean temperature was 40.2°C. Patients admitted to the hospital because of complications (e.g. meningitis, status epilepticus, facial cellulitis, and reactions to DPT vaccine) were excluded from the analysis. The authors recommend that the indications for blood culture are the same in patients with fever, with or without seizures. (Chamberlain JM, Gorman RL. Occult bacteremia in children with simple febrile seizures. *AJDC* Oct 1988; *142*:1073-1076).

COMMENT. It is interesting that the American Academy of Pediatrics Consensus statement from 1980 regarding the workup for febrile seizures did not include mention of blood culture. The authors of the paper reviewed here point out that patients with fever complicated by seizure are at the same risk for occult bacteremia as patients with fever alone, and should receive the same attention with regard to blood cultures. My colleague, Dr. Subhash Chaudhary, Head of the Division of Pediatric Infectious Disease at SIU School of Medicine, commented on the indications for blood culture in young children with fever but with no recognized focus of infection: "a child who looks sick and/or has a WBC of 20,000 or more should receive a blood culture and initial treatment with an antibiotic effective against pneumococcus and H influenza type b pending the isolation of an organism". - Editor. *Ped Neur Briefs* September 1988.

Bacterial Meningitis and Deafness: Dexamethasone Therapy

Dexamethasone (0.15 mg/kg/bwt q6 hr for 4 days) was considered beneficial in the treatment of infants and children with bacterial meningitis, particularly in preventing deafness, in two double blind, placebo-controlled trials involving 200 patients treated in the Dept of Pediatrics, University of Texas at Southwestern Medical Center, Dallas, TX. As compared to 98 patients receiving placebo, 102 treated with dexamethasone became afebrile earlier (1.6 vs 5 days; P < 0.001) and were less likely to acquire bilateral sensorineural hearing loss (15.5 vs 3.3%; P < 0.01). Twelve patients in the 2 placebo groups (14%) had severe bilateral loss as compared with 1 (1%) in the 2 dexamethasone groups (P < 0.001). (Lebel MH et al. Dexamethasone therapy for bacterial meningitis. Results of 2 double-blind, placebo-controlled trials. *N Engl J Med* Oct 13, 1988; *319*:964-71).

COMMENT. An editorial in the same issue (Smith AL. Neurological sequelae of meningitis. *N Engl J Med* 1988; *319*:1012) applauds the investigators for undertaking a difficult and complex study but notes that enthusiasm for the findings is dampened by the lack of follow-up of all patients enrolled in the study. The patients may have been restudied too early to detect improvement in auditory acuity of controls, and the dexamethasone group may have been less severely ill than the controls. An assessment of higher cortical function one year after discharge revealed no significant difference in treatment and control groups. Dexamethasone in the treatment of a severely ill child with meningitis may be recommended but a confirmatory study documenting safety is advised to determine its necessity in mild cases. Dexamethasone may save the hearing but worsen cerebral cortical function by ischemic injury and may induce gastrointestinal bleeding. - Editor. *Ped Neur Briefs* October 1988.

Neonatal Meningitis

The overall mortality and survival without handicap of babies with meningitis have been reviewed over a 14 year period, 1973-1986, at the Royal Maternity Hospital, and Department of Child Health, Queen's University, Belfast, Ireland. Of 41 patients treated 24 were born at the Royal Maternity Hospital giving an incidence of 0.54/1000 live births. The incidence fell progressively from 1979 (1.11/1000 live births) to 0.56/1000 in 1984. Antenatal risk factors were rupture of the membranes longer than 24 hours (n=8) and maternal infection (n=6). Signs and symptoms were vague with apnea being the most common. Only four of the 41 patients had a full or bulging fontanel and none had fever. Diagnosis was made at autopsy in five infants. The median age at presentation was nine days (range 1-57). Escherichia coli was the commonest organism. Twenty babies died (49%) and 13 (32%) survived without handicap. Of eight with handicaps three have hydrocephalus, three spastic quadriplegia, and two monoplegia. Factors associated with poor outcome were low birth weight and positive cerebrospinal fluid. The outcome for babies with more unusual organisms (Candida albicans and Serratia marcescens) was uniformly fatal. (Bell AH et al. Meningitis in the newborn - a 14 year review. *Arch Dis Child* June 1989; *64*:873-4).

COMMENT. The authors observed that failure to improve the prognosis of neonates with meningitis during a period when overall perinatal mortality fell rapidly is because smaller babies are being affected and different more unusual organisms are being cultured. Improved methods of diagnosis and management are needed with this change in epidemiology. In infants with apnea meningitis should be suspected. It is noteworthy that the diagnosis was made only at autopsy in 12% of patients. - Editor. *Ped Neur Briefs* June 1989.

Infantile Botulism

A case of a four month old boy with botulism is reported from the Department of Microbiology, Bristol Royal Infirmary and Bristol Royal Hospital for Sick Children, England. For the week before admission he had profuse rhinorrhea, and for 24 hours there was difficulty in feeding, hypotonia, and respiratory distress. On admission, he was profoundly hypotonic and had bilateral ptosis, impassive facies, depressed deep tendon reflexes and gag reflex, and pharyngeal pooling of saliva. He was mentally alert and responded to painful stimuli. Intravenous edrophonium (0.1 mg/kg) had no effect. EMG showed reduced amplitude of motor action potentials. EEG showed generalized high amplitude slow wave activity. Intermittent positive pressure ventilation was required and he began to show improvement by day 18 and was extubated on day 24. Clostridium botulinum and its toxin were isolated from the feces. (Smith GE et al. Infantile botulism. *Arch Dis Child* June 1989; *64*:871-2).

COMMENT. Infantile botulism is rare, this being only the second case in the United Kingdom. The diagnosis should be entertained in infants with an acute onset of hypotonia and respiratory distress. Honey has been implicated in several cases from the United States. (Arnon, SS. *Annu Rev Med* 1980; *31*:541). Fortunately, almost all infants recover completely, the illness lasting between 3 and 20 weeks, but supportive therapy is necessary and the differentiation from neonatal myasthenia gravis, septicemia, and infectious polyneuritis is important.

Botulinum toxin is not all bad! Local intradermal injections of botulinum A toxin may be useful in the treatment of eyelid and facial spasms in patients with generalized dystonias according to a report from the University of California School of Medicine, San Francisco (Sieff SR. Use of botulinum toxin to treat blepharospasm in a 16 year old with dystonic syndrome. *Pediatr Neurol* Mar/Apr 1989; *5*:121-3). Very small doses of botulinum A toxin are required but the effect is limited to a few months. - Editor. *Ped Neur Briefs* June 1989.

Relapsing Infant Botulism

Three infants with a relapsing form of infant botulism are reported from the Division of Child Neurology, The Children's Hospital of Philadelphia, PA. Between Jan 1, 1976 and Jan 1, 1989, 63 infants with confirmed infant botulism presented with the characteristic complaints of constipation followed by hypotonia, bulbar signs, and weakness. The diagnosis of infant botulism was confirmed by toxin identification in stool. The median age was 13.5 weeks (range 2-33 weeks of age) and the median length of hospitalization was four weeks. Three infants (5%) relapsed after a 1-2 week normal interval at home. None had been re-exposed to honey. Electrophysiological testing showed incremental response in compound motor action potential to high rates of repetitive stimulation. Recovery from relapse was complete but the authors recommend careful follow-up of infants after discharge. (Glauser TA et al. Relapse of infant botulism. *Ann Neurol* August 1990; *28*:187-189).

COMMENT. The mechanism underlying this relapse was unknown. Over 600 cases have been reported in the past 14 years and the disease is endemic in California, Utah, and Pennsylvania. Risk factors are breast-feeding and possibly honey. The differential diagnosis includes systemic infection, tic paralysis, myasthenia gravis, congenital myopathies, and myasthenic syndromes, Guillain-Barre syndrome, and organic phosphate intoxication. There is no specific treatment. Some antibiotics such as aminoglycosides may impair neuromuscular transmission and may exacerbate the paralysis and hypotonia. (Gay CT, Bodensteiner JB. *Pediatric Clinics* August 1990; *8*:722). - Editor. *Ped Neur Briefs* September 1990.

Nontraumatic Lumbar Puncture

A technique and formula for avoiding the traumatic spinal tap is reported from the Medical College of Wisconsin, Milwaukee, WI. To increase the accuracy and to minimize the frequency of traumatic puncture, the authors conducted a 12-month prospective analysis of 158 children of various ages in whom this diagnostic procedure was performed during the evaluation of an acute illness. The right lateral decubitus position was used and the needle was inserted perpendicularly in the L-3 to L-4 vertebral interspace. After CSF was collected, the needle

was marked at the skin line and the length inserted was measured. The patient's age, weight, and height were used to calcu-
late the body-surface area in square meters. The body-surface
area showed the highest correlation with the depth of lumbar
puncture. Linear regression for surface area provided a simple
formula to estimate the depth of puncture to within 5 mm in
young children of all ages: Depth = 0.77 cm + 2.56 (m²)
(Bonadio WA et al. Estimating lumbar-puncture depth in children. *N Engl J Med* Oct 6, 1988; *319*:952-953).

COMMENT. Insertion of the needle too deeply with
puncture of venous plexuses in the anterior wall of the vertebral wall is the most common error. The avoidance of
traumatic lumbar puncture by the use of this simple calculation and formula should facilitate the diagnosis of meningitis and reduce the risk of iatrogenic meningitis resulting
from blood contamination of a previously sterile CSF in the
patient with bacteremia. The authors are to be congratu-
lated on their attempt to introduce some mathematical
accuracy into a commonly "hit or miss" procedure. -
Editor. *Ped Neur Briefs* September 1988.

CHAPTER **14**

TOXIC DISORDERS

Harmful Effects Of Lead On Learning

Members of the Depts. Community Medicine, Education, Geology, and Med. Statistics Unit, Univ. Edinburgh, have investigated the effect of blood-lead on cognitive ability and educational attainment in a sample of 855 boys and girls aged 6-9 years from 19 primary schools in central Edinburgh. The mean blood-lead level was 10.4 ug/dl. Multiple regression analyses of individual test scores showed a significant negative relation between blood-lead and British Ability Scales combined scores, number skills, and word reading, with 33 possible variables accounted for. The dose-response relation between blood-lead and test scores showed no evidence of a threshold or safe level. It was concluded that lead at low levels of exposure probably has a small harmful effect on the performance of children in cognitive ability and attainment tests. (Fulton M et al. *Lancet* 1987; *1*:1221).

> COMMENT. This finding is in agreement with that of a previous study in the USA (Needleman et al. *N Engl J Med* 1979; *300*:689-95) showing lead-related deficits in

neuropsychological and classroom performance of children with elevated dentine lead levels. Exposure levels in the UK were lower than in the US study. Water and dust were the main sources of lead, attributed to a plumbosolvent water supply and lead plumbing in Edinburgh. Reports of research (1979-83) on the neuropsychological effects of lead in children are reviewed by the Medical Research Council, London, 1984.

A case of schizophrenic-like psychosis is an unusual manifestation of moderate lead intoxication (blood level of 60 ug/dl) reported in a 14 year old boy who had sniffed gasoline for 3 months. He was treated at Duke Univ Med Cntr, Durham, N Carolina, using a Ca EDTA challenge and 4 days chelation with dramatic clearing of agitation and psychotic symptoms. He had a history of dyslexia, visual-motor incoordination and conduct disorder. His IQ was 83 at 9 years of age and 69 on recovery from the lead intoxication. A possible psychobiological vulnerability to lead intoxication in children with learning problems, ADD, or mental retardation is proposed. (McCracken JT. *J Amer Acad Child Adol Psychiat* 1987; 26:274-276). - Editor. *Ped Neur Briefs* August 1987.

Low Dose Lead And CNS Long-Term Deficits

The long term effects of exposure to low doses of lead in childhood have been examined in 132 of 270 young adults who had initially been studied as primary school children in 1975-1978 and the results of an 11 year follow-up are reported from the School of Medicine, University of Pittsburgh; Boston University; and the Neuroepidemiology Unit, Children's Hospital and Harvard Medical School, Boston, MA. Neurobehavioral functioning in the earlier study of school children was found to be inversely related to dentin lead levels. In the subjects reexamined as adults, impairment in neurobehavioral function was still related to the lead content of teeth shed at the ages of six and seven. The persistent toxicity of lead was seen to result in significant and serious impairment of academic success, specifically a sevenfold increase in failure to graduate from high school, lower class standing, greater absenteeism, impairment of reading skills, and deficits in vocabulary, fine motor skills, reaction time, and hand-eye coordination. A dose response relation was demonstrated between exposure and numerous outcome variables. Young people with dentin lead levels greater than 20 PPM had a markedly higher risk of dropping out of high school and of having a reading disability as compared with those with dentin lead levels less than 10 PPM. (Needleman HL et al. The long-term effects of exposure to low doses of lead in childhood: An ll-year follow-up report. *N Engl J Med* Jan 11, 1990; *322*:83-88).

COMMENT. Exposure to lead even in children who remain asymptomatic may have an important and enduring effect on brain function and learning. Since 16% of children in the United States are reported to have elevated blood lead levels (greater than 15 mcg/dl), the early detection and attention to lead in the environment might prevent school failure in a significant number of children in the USA. The agency for Toxic Substances and Disease Registry has defined the threshold for neurobehavioral toxicity for lead as 10-15 mcg/dl. The mean blood level among the subjects reported with high tooth lead levels was 34 mcg/dl.

In the Sydney Lead Study, a prospective investigation of the relationship between low level lead exposure and neurobehavioral development during the first five years of life, average blood lead levels at the fourth year were approximately 10 mcg/dl and this degree of lead exposure was not associated with mental or motor deficits. (Cooney GH et al. Low-level exposures to lead: The Sydney Lead Study. *Dev Med Child Neurol* 1989; *31*:640-649). A meta-analysis of 24 modern studies of childhood exposures to lead in relationship to IQ inferred that low dose lead exposure is closely associated with deficits in psychometric intelligence (Needleman HL, Gatsonis CA. Low-level lead exposure and the IQ of children. A meta-analysis of modern studies. *JAMA* Feb 2, 1990; *263*:673-678). The level of lead exposure in these studies may have been higher than that in the Sydney Lead Study.

In another current study of lead exposure in preschool children, the calcium status of 64 black urban children aged 18-47 months was evaluated in relation to blood lead levels and behavior, particularly pica. Children with blood levels less than 30 mcg/dl were compared with a group having blood levels greater than 30 mcg/dl. The study verified the positive association between blood lead levels and pica, an association recognized for many years. Decreased calcium intake and three other calcium measures were not related to blood lead levels and calcium intake was not associated with pica scores. (Laraque D et al. Blood lead, calcium status and behavior in preschool children. *AJDC* Feb 1990; *144*:186-189). Pica has been emphasized as a common prelude to plumbism (Millichap JG et al. Lead paint: A hazard to children. *Lancet* 1952; *2*:360) and should prompt the early diagnosis of lead exposure and prevention of neurobehavioral deficits. The identification of children with lead poisoning in need of chelation is possible using unstimulated urinary lead excretion without the necessity of the CaNa2EDTA provocative test. (Berger OG et al. Using unstimulated urinary lead excretion to assess the need for chelation in the treatment of lead poisoning. J *Pediatr* 1990; *116*:46-51). - Editor. *Ped Neur Briefs* January 1990.

Neuropsychological Sequelae Of Reye's Syndrome

The author, a pediatric neurologist at the U. of Kansas School of Medicine, Wichita, Kansas, reviews the sequelae and risk factors in survivors of Reye's syndrome. He reports a mortality rate of less than 20-30% but significant psychological sequelae in up to 64%, neurologic deficits in 54%, and major handicaps in 42% that include blindness, spasticity, mental retardation, and occasionally, seizures. Mild residual problems involve speech and language (30%), learning (30%), and behavior and emotion (50-70%). Factors that predict sequelae are 1) severe symptoms, 2) prolonged coma, and 3) young age group. Ammonia and SGOT levels do not correlate with prognosis. (Svoboda WB. *J Nat Reye's Syndrome Foundation* 1987; 7:34-37).

COMMENT. This report was one of 10 invited papers presented at the 12th annual meeting of the Nat Reye's Syndrome Foundation. The author points out that in the 1960s the question was "What is Reye's Syndrome?", in the 1970s "Will the child survive?", and in the 1980s, "What sequelae may be expected and how should these be managed?"

In one report of 16 survivors of Reye's syndrome (Benjamin PY et al. *Crit Care Med* 1982; *10*:583) significant emotional problems in 56% of the children and 94% of their mothers contrasted with relatively good intellectual and academic recovery. None had severe neurologic sequelae and 14 (88%) had IQs within the normal range. The decreasing mortality rate of Reye's syndrome has focused attention on the quality of life of survivors and their parents. - Editor. *Ped Neur Briefs* August 1987.

Reye Syndrome And Aspirin

Twenty-six cases of Reye syndrome occurring between 1973 and 1982 have been reviewed in relation to aspirin ingestion at the Children's Hospital, Camperdown, Australia (formerly the Royal Alexandra Hospital for Children in Sydney), where Reye first described his syndrome of encephalopathy and fatty degeneration of the viscera in 1963. The ages ranged from 3 mos to 7 yrs (median 22 mos). Only 5% of patients had ingested aspirin and 30% acetaminophen. For the period of this study, aspirin accounted for 0.3% and acetaminophen for 99.7%

of all pediatric analgesic/antipyretic sales. Despite this lack of association of Reye syndrome with aspirin use, Reye syndrome has been as common in Australia as in the US (9 cases per/million children c.f. 10-20 cases/mil in US and 3-7/mil in UK). The authors conclude that the purported association of Reye syndrome with aspirin use in the US is coincidental. (Orlowski JP et al. A catch in the Reye. *Pediatrics* 1987; *80*:638-642.

> COMMENT. Rupert Murdoch, the Australian journalist and publisher, would approve of this apt title, a refreshing innovation for our generally plain medical style of writing. Despite the conclusions drawn here and supported by a study from Japan, which also failed to show an association between aspirin and Reye syndrome, it is unlikely that the pediatric usage of aspirin will be resumed in the US. The massive public education campaign launched by the Government in 1982 to caution parents against aspirin use for colds, influenza or chicken pox has been very successful, notwithstanding the persisting mystery regarding the true cause or causes of Reye syndrome. - Editor. *Ped Neur Briefs* November 1987.

Neurotoxic Complications Of Contrast CT

Four children, ages 4-10 yrs, with brain tumors treated at the Univ of Calgary, Alberta, Canada, developed alterations in consciousness and vital signs after contrast-enhanced cranial computed tomography (CT). Each had increased intracranial pressure but was alert and coherent before the IV injection of diatrizoate meglumine 60%, 2 to 2.5 ml/kg. Two children had generalized seizures and two died immediately after the procedure. The authors caution that CT with contrast should be reserved for children who warrant the additional procedure and when the necessity for urgent neurosurgical intervention is not resolved after the nonenhanced scan. (Haslain RHA et al. Neurotoxic complications of contrast computed tomography in children. *J Pediat* 1987; *111*:837-40).

COMMENT. Reactions to contrast enhanced CT are sufficiently frequent to avoid its use as a routine neurodiagnostic procedure, especially in children with brain tumor and raised intracranial pressure. Neurologists requesting a CT in nonsurgical cases will usually specify a pre-infusion scan only, unless the diagnosis suspected requires enhancement of the lesion. Magnetic resonance imaging is a noninvasive technique that provides images of comparable or superior quality without exposure to contrast effects or ionizing radiation. When available, MRI should be used in preference to contast-enhanced CT, particularly in children. - Editor. *Ped Neur Briefs* December 1987.

Polychlorinated Biphenyls (PCBs) And Cognitive Deficits

The effects of prenatal exposure to polychlorinated biphenyls (PCBs) and related contaminants on the CNS function of infants born to women who had consumed Lake Michigan sports fish have been investigated in 236 children previously evaluated for PCB-related deficits in infancy and reassessed at four years of age in the Psychology Department, Wayne State University, Detroit, MI and the Michigan Department of Public Health, Lansing, MI. Prenatal exposure, indicated by umbilical cord serum PCB levels, was associated with poorer short term memory function on both verbal and quantitative tests and the adverse effects were dose dependent and not attributed to other variables. Exposure from nursing was unrelated to cognitive performance. The study demonstrates continuation of toxic effects through early childhood. (Jacobson JL et al. Effects of in utero exposure to polychlorinated biphenyls and related contaminants on cognitive functioning in young children. *J Pediatr* Jan 1990; *116*:38-45).

COMMENT. Polychlorinated biphenyls were once used in industrial products and were banned in the United States in 1970. Residues persist in air, soil, water and sediments in lakes and can be detected in residents of industrialized countries. PCB levels are unusually high in sports fish from Lake Michigan and transplacental exposure to PCBs has been documented. - Editor. *Ped Neur Briefs* January 1990.

Fetal Alcohol Syndrome And Hearing Deficits

Hearing and speech and language development in 14 children with fetal alcohol syndrome were evaluated at the Fetal Alcohol Research Center, Wayne State University School of Medicine, Detroit, MI, and the Audiology Division, School of Medicine, University of Colorado Health Sciences Center, Denver, CO. Recurrent serous otitis media with hearing loss and speech and language problems occurred in 13, and 4 also had sensorineural hearing loss. The IQ was 70-85 in 7 children and below 69 in 7. The authors conclude that hearing disorders are a significant complication of fetal alcohol exposure, probably contributing to the speech and language and learning disabilities commonly associated with the syndrome. (Church MW, Gerkin KP. Hearing disorders in children with fetal alcohol syndrome: findings from case reports. *Pediatrics* Aug 1988; *82*:147-154).

COMMENT. As a cause of mental retardation, fetal alcohol syndrome is as prevalent as Down's syndrome and occurs in at least one in 1000 births. Postmortem examination of the brain reveals extensive developmental defects, mostly the consequence of migration anomalies. Heterotopias, lissencephaly, and agenesis of the corpus callosum have been described. Migration anomalies may involve the brain stem as well as the cerebrum, thus accounting for the sensorineural deafness noted in the above study. - Editor. *Ped Neur Briefs* August 1988.

Fetal Alcohol Syndrome And Growth Retardation

The relationship between prenatal maternal alcohol use and growth and morphologic abnormalities in the offspring of 650 women studied prospectively is reported from the School of Medicine and Department of Mathematics and Statistics, University of Pittsburg, PA. Low birth weight, decreased head circumference and length, and an increased rate of fetal alcoholic effects were all found to be significantly correlated with exposure to alcohol during the first two months of the first trimester. The average amounts of alcohol consumed in the first trimester for women who were delivered of infants with no, one, or multiple minor physical anomalies were 0.67, 0.98, and 1.07 drinks per day, respectively (P=0.5). The corresponding average daily volumes for mothers of babies exhibiting no, one, or multiple fetal alcohol effects were 0.69, 0.85, and 1.28 (P=0.13). The time of greatest impact of drinking was in the early part of the first trimester. (Day NL et al. Prenatal exposure to alcohol: Effect on infant growth and morphologic characteristics. *Pediatrics* Sept 1989, *84*:536-541).

COMMENT. Data from this study have also demonstrated an effect of alcohol use on the sleep electroencephalographic patterns of newborns and on growth at eight months of age. (Scher M et al. *Pediatrics Res* 1988; *24*:101). This study identifies and emphasizes the importance of exposure to alcohol early in the first trimester as a cause of intrauterine growth retardation and/or morphologic abnormalities in newborn infants. The infant is also at risk if mother drinks alcohol during the breast-feeding period. - Editor. *Ped Neur Briefs* September 1989.

Alcohol During Breast-Feeding And Infant Development

The relation of the mother's use of alcohol during breast feeding to the infant's development at one year of age has been investigated in 400 infants studied in the Department of Epidemiology, University of Michigan, Ann Arbor, Department of Epidemiology and Pediatrics, University of Washington, Seattle. Mental development, as measured by the Bayley Mental Development Index, was unrelated to maternal drinking during breast-feeding. However, motor development, as measured by the Psychomotor Development Index, was significantly lower in infants exposed regularly to alcohol in breast milk with a dose response relation. (Little RE et al. Maternal alcohol use during breast-feeding and infant mental and motor development at one year. *N Engl J Med* Aug 17, 1989; *321*:425-30).

> COMMENT. Nursing mothers can no longer enjoy a glass of beer as a prescribed method for sedating a sleepless baby without risking a detrimental effect on the infant's development. The practice of offering the parents a complimentary dinner with champagne at the time of discharge from maternal units will have to cease, or if continued, with moderation and caution. It may be argued that the results of this study are suggestive but the detrimental effects on the development are not sufficiently severe to be clinically important for the individual child. The finding that the mental development of infants exposed to alcohol through breast feeding was not affected is of interest and might be explained by the timing of the exposure and the age at which the child was tested. - Editor. *Ped Neur Briefs* September 1989.

Hyperbilirubinemia
And Neurodevelopmental Outcome

The results of the Collaborative Project on Preterm and Small for Gestational Age Infants in the Netherlands, 1983, in regard to hyperbilirubinemia and neurodevelopmental outcome at two years of age are reported from the Division of Neonatology, Department of Pediatrics, University Hospital, Leiden, the Netherlands.

Children with minor and major handicaps had significantly greater maximal serum total bilirubin concentrations than children with a normal neurodevelopmental outcome (P = 0.02). An increase in prevalence of handicaps was found for each 50 mmol/L (2.9 mg/dL) increase of maximal serum total bilirubin concentration. The neurological abnormalities included cerebral palsy, seizures, hearing defects as well as retinopathy of prematurity. The risk of a handicap increased by 30% for each 2.9

mg/dL increase of maximal serum total bilirubin concentration
(P = 0.02) suggesting a causal relationship. (van de Bor M et al.
Hyperbilirubinemia in preterm infants and neurodevelopmental
outcome at 2 years of age: Results of a national collaborative
survey. *Pediatrics* June 1989; *83*:915-920).

COMMENT. In the same issue, Newman TB and Maisels
MJ comment that the strength of the association between
bilirubin levels and brain damage in the present study was
insufficiently precise to provide evidence of a strong causal
relationship. The 95% confidence interval was wide, the
association has not been consistent in other studies, and
panic about bilirubin in the 6-12 mg/dL range is premature. They note that the NICHD collaborative phototherapy
trial showed that bilirubin levels were reduced significantly by 4 mg/dL but this did not reduce the incidence of
motor deficits or cerebral palsy and there was no effect on
IQ scores. They estimate that even if the hyperbilirubinemia was toxic and causally related to neurologic damage,
about 33 premature infants would need to be treated to
prevent one case of neurologic handicap. To achieve similar benefit in term infants the number to be treated would
be 333. Further studies are suggested. - Editor. *Ped Neur
Briefs* June 1989.

Dystonia And Cocaine Withdrawal

An acute dystonic episode in a 15-year-old girl during cocaine
withdrawal is reported from the Departments of Neurology and
Psychiatry, Albert Einstein College of Medicine, Bronx, NY. After
16 hours of observation in the hospital without receiving any
drugs, she developed generalized dystonia, torticollis, extensor
posturing, and high-pitched vocalizations. The episode subsided
after administration of 50 mg IV diphenhydramine. She was discharged nine days later with diagnosis of adjustment disorder with
depressed mood, and cocaine abuse. (Choy-Kwong M, Lipton
RB. Dystonia related to cocaine withdrawal: a case report and
pathogenic hypothesis. *Neurology* July 1989; *39*:996-997).

COMMENT. There is a high frequency of neuroleptic-induced dystonia reported in cocaine users. Cocaine may lower the threshold to these reactions. This report indicates that dystonic reactions to cocaine withdrawal can occur in the absence of other drugs. - Editor. *Ped Neur Briefs* September 1989.

Cocaine And Heroin In Utero Effects

A study of 86 infants who were born to women with a history of cocaine and/or heroin use during pregnancy is reported from the Department of Pediatrics, Highland General Hospital, and the Division of Neonatology, Children's Hospital, Oakland, CA. The newborns were observed over a five day hospital period using a standardized abstinence scoring system and urine drug screening of both mother and infant. Urine tests were positive for cocaine only in 35, heroin only in 14, cocaine and heroin in 17, and 20 were negative. In the cocaine group 17% of the newborns had growth retardation and 27% were microcephalic. Microcephaly occurred in 17% of 12 infants in the heroin group, 20% of the 15 infants in the cocaine/heroin group, and in none of 20 infants in the urine negative cocaine history group. Of 985 newborns in the no drug group, 4% were microcephalic. The incidence of microcephaly was significantly higher in the cocaine group and in the cocaine/heroin group than in the no drug group. Cocaine and heroin were synergistic in causing abnormal behavior of withdrawal as assessed by the Finnegan scoring system which includes hypertonia, tremulousness, tachypnea, decreased sleep and feeding disturbances. (Fulroth R et al. Perinatal outcome of infants exposed to cocaine and/or heroin in utero. *AJDC* August 1989; *143*:905-910).

COMMENT. The authors conclude that infants exposed to cocaine and/or heroin in utero should be followed up closely after discharge from the nursery since growth retardation, microcephaly, and abnormal behavior may be suggestive of potential long-term neurologic or developmental problems. The cocaine induced microcephaly might be explained by impaired maternal nutrition, vasoconstriction in the placenta, and reduced fetal blood flow and fetal hypoxia. In this study 85% of mothers using cocaine reported the abuse of free base "crack" cocaine which causes significantly more vasoconstriction than that taken intranasally. None of the infants studied had the features of fetal alcohol syndrome. - Editor. *Ped Neur Briefs* September 1989.

Mercury Poisoning And Latex Paint

Mercury poisoning manifested as acrodynia, reported in a four year old boy in Michigan ten days after the inside of his home was painted with 64 liters of interior latex paint containing phenylmercuric acetate, prompted an investigation by the Division of Environmental Hazards and Health Effects, Centers for Disease Control, Atlanta, GA. Nineteen families were recruited from a list of more than 100 persons who called the Michigan Department of Public Health after a press release announced that some interior latex paint contained more than the recommended limit of mercury of 1.5 mmol per liter. The median mercury content of the paint in 29 cans sampled from the exposed households was 3.8 mmol per liter. The concentrations of mercury in the air samples obtained from homes of exposed families were significantly higher than in the unexposed households. Urinary mercury concentrations were significantly higher among the exposed persons than among unexposed persons (4.7 nmol of mercury per millimole of creatinine compared to 1.1 nmol per millimole). These mercury concentrations in exposed persons have been associated with symptomatic mercury poisoning. (Agocs MM, Etzel RA et al. Mercury exposure from interior latex paint. *N Engl J Med* Oct 18, 1990; *323*:1096-1101).

COMMENT. Exposed children had the highest urinary mercury concentrations and young children may be at increased risk since vapors containing mercury are heavier than indoor air and tend to settle toward the floor. Individual exposure to mercury varies with the time spent in painted rooms, the depth and frequency of inhalation, the degree of ventilation in the room, and the likely decrease in mercury vapors over time. Opening all windows and doors decreased the concentration of mercury but it returned to the unventilated value within three hours of closing doors and windows. Mercury is released from surfaces coated with a paint containing mercury after the paint has dried. In the body phenylmercuric acetate is broken down to form inorganic mercury which accumulates in the kidney, the brain, and the fetus, and is excreted in the urine. A urinary mercury concentration of less than 100 nmol per liter is considered acceptable for adults but a background urinary mercury concentration for children has not been established.

In the four year old boy who developed acrodynia, a 24 hour urine sample contained 324 nmol of mercury per liter. The clinical manifestations of acrodynia in this child included leg cramps, a generalized rash, pruritus, sweating, tachycardia, an intermittent low-grade fever, marked personality change, erythema and desquamation of the hands, feet, and nose, weakness of the pelvic and pectoral girdles, and lower extremity nerve dysfunction developing sequentially.

On June 29, 1990 the Environmental Protection Agency announced that compounds containing mercury could no longer be lawfully added to interior latex paint after August 20, 1990. If paint containing mercury is employed then proper ventilation must be insured. The history of mercury poisoning and its manifestation as acrodynia in children is reviewed in an editorial (Clarkson TW. Mercury - An element of mystery. *N Engl J Med* Oct 18, 1990; *323*:1137-39). Dimercaptosuccinic acid given orally is the most promising therapy. - Editor. *Ped Neur Briefs* November 1990.

CHAPTER **15**

METABOLIC DISORDERS

Neonatal Hypoglycemia Definition

The definition of neonatal hypoglycemia has been surveyed at the Department of Child Health, University of Newcastle upon Tyne by reference to 36 textbooks of pediatrics and answers to questionnaires from 178 pediatricians in charge of nurseries with 4 or more intensive care cots. In textbooks there was a wide variation in definition ranging from a glucose concentration of < 1 mmol/l to < 2.5 mmol/l with a modal value of < 1.7 mmol/l for term babies of appropriate weight, and < 1.1 mmol/l for babies who were preterm or small for gestational age. Among practicing pediatricians the definitions showed an even greater range from a glucose concentration of < 1 mmol/l to < 4 mmol/l with a modal value of < 2.0 mmol/l for term babies of appropriate weight and < 1.1 mmol/l for babies who were preterm or small for gestational age. The site of sampling, whether capillary, venous, or arterial blood, was not included in the definition of hypoglycemia obtained from textbooks nor from pediatricians surveyed. There appeared to be no accepted definition of the lower limit of normality for circulating blood glucose concentrations. (Koh THHG, Eyre JA, Aynsley-Green A. Neonatal hypoglycemia — the controversy regarding definition. *Arch Dis Child* Nov 1988; *63*:1386-1398).

> COMMENT. A functional definition of hypoglycemia was suggested by the authors to be based on a correlation between objective measurements of neurophysiological function and blood glucose concentrations. The "safe" blood glucose concentration may vary according to the clinical situation, e.g. during hypoxia, polycythemia, or convulsions, and may be independent of the gestational and postnatal age and birth weight. Clinical signs of hypo-glycemia in the neonate are not well established and the question of neural dysfunction or damage with asymp-tomatic hypoglycemia is addressed in the following paper. - Editor. *Ped Neur Briefs* November 1988.

Hypoglycemia And
Neural Dysfunction: Evoked Potentials

Evoked potentials were used to measure neural function in relation to blood glucose concentration in 17 children at the Department of Child Health, University of Newcastle upon Tyne, UK. Thirteen children were admitted for investigation of metabolic or endocrine disorders and hypoglycemia was pro-voked by fasting or insulin administration; 4 had recurrent episodes of spontaneous hypoglycemia. Abnormal brainstem auditory evoked potentials were recorded in 9 and abnormal somatosensory evoked potentials in 1 of the 11 children whose blood glucose concentration remained about 2.6 mmol/l; 5 of these 10 children were asymptomatic and 5 became drowsy. No change in evoked potentials was recorded in the 6 children whose blood glucose concentration remained about 2.6 mmol/l. Of the 10 children with abnormal evoked potentials, 6 had normal latencies immediately after the IV administration of 25% dextrose (2 ml/kg) or the IM administration of glucagon (20 ug/kg), whereas 4 had persistently prolonged I-V latencies or absent wave V for 1 hr, 1.5 hrs, 16 hrs, and 2 days. The authors suggest that blood glucose concentration should be maintained above 2.6 mmol/l to ensure normal neural function in newborns and children irrespective of the presence or absence of abnormal clinical signs. (Koh TTHG, Aynsley-Green A, Tarbit M, Eyre JA. Neural dysfunction during hypoglycemia. *Arch Dis Child* Nov 1988; *63*:1353-1358).

COMMENT. A prospective controlled study of neonates with episodes of hypoglycemia has shown that long term follow-up may reveal impairments in intellectual function (Pildes et al. *Pediatrics* 1974; *54*:5). Short term follow-up studies of infants who have suffered hypoglycemia may be misleading. Clinical signs of hypoglycemia and disturbances of neural function in the newborn baby may be subtle and difficult to recognize, and the distinction between "symptomatic" and "asymptomatic" hypoglycemia may require recordings of evoked potentials to demonstrate neural dysfunction. Whether the transient abnormalities in evoked potentials demonstrated in the above study can be predictive of permanent neural damage remains to be determined. The neurological signs resulting from abnormal cerebral metabolism secondary to hypoglycemia may depend on the rate of fall of blood sugar, the duration and degree of hypoglycemia, and the age of the patient. (Etheridge JE. Hypoglycemia and the central nervous system. In *Symposium on Pediatric Neurology*, Ed. Millichap JG. *Ped Clin N Amer* Nov 1967; *14*:865). Alternative substrates, particularly ketone bodies, can be used for energy by the brain and may have a protective effect during episodes of hypoglycemia. (Persson B et al. *Acta Paediatr Scand* 1972; *61*:273). - Editor. *Ped Neur Briefs* November 1988.

Hypoglycemia And Brain Damage

The neurochemical effects, patterns of cerebral blood flow derangement, time course and distribution of brain tissue damage, and selective neuronal necrosis resulting from hypoglycemia are compared to the biological effects of ischemia and epilepsy in a neurological progress report from the Departments of Pathology and Clinical Neurosciences, University of Calgary, Alberta, Canada, and the Laboratory for Experimental Brain Research, University Hospital, Lund, Sweden. Hypoglycemia interferes with cerebral energy production, causing membrane depolarization, loss of ion homeostasis, and lipolysis with accumulation of free fatty acids. Tissue aspartate and quinolinic acid levels rise and glutamate levels in CNS tissue fall during hypoglycemia. Cerebral blood flow is increased during the insult and decreased following the insult. Energy failure is moderate in degree with ATP levels dropping to 25 to 30% of control. Unlike ischemia and epilepsy, hypoglycemia is not accompanied by lactic acidosis. The duration of hypoglycemic insult required to produce selective neuronal necrosis is 10-20 min and neuronal death occurs within 1-8 hrs. (Auer RN, Siesjo BK. Biological differences between ischemia, hypoglycemia, and epilepsy. *Ann Neurol* Dec 1988; 24:699-707).

> COMMENT. Ischemia, hypoglycemia, and epilepsy, long thought to produce similar or identical brain damage, apparently have different mechanisms and effects on brain tissue. Insults of equal duration are not equipotent in causing brain damage. Ischemia is much more potent than hypoglycemia, and hypoglycemia is more potent than status epilepticus per minute of insult. The timing of neuronal necrosis evolves over hours to days in ischemia, minutes to hours in hypoglycemia, and during or very shortly after the insult of status epilepticus. - Editor. *Ped Neur Briefs* November 1988.

Focal Neurologic Deficits
With Hypoglycemia And Diabetes

Focal neurologic deficits on 19 occasions in seven children with diabetes are reported from Children's Hospital, Winnipeg, Manitoba, Canada. None had a history of a seizure disorder or a febrile seizure prior to onset of diabetes. One had generalized seizures attributed to hypoglycemia. Two had a parent with migraine. The neurological examination was normal between events, all of which occurred during sleep. All seven patients had at least one episode of a focal motor deficit. Two children had separate episodes of right and left-sided hemiparesis, two had focal motor seizures followed by ipsilateral paresis, and two had headache beginning after the onset of the acute neurologic event. Hypoglycemia was demonstrated on the three occasions that blood glucose was measured at the outset of hemiparesis or focal seizures. (Wayne EA et al. Focal neurologic deficits associated with hypoglycemia in children with diabetes. *J Pediatr* Oct 1990; *117*: 575-577).

COMMENT. The authors consider that focal seizures induced by hypoglycemia are the most likely cause of these transient neurologic deficits and that the paretic episodes are examples of Todd paralysis. The administration of sugar did not always result in reversal of the neurologic deficit and the neurological symptoms were not a direct consequence of hypoglycemia. Hemiplegic migraine seemed to be an unlikely explanation. The anticonvulsant phenytoin has a hyperglycemic effect (Belton NR, Etheridge JE, Millichap JG. *Epilepsia* 1965; *6*:234) and may be beneficial in the treatment of seizures and transient hemiparesis associated with hypoglycemia in diabetic children. - Editor. *Ped Neur Briefs* December 1990.

Hereditary Fructose Intolerance

Symptoms of neurological impairment in five children with hereditary fructose intolerance are described from the Service de Pediatrie, Hopital Antoine Beclere, Clamart, France. The diagnosis was proved by the deficiency of fructose-1-phosphate aldolase hepatic activity. Neurological symptoms during or after the acute phase of fructose intoxication included seizures, intracranial hypertension, tetraplegia, mental retardation, and deafness. Roentgenographic examination showed hydrocephalus, intraparenchymatous hemorrhage, cortical atrophy with ventricular dilatation, and ischemic or hypoxic cerebral lesions. In three patients cerebral impairment was secondary to cardiovascular collapse, prolonged hypoglycemia, or hemorrhagic diathesis related to liver insufficiency. Improvement followed treatment with a fructose-free diet but seizures necessitating anticonvulsant treatment persisted in three patients. (Labrune P et al. Unusual cerebral manifestations in hereditary fructose intolerance. *Arch Neurol* Nov 1990; *47*:1243-1244).

> COMMENT. Hereditary fructose intolerance is a metabolic disease of autosomal recessive inheritance that is due to a deficiency of aldolase B, the enzyme which catalyzes the catabolism of fructose-1-phosphate. The main symptoms are abdominal pain, vomiting, hypoglycemia, and liver dysfunction following the ingestion of fructose. Central nervous system involvement is unusual and serious sequelae may develop in cases that present with hemorrhage or hypoglycemia. - Editor. *Ped Neur Briefs* December 1990.

Skin Biopsy In Glycogenosis Type III

Electron microscopy of skin specimens of five patients with glycogenosis type III were correlated with clinical, biochemical, and electrophysiological findings from the Divisions of Neuropathology and Neuropediatrics, Ciudad Sanitaria Valle de Hebron, Barcelona, Spain. The disease began in infancy in four patients and at 38 years of age in one adult patient. Massive glycogen storage was observed in epithelial secretory cells of eccrine sweat glands and other cells, including Schwann cells of myelinated and unmyelinated fibers, were not affected. The changes differed clearly from those in glycogenosis II where glycogen storage is membrane bound and is found in most skin cells including fibroblasts, sweat glands, smooth muscle fibers, endothelial cells, and Schwann cells. Skin biopsy appeared to be useful in diagnosis of glycogenosis III and its differentiation from other glycogen storage disorders. (Sancho S et al. Skin biopsy findings in glycogenosis III: Clinical, biochemical, and electrophysiological correlations. *Ann Neurol* May 1990; *27*:480-486).

COMMENT. Glycogen storage disease type III (debrancher deficiency, Cori-Forbes disease) is an autosomal recessively inherited disease with a deficiency in amyl-1,6-glycosidase or debrancher enzyme. Enzyme deficiencies occur in liver, muscle, heart, leukocytes, erythrocytes, fibroblasts, and muscle cultures. Abnormal glycogen storage is found in liver, muscle, and erythrocytes. Clinically there are three types, 1) infantile, 2) childhood, 3) adult type. The infantile type is associated with hypoglycemia, failure to thrive, and hepatomegaly. Symptoms usually remit partially with growth. Childhood types present with heart failure and exercise intolerance. Adults develop gradual weakness and wasting of distal muscles and may have a history of abdominal enlargement with hepatic dysfunction in early childhood. EMG shows diffuse myopathic changes. Growth failure and hepatic dysfunction including hypoglycemia have been improved by the administration of cornstarch (Borowitz SM, Greene HL. *J Pediatr Gastroenterol Neutr* 1987; 6:631). - Editor. *Ped Neur Briefs* May 1990.

Lesch-Nyhan Syndrome

Five boys with Lesch-Nyhan syndrome and varying degrees of dystonia, chorea, spasticity, ataxia, dysarthria, and mental retardation were studied at the Depts of Neurology and Medicine, Baylor College of Medicine, and Depts of Neurology and Pediatrics, University of Texas Health Science Center, Houston, TX. Four showed reduction of homovanillic acid (HVA) in the CSF and all had low CSF phenethylene glycol, indicating reduced dopamine and norepinephrine turnover. Three children had high CSF 5-hydroxyindoleacetic acid (HIAA), suggesting increased serotonin turnover. The patient with the most severe chorea had the lowest CSF HVA value, whereas the patient with the least amount of self-multilation had the highest CSF 5HIAA. Only one patient improved with carbidopa-levodopa, whereas all 5 showed some lessening of self-mutilatory or hyperkinetic behavior in response to tetrabenazine, a monoamine-depleting agent. The study was thought to support the theory of abnormal central monoamine metabolism in Lesch-Nyhan syndrome. (Jankovic J et al. Lesch-Nyhan syndrome: a study of motor behavior and cerebrospinal fluid neurotransmitters. *Ann Neurol* May 1988; 23:466-469).

> COMMENT. Lesch-Nyhan syndrome is an X-lined recessive disorder of purine metabolism characterized by hypotonia followed by spasticity, chorea, athetosis, dystonia, growth and mental retardation, self-mutilatory behavior, hyperuricemia, and nephrolithiasis (Lesch M, Nyhan WL. *Am J Med* 1964; 36:561). The phenotypical expression is the result of a deficiency of hypoxanthineguanine phosphoribosyl-transferase enzyme, the gene located on the long arm of the X chromosome. Response to medications is variable but self-mutilation can sometimes be ameliorated (Herman BH et al. Naltrexone decreases self-injurious behavior. *Ann Neurol* 1987; 22:550). Editor. *Ped Neur Briefs* May 1988.

Methylmalonic Acidemia And Extrapyramidal Disease

Four children, 4-13 yrs old, with methylmalonic acidemia who developed acute dystonia after metabolic decompensation with ketoacidosis are reported from the Department of Pediatrics, University of Pennsylvania School of Medicine, and the Children's Hospital of Philadelphia, PA, and other collaborating institutions. The neurological complications were the result of acute necrosis of the globus pallidus and some involvement of internal capsules. One patient, aged 5 yrs, was a poor feeder and had vomited soon after birth. She was hospitalized at 1 wk of age with lethargy and ketoacidosis, and had massive amounts of methylmalonic acid in the urine that were not reduced by IM cyanocobalamin. Treatment with long-term oral alkali, and a diet restricted in isoleucine, valine, methionine, and threonine resulted in improvement and normal growth and development up to 2 yrs of age when she had an acute "metabolic stroke" precipitated by otitis media. Subsequently, she developed dystonia, dysarthria, dysphagia, and spastic quadriplegia. A CT scan showed bilateral symmetric lucencies of the globus pallidus and internal capsules. The lesions were thought to result from deranged organic acid metabolism and accumulation of toxic metabolites in the brain. (Heidenreich R et al. Acute extrapyramidal syndrome in methylmalonic acidemia: "Metabolic stroke" involving the globus pallidus. *J Pediatr* Dec 1988; *113*:1022-7).

COMMENT. Lesions of the basal ganglia have been noted in other inborn errors of organic acid metabolism, including propionic acidemia, and glutaric aciduria type 1, in Leigh syndrome and the mitochondrial encephalomyopathies including Kearns-Sayre and MELAS syndromes, and in several other hereditary diseases involving the CNS. - Editor. *Ped Neur Briefs* November 1988.

Infantile Glutaric Acidemia And Dystonia

Glutaric acidemia, an autosomal recessively inherited disease caused by deficiency of glutaryl-CoA dehydrogenase, was manifested by acute dystonia in 3 infants reported from the Children's Hospital of Pittsburgh, PA. Onset of symptoms was at 6, 9, and 21 months, the earlier history being entirely normal. Two infants developed dystonic posturing and hypertonia and one had choreoathetosis and hypotonia. Treatment with a low lysine diet, vitamin B and carnitine supplements, and baclofen resulted in some improvement in one infant, no change in one, and the third infant died at 13 months of age. Pathological findings included cerebral and cerebellar atrophy, shrinkage of the putamen, and white matter vacuolation. CT scans and MRI showed prominent Sylvian fissures, progressive loss of cerebral volume, especially temporal lobes and caudate nuclei, and increased ventricular and subarachnoid spaces. Unusual features of the disease in these patients included the acute onset of symptoms, absence of metabolic acidosis, and late onset at 21 months in one. Analysis of glutaryl-CoA dehydrogenase in skin fibroblasts is the only definite diagnostic test for glutaric acidemia. The authors stress that the enzyme should be measured in any infant with persistent dystonia and/or choreoathetosis and CT evidence of atrophic changes around the temporal lobes and Sylvian fissures, even when urine organic acid analysis for excess glutaric acid is negative. (Bergman I et al. Acute profound dystonia in infants with glutaric acidemia. *Pediatrics* Feb 1989; *83*:228-234).

> COMMENT. Glutaric acidemia, first described 14 years ago (Goodman SI et al. *Biochem Med* 1975; 1212), is now considered a relatively common metabolic disorder with an estimated frequency in the Swedish population about equal to phenylketonuria or 1/30,000 newborns (Kyllerman M, Steen G. *Arch Fr Pediatr* 1980; *37*:279). - Editor. *Ped Neur Briefs* January 1989.

CNS Complications Of Cystinosis

Fourteen patients with cystinosis, eight males and six females ranging in age from 13 to 24 years (mean 18.1 years) were examined for neurological involvement at the National Institute of Neurology and Communicative Disorders and Stroke, the National Institutes of Health Clinical Center, Bethesda, MD. Two patients had neurological symptoms, including bradykinesia, dementia and spasticity, and behavioral and cognitive disturbances; 12 patients had CT evidence of generalized cerebral atrophy; two had multifocal intracerebral mineralization on CT scan; two had abnormal electroencephalograms; and only one patient was entirely normal. Patients with neurologic symptoms or markedly abnormal CT scans were older and had a longer interval between their initial renal transplantation and the examination at follow-up than those patients who were normal or who had only mild cerebral atrophy. The neurologic and neuropsychometric abnormalities correlated with the degree of roentgenographic abnormality. The patients with nervous system abnormalities were not distinguished by patterns of medication use or the relative severity of cystinosis. The differential diagnosis included other complications from renal failure, dialysis and immunosuppression. (Fink JK et al. Neurologic complications in long-standing nephropathic cystinosis. *Arch Neurol* May 1989; *46*:543-548).

COMMENT. The central nervous system involvement in nephropathic cystinosis has not been implicated until recently. Survival into adulthood following renal dialysis and transplantation has drawn attention to the sequelae of long-standing cystinosis. Cystinosis is a rare autosomal recessive disorder of children and adults characterized biochemically by the intracellular accumulation of cystine crystals in the kidneys, bone marrow, and cornea as well as the reticuloendothelial system. With increasing longevity, involvement of other organs such as the thyroid, pancreas, and central nervous system has become apparent.

Three different patterns of the disease are recognized depending on the degree of cystine accumulation: Infantile nephropathic form, intermediate or late onset adolescent form, and a benign adult form. The clinical manifestations of infantile cystinosis include recurrent episodes of dehydration, the Fanconi renal tubular syndrome, retarded growth, anemia, photophobia, retinopathy, and vitamin D resistant rickets. Long-term treatment with Cysteamine may delay or prevent the accumulation of cystine crystals in various organs and may alter the prognosis. (daSilva VA et al. *N Engl J Med* 1985; *313*:1460). Biopsy specimens of cerebral cortex and meninges have revealed cystine crystals in the walls of arachnoidal blood vessels and in the cytoplasm of cortical neurons, basal ganglia, thalamus, cerebellum and posterior pituitary. The relationship of these crystalline deposits to neurological abnormalities has not been determined. Editor. *Ped Neur Briefs* May 1989.

Mannosidosis And Cognitive Functioning

Longitudinal assessments of the biochemistry and cognitive functioning in three brothers with mannosidosis are reported from the Department of Pediatrics in Human Development; Michigan State University, East Lansing, MI. The patients were followed from three or four years of age. The biochemical findings demonstrated profound deficits of leukocyte alpha mannosidase that remained stable over time and were very similar to levels of the same enzyme activity in fibroblasts. Cognitive tests including general intelligence, language, visual spatial skills, and overall adaptive abilities, were generally uniform with no signs of progressive deterioration except for receptive language abilities. When examined initially the patients were mildly retarded. Loss of receptive vocabulary abilities seen above the age of six years may have been related to a conductive hearing loss of 30-40 dB and frequent otitis media. There was a lack of correspondence between the level of enzyme deficiency and the degree of mental dysfunction. Sequential data were obtained for six years for the oldest brother, five years for the middle brother, and four years for the youngest brother. The authors suggest that hearing should be constantly examined to address potential sensory deprivation as it affects cognitive functioning in children with mannosidosis. (Noll RB et al. Long-term follow-up of biochemical and cognitive functioning in patients with mannosidosis. *Arch Neurol* May 1989; *46*:507-509).

COMMENT. Children with mannosidosis have coarse features, slight hepatosplenomegaly and psychomotor retardation. After two years of age, growth slows down, the tongue enlarges and a lumbar kyphosis and prominent forehead develop. Based on the findings in this study, overall intellectual functioning was low but showed no evidence of progressive deterioration except for receptive language skills. - Editor. *Ped Neur Briefs* May 1989.

Hereditary Tyrosinemia And Peripheral Neuropathy

Neurologic crises in 48 children with tyrosinemia identified on neonatal screening since 1970 are described from the Departments of Genetics, Hopital Sainte Justine, Hopital de Chicoutimi; and Universite Laval, Quebec, Canada. Neurologic crises had occurred in 20 (42%) and began at a mean age of one year leading to 104 hospital admissions. Abrupt episodes of peripheral neuropathy were characterized by severe pain with extensor hypertonia (75%), vomiting or paralytic ileus (69%), muscle weakness (29%), and self-mutilation (8%). Fourteen patients died due to complications of respiratory insufficiency or mechanical ventilation. In 5 patients undergoing hepatic transplantation none had neurologic crises. Urinary excretion of gamma aminolevulinic acid, an intermediate of porphyrin biosynthesis, was elevated during crises and during asymptomatic periods. Axonal degeneration and demyelination were demonstrated by EMG, NCS and neuromuscular biopsies. (Mitchell G et al. Neurologic crises in hereditary tyrosinemia. *N Engl J Med* Feb 15, 1990; *322*:432-437).

COMMENT. This study indicates that episodes of acute severe peripheral neuropathy are common in hereditary tyrosinemia and resemble crises of the neuropathic porphyrias. Hepatic transplantation eliminated the neurologic crisis, the major cause of mortality in these patients.

Abnormal porphyrin metabolism appears to underlie the neurologic crisis of tyrosinemia and is associated with elevated gamma aminolevulinic acid excretion. Therapy for the neurologic crises included adequate caloric intake, respiratory support, and control of pain, hypertension, hyponatremia, and self-mutilation. Gavage with high carbohydrate, high calorie feeds without phenylalanine or tyrosine were employed. Barbiturates and other agents contraindicated in porphyria were avoided. - Editor. *Ped Neur Briefs* March 1990.

Maternal Phenylketonuria And
Congenital Malformation

Infants born to women with PKU are frequently mentally retarded, microcephalic, of low birth weight, and have various malformations. The results of an international collaborative study (in UK, Europe, Australia) by the MRC/DHSS Phenylketonuria Register concerning the diet of pregnant women with PKU are reported from the Institute of Child Health, London: 1) Normal birth weights and head circumferences and no malformations in 17 infants whose mothers received a strict low phenylalanine diet at conception; 2) below average birth weights and head circumferences and excess malformations a) in 29 infants whose mothers were on a relaxed or normal diet at conception and a strict diet during pregnancy, and b) in 18 infants whose mothers received no dietary treatment during pregnancy. Birth weights and head circumferences of the 64 infants were inversely related to the maternal phenylalanine concentrations at conception, and hyperphenylalaninemia in early gestation had a dose-dependent effect on the fetus. The authors estimate 2000 women with PKU of fertile age by 1990 in the UK and unless monitored closely through their reproductive lives, a substantial number of microcephalic and mentally retarded children will be expected. (Drogari E, Smith I (for correspondence), Beasley M, Lloyd JK. Timing of strict diet in relation to fetal damage in maternal phenylketonuria. *Lancet* 1987; 2:927-930).

COMMENT. A National Collaborative Study of Maternal PKU was initiated in the US in 1984 and initial findings will be evaluated in 1991. Female PKU patients of fertile age receive education concerning risks to offspring and need for dietary and blood phenylalanine monitoring during pregnancies (O'Flynn M, Director PKU Clinic, Children's Memorial Hospital, Chicago, personal communication).

Levy HL and Waisbren SE (*N Engl J Med* 1983; *309*:1269) studied the effects of maternal PKU and hyperphenylalaninemia on 53 offspring from untreated pregnancies. Decreases in IQ, head circumference, and birth weight of the infants were correlated directly with the maternal IQ and inversely with maternal blood phenylalanine level. These authors concluded that maternal PKU has a substantial adverse effect on the fetus, and less severe maternal PKU may have subtle effects, resulting in slight reduction in IQ and intrauterine head growth. The UK report demonstrates that mothers with PKU who start a low phenylalanine diet before conception can give birth to normal infants despite variable phenylalanine blood levels during pregnancy. Congenital malformations and irreversible impairment of brain and body growth are determined within the first trimester of pregnancy. - Editor. *Ped Neur Briefs* November 1987.

New Treatment For Phenylketonuria

Sixteen adolescents and young adults with phenylketonuria were treated with a mixture of valine, isoleucine, and leucine for four 3-month periods, and biochemical and neuropsychological tests were carried out before and after treatment at the Metabolic Disease Center, Children's Hospital Medical Center, University of Cincinnati College of Medicine. The performance of timed attentional tests and a continuous performance test was improved during the valine, isoleucine, and leucine periods compared to the control mixture periods. The attention diagnostic method, a test with strong attentional components, showed significant improvements. These results were consistent with earlier reports of improvement in specific cognitive processes with valine, isoleucine, and leucine treatment in patients who were unable to maintain low serum phenylalanine levels. (Berry HK et al. Valine, isoleucine, and leucine. A new treatment for phenylketonuria. *AJDC* May 1990; *144*:539-543).

COMMENT. Phenylalanine and other large neutral amino acids share common receptocytes on a blood brain barrier transport system. The administration of other large neutral amino acids to patients with elevated plasma phenylalanine may reduce the amount of phenylalanine reaching the brain and prevent further deficits in cognition. The amino acid mixture consisted of 150 mg/kg Valine, 150 mg/kg Isoleucine, and 200 mg/kg Leucine. This mixture was prescribed as a supplement to the low phenylalanine formula. - Editor. *Ped Neur Briefs* May 1990.

PEROXISOMAL DISORDERS

Cerebro-Hepato-Renal (Zellweger) Syndrome

Selective neuronal lipidosis and neuroaxonal dystrophy of the dorsal nucleus of Clarke and lateral cuneate nucleus were the neuropathological findings in 3 males with Zellweger syndrome examined at the Medical Unit S. Carolina, Charleston, SC; the John F. Kennedy Institute, Johns Hopkins Univ, Baltimore, MD; and the Philadelphia Children's Hosp. Large amounts of abnormal cholesterol esters containing saturated and monosaturated very long-chain fatty acids were demonstrated in the striated neurons of the dorsal thoracic cord. The CNS neurons of these patients manifested the same morphological alteration as adrenocortical cells of adreno-leukodystrophy, and many of the striated neurons were degenerate or necrotic. It is suggested that a more generalized defect in neuronal fatty acid metabolism may explain the neuronal migration defects characteristic of Zellweger syndrome. These consist of pachygyria, micropolygyria and cerebral and cerebellar heterotopia. (Powers JM et al. Neuronal lipidosis and neuroaxonal dystrophy in cerebro-hepato-renal (Zellweger) syndrome. *Acta Neuropathol (Berl)* 1987; *73*:333-343).

COMMENT. CHR (Zellweger) syndrome, transmitted as an autosomal recessive, is invariably fatal within a few months after birth. Prenatal diagnosis may be made by amniocentesis and the production of very-long-chain fatty acids (VLCFA) from cultured amniocytes (*Lancet* 1984;

*1:*1234. Mosher AE et al. *N Engl J Med* 1984; *310*:1141).
The determination of VLCFA in the blood permits prompt
diagnostic confirmation of CHRS in the infant with dysmorphic facial and skull features, liver enlargement and
fibrosis, renal cysts, stippled calcifications of the patellae,
Brushfield's spots, optic atrophy and retinal pigmentation.
Zellweger syndrome is a peroxisomal disorder. The lacking
peroxisomes are cytoplasmic organelles containing oxidases
and catalase and are involved in metabolism of hydrogen
peroxide, fatty acids and bile acids. - Editor. *Ped Neur
Briefs* October 1987.

Infantile Refsum Disease

Two patients with infantile Refsum (phytanic acid storage)
disease were treated at 9 mos and 5-1/2 years of age with a low
phytanic acid diet and the effects studied over a 2-yr period or
longer in the Depts of Chemical Pathology, Neurology and
Histopathology, Adelaide Children's Hospital, and the Dept of
Neurology, Prince of Wales Children's Hospital, New South
Wales, Australia. Elevated phytanic and pipecolic acid plasma
levels were significantly decreased but very long chain fatty acids
remained grossly abnormal after 6 weeks or longer on the diet
consisting of skimmed milk powder, white meats, fish, root vegetables, some fruits and supplementary vitamins. Growth, motor
skills, self-mutilating behavior, intention tremor and nystagmus
improved, although ataxia and hypotonia persisted in the older
child who developed peripheral neuropathy with slowed motor
and sensory nerve conduction velocities. Impaired visual acuity
with optic atrophy and retinitis pigmentosa and sensorineural
deafness persisted. Head growth continued at the original 25th
and 3rd low percentiles. Electronmicroscopy of liver biopsies
before and after dietary treatment showed an increase in inclusion bodies, and peroxisomes and lysosomes were present.
(Robertson EF et al. Treatment of infantile phytanic acid storage disease: clinical, biochemical and ultrastructural findings in
two children treated for 2 years. *Eur J Pediatr* Feb 1988;
147:133-42).

COMMENT. Infantile Refsum syndrome is characterized by retinitis pigmentosa, sensorineural deafness, developmental delay, hepatomegaly and dysmorphic features. The older of the 2 present cases showed chronic polyneuropathy, ataxia and intention tremor, typical of the classical form of Refsum disease-heredopathia atactica polyneuritiformis. The exclusion of phytanic acid from the diet of affected adults has been successful in lowering plasma phytanic acid levels, improving peripheral nerve function and arresting the progress of visual and hearing defects. - Editor. *Ped Neur Briefs* March 1988.

Peroxisomal Disorders — Classification

Generalized peroxisomal disorders are classified in three main groups in a review article from the Kennedy Institute and the Departments of Neurology and Pediatrics, Johns Hopkins University, 707 N. Broadway, Baltimore, MD.

Group 1 includes Zellweger (cerebro-hepato-renal) syndrome, neonatal adrenoleukodystrophy, infantile Refsum disease, and hyperpipecolic acidemia, all characterized by a reduction in the number of peroxisomes and deficiency of multiple peroxisomal enzymes.

Group 2 contains only one rare disorder, rhizomelic chondrodysplasia punctata, characterized by stippled calcifications of hyaline cartilage, dwarfing, cataracts, multiple malformations with contractures, koala bear facies, and severe mental retardation. Peroxisomes are normal in number but functionally impaired.

Group 3 includes Refsum disease, X-linked adrenoleukodystrophy, pseudo-Zellweger syndrome, hyperoxaluria type 1, acatalasemia and an undescribed variant. All have a normal number of peroxisomes and the activity of only one peroxisomal enzyme is reduced.

Peroxisomal disorders are a newly recognized and heterogeneous group of diseases with variable manifestations transmitted as autosomal recessive or sex-linked recessive traits and have in common one or more peroxisomal enzyme defects. The term peroxisome is coined from the hydrogen peroxide-forming enzymes found within the subcellular organelle. More than 40 enzymes have now been localized to the peroxisomes. (Naidu S, Moser AE, Moser HW. Phenotypic and genotypic variability of generalized peroxisomal disorders. *Pediatr Neurol* Jan/Feb 1988; 4:5-12).

COMMENT. This is an excellent review of the various entities now classified as generalized peroxisomal disorders. See *Ped Neur Briefs* March 1988; 2:22-23, and Oct 1987; 1:32) for case reports of infantile Refsum and Zellweger syndromes. - Editor. *Ped Neur Briefs* April 1988.

Peroxisomal Disorders — Diagnostic Features
The biochemical and clinical diagnostic characteristics of peroxisomal disorders are reviewed by authors from the Department of Pediatrics, Medical University of South Carolina, Charleston, SC. Two major groups are recognized: 1) those that represent a diffuse peroxisomal dysfunction due to (a) a reduction in number of peroxisomes (Zellweger's syndrome, neonatal adrenoleukodystrophy, infantile Refsum's disease, and hyperpipecolic acidemia); and (b) normal numbers but reduced activities of multiple enzymes (rhizomelic chondrodysplasia punctata); and 2) those disorders with specific single peroxisomal enzymatic defects (childhood adrenoleukodystrophy-X-linked, adult Refsum's disease, hyperoxaluria, acatalasemia, and pseudo-Zellweger's syndrome).

Peroxisomal disorders should be considered in any infant with hypotonia and delays in psychomotor development, and especially in those with facial dysmorphisms (high and prominent forehead), hepatomegaly, cataracts, retinitis, calcific stippling, short limbs, failure to thrive, seizures, and hearing deficit.

In childhood, loss of motor skills, progressive dementia, and skin bronzing should suggest the diagnosis. Measurement of very long chain fatty acids is used to confirm the biochemical defect, and other tests including bile acid, phytanic acid, and plasmalogen are included for specific diagnoses. (Singh I et al. Peroxisomal disorders. Biochemical and clinical diagnostic considerations. *AJDC* Dec 1988; *142*:1297-1301).

COMMENT. Peroxisomal disorders are rare but important because clinical sequelae can be related to specific biochemical deficits and some may be identified prenatally and their recurrence prevented. Dietary restriction of very long chain fatty acids and plasmapheresis are helpful in treatment by controlling the accumulation of toxic metabolites in some peroxisomal disorders, and the addition of glycerol trioleate, a lipid containing unsaturated fatty acid, is a promising new therapy that reduces the synthesis of C22-26 fatty acids. For further information on peroxisomal disorders, refer to a special article by Moser HW (*Neurology* Oct 1988; *38*:1617).

A family with Refsum's disease (heredopathia atactica polyneuritiformis) in whom 4 out of 6 siblings were affected is reported from the Department of Neurology, Westminster Hospital, London (Britton TC, Gibberd FB. *JR Soc Med* Oct 1988; *81*:602-3). Retinitis pigmentosa was the presenting diagnostic sign in the index case, and other affected members of the family were detected by screening for raised plasma phytanic acid levels. Early diagnosis is important because dietary treatment will prevent the development of neuropathy, ataxia, cardiac arrhythmias, and ichthyosis. Retinitis pigmentosa, anosmia, and ataxia should suggest the diagnosis. - Editor. *Ped Neur Briefs* November 1988.

Adrenoleukodystrophy Dietary Therapy

The biochemical and clinical efficacy of dietary erucic acid (C22:1) therapy for X-linked adrenoleukodystrophy (ALD) was investigated at the Departments of Pediatrics, Human Genetics, Neurology, Medical College of Virginia, Virginia Commonwealth University, Richmond, VA, and the Department of Neurology, University of California, Davis, Sacramento, CA. Twelve patients, aged six to 12 years, were treated with a diet enriched with erucic acid and oleic acid for 2-19 months. The mean plasma C26:0 concentration decreased to normal by four weeks, and the C26:0 composition of plasma sphingomyelin and phosphatidylcholine became normal by four months. Two mildly affected patients remained clinically stable whereas six with moderate to advanced disease deteriorated. The diet may prevent further demyelinization in some mildly affected boys with X-linked adrenoleukodystrophy. (Rizzo WB et al. Dietary erucic acid therapy for X-linked adrenoleukodystrophy. *Neurology* November 1989; *39*: 1415-1422).

COMMENT. X-linked adrenoleukodystrophy is an inborn error of metabolism characterized by adrenal insufficiency and progressive demyelinization. ALD is usually fatal within several years after onset of neurologic abnormalities. A clinically milder form of ALD, *adrenomyeloneuropathy*, has a later age of onset and slower progression. The authors consider that the dietary erucic acid therapy may be more useful in patients with this milder form of ALD and in presymptomatic boys who express the biochemical defect of ALD.

The possibility of adrenomyeloneuropathy should be considered in any boy with Addison's disease. (Sadeghi-Nejad A, Senior B. *N Engl J Med* 1990; *322*:13-16). These authors measured the plasma concentrations of very long chain saturated fatty acids in eight patients with adrenal insufficiency; five had elevated plasma hexacosanoic acid confirming the presence of adrenomyelo-neuropathy.

MRI showed brain involvement in all five patients. It was concluded that adrenomyeloneuropathy may present as Addison's disease in childhood.

In a further recent study from the Departments of Pediatric Endocrinology and Radiology, Hopital Saint Vincent de Paul, Paris, France, the MRI detected white matter lesions in two of seven patients with biochemically proven ALD but without neurologic manifestations. The ages at the time of MRI diagnosis were 14 and 21 years. (Auborg P et al. *Neurology* December 1989; 39:1619-1621). Six of the seven neurologically asymptomatic ALD patients in this study had adrenal insufficiency. - Editor. *Ped Neur Briefs* December 1989.

Zellweger's Syndrome: Tissue Chemistry

The total fatty acid and aldehyde composition in the brain, liver, and kidneys of two infants with Zellweger's syndrome and one with pseudo-Zellweger's syndrome and the fatty acid patterns expressed as percent values are reported from the Autonomous University of Barcelona, Hospital Infantil Vall d'Hebron, Barcelona, Spain. In confirmation of previous findings, patients with Zellweger's syndrome had extremely low levels of docosahexaenoic acid in the brain, liver, and kidneys. In both Zellweger's and pseudo-Zellweger's syndrome the ratio of the polyunsaturated fatty acids 22:6w3/22:4w6 was markedly decreased in all tissues. The findings reinforced the hypothesis of an enzymatic defect in peroxisomal disorders involving the desaturation of long polyunsaturated fatty acids. (Martinez M. Severe deficiency of docosahexaenoic acid in peroxisomal disorders: A defect of delta 4 desaturation? *Neurology* August 1990; 40:1292-1298).

COMMENT. In an excellent review of peroxisomal disorders (Naidu S, Moser HW. *Neurologic Clinics* August 1990; 8:507. W. B. Saunders Company, Philadelphia) the clinical signs of Zellweger's syndrome and other group I peroxisomal disorders are listed as follows: dysmorphism, hypotonia and retardation, early onset seizures, sensorineural hearing loss, retinal pigmentary degeneration, cataract, hepatomegaly. The biochemical and morphologic abnormalities include plasma increased very long chain fatty acids, phytanic acid, pipecolic acid; RBCs reduced plasmalogens, x-ray bony stippling, MRI central demyelination, liver absent peroxisomes, fibrosis and cirrhosis; kidney renal cortical cysts. Dietary treatment which effectively reduces plasma VLCFA levels is now available and bone marrow transplant has been partially effective in two patients. - Editor. *Ped Neur Briefs* September 1990.

CHAPTER **16**

HEREDO-DEGENERATIVE AND DEMYELINATING DISORDERS

Degenerative Ataxic Disorders

Harding AE at the Institute of Neurology, London, author of the *Hereditary Ataxias and Related Disorders* (Edinburgh, Churchill Livingstone, 1984) reviews the classification, causes, clinical characteristics and treatment of degenerative ataxias. A combination of genetic and environmental factors is the most common origin for this complex group of over 50 distinct diseases, subdivided according to clinical and genetic features. Metabolic defects such as arylsulfatase-A in metachromatic leukodystrophy are recognizable but untreatable but some deficiency diseases (e.g. Vitamin E) are amenable to treatment with supplements. The cause of Friedreich's ataxia, an autosomal recessive disorder, is unknown and reported deficiencies of pyruvate dehydrogenase and mitochondrial malic enzymes have not been confirmed. Similarly, in olivopontocerebellar atrophy, a late onset ataxia, recent studies have not confirmed an earlier report of reduced leucocyte glutamate dehydrogenase activity. Most attempts at treatment of degenerative ataxias have been disappointing but promising results using thyrotrophin releasing hormone have been reported from Japan. (Harding A. Degenerative ataxic disorders, still perplexing. *BMJ* 1987; *295*:1223-4).

COMMENT. Degenerative ataxias resembling Friedreich's ataxia that may be amenable to treatment include Vitamin E, B12, folate and biotin deficiencies and Refsum's disease, responsive to a diet low in phytol and phytanic acid. - Editor. *Ped Neur Briefs* December 1987.

Spinocerebellar Degeneration And Mitochondrial Inclusions

Two children, an 8-year old boy and a 6-year old girl, with progressive ataxia, dysmetria, hypoactive or absent deep tendon reflexes, equivocal plantar response, and sensory impairments, were investigated by pathologists and neurologists at the University of Vermont, Burlington, VT, and University of Saskatchewan, Saskatoon, Canada. The diagnosis of SCD was established by the clinical course and laboratory tests that were normal for arylsulfatase, amino acids, phytanic acid, etc.

Rectal biopsy specimens were examined ultrastructurally by electron microscope and by a laser microprobe mass analyzer (LAMMA). Clusters of acicular osmophilic inclusions in the mitochondria of neuronal somata was consistent with crystals of calcium hydroxyapatite (CHA). The calcific nature of the deposits was confirmed by LAMMA. Similar mitochondrial inclusions were found in 10% of smooth muscle cells but not in skeletal muscle and nerve biopsy specimens. Tissue from control subjects had no mitochondrial acicular deposits. It has been suggested that the calcium overload may interfere with mitochondrial enzyme activity by disrupting oxidative phosphorylation. (Munoz DG, Emery ES III, Highland RA. Mitochondrial hydroxyapatite deposits in spinocerebellar degeneration. *Ann Neurol* 1987; *22*:258-263).

COMMENT. An abnormal oxidative phosphorylation in muscle mitochondria of patients with Friedreich's ataxia (FA) was previously demonstrated by Stumpf DA et al (*Neurology* 1982; *32*:221); mitochondrial malic enzyme activity was 10% of control level in FA fibroblasts. Also, glutamate dehydrogenase deficiency has been noted in cultured skin fibroblasts and leukocyte homogenates of patients with spinocerebellar syndrome (Plaitakis A et al. *Ann Neurol* 1980; *7*:297). These studies and the present report may eventually lead to carrier detection and possible specific therapies for spinocerebellar degenerative disease. - Editor. *Ped Neur Briefs* September 1987.

Friedreich's Ataxia And Glucose Metabolism

Glucose metabolism was investigated in 21 patients with FA at the Instituto Neurogico, Cattedra di Clinica Medica, Milan, Italy. Abnormalities of glucose tolerance occurred in 5 (23.8%) and 4 were diabetic (19%). By oral glucose tolerance tests, the plasma glucose levels of 5 patients were 140-200 mg/ml 2 hours after glucose ingestion. Plasma insulin levels of glucose-intolerant patients were significantly higher than controls after 180 minutes following glucose ingestion. Plasma glucagon levels of FA patients were higher than controls, and plasma lactate levels of glucose intolerant FA patients were higher than controls. By intravenous glucose load, glucose responses did not differ significantly between patients and controls. The results showed that FA is associated with insulin resistance, B-cell deficiency, and type I diabetes. The alterations might be genetically linked or metabolically related to the primary defect in FA. (Finocchiaro G et al. Glucose metabolism alterations in Friedreich's ataxia. *Neurology* Aug 1988; *38*:1292-96).

COMMENT. Friedreich's ataxia, the most common heredodegenerative ataxia, is recessively inherited. The incidence of diabetes in FA patients is high, glucose intolerance during oral glucose tests have been reported previously, but the abnormalities of glucose metabolism have not previously been studied in detail. The abnormalities of glycemic control in FA may be due to the interplay of insulin resistance and B-cell dysfunction or their independent effects. - Editor. *Ped Neur Briefs* August 1988.

Spinocerebellar Degeneration And Ceroid Lipofuscinosis

Neuronal ceroid lipofuscinosis (NCL) presenting in two different forms within a family is reported from the New York State Office of Mental Retardation and Developmental Disabilities, Institute for Basic Research, 10560 Forest Hill Rd, Staten Island, NY and the Dept of Neurology, Albert Einstein Coll of Med, Bronx, NY. In the proband, the clinical course was compatible with an atypical juvenile form of NCL, beginning with ataxia and spasticity at 4 to 5 yrs, and followed by blindness with optic atrophy, intractable seizures, dementia, and death at 14 yrs. Areflexia, hypotonia, and ataxia were atypical manifestations, suggesting peripheral nervous system involvement similar to that in her two affected siblings. The illness in the siblings, a brother and a sister, showed a more protracted course, a later age of onset (8.5 and 10.5 yrs), more severe cerebellar and cortico-spinal signs, and sensorimotor neuropathy; seizures, dementia and visual loss were lacking. All 3 siblings had cytoplasmic inclusion bodies characteristic of the juvenile form of NCL and increased excretion of urinary dolichol. The authors propose that either variability of gene expression or two different recessive genes in this consanguineous family may account for the divergent phenotypes in the proband and siblings. (Wisniewski KE et al. Spino-cerebellar degeneration with polyneuropathy associated with ceroid lipofuscinosis in one family. *J Child Neurol* Jan 1988; 2:33-41).

COMMENT. The diagnosis of neuronal ceroid lipofuscinosis (Batten's disease, Spielmeyer-Vogt-Sjogren syndrome, Kufs' disease) is based on characteristic clinical manifestations, ultrastructural fingerprint cytoplasmic inclusion bodies in the rectal biopsy, punch skin biopsy, and buffy coat of lymphocytes, and elevated urinary dolichol excretion as a biochemical marker. Although the clinical course and manifestations were atypical, the patients in this study exhibited the cytoplasmic inclusions seen in the juvenile variant of ceroid lipofuscinosis. These cases include an unusual presentation as a spinocerebellar degeneration. - Editor. *Ped Neur Briefs* April 1988.

Spinocerebellar Ataxia — Autosomal Dominant Type

The onset below 15 years of age of autosomal dominant spinocerebellar ataxia (SCA) in 6 of 41 affected patients is reported from the Dept of Pediatrics, Baylor College of Medicine, Houston, TX. Linkage analysis was performed on 93 individuals in a seven-generation kindred, and strong evidence of linkage of the SCA to the human leukocyte antigen loci on the short arm of chromosome 6 was documented. Age at onset was 6 to 15 years, and clinical findings included ataxia, dysmetria, dysdiadochokinesia, intellectual deficit, ophthalmoparesis, dysarthria, dysphagia, amyotrophy, and cerebellar atrophy on CT scan. Progression was rapid, 1 patient dying 3 years after the onset of symptoms at age 12 years, and 2 patients aged 15 to 26 years are terminally ill. None had seizures, retinal degeneration or optic atrophy. Poor intellectual performance preceded other neurological abnormalities in 5 children. Of the 6 patients with juvenile onset, 5 were offspring of affected males. This was the first report of childhood onset in the HLA-linked form of SCA. (Zoghbi HY et al. Spinocerebellar ataxia: variable age of onset and linkage to human leukocyte antigen in a large kindred. *Ann Neurol* June 1988; *23*:580-584).

COMMENT. The authors comment that all families with dominantly inherited SCA should undergo genetic studies to determine linkage to HLA. Families with the HLA-linked form of SCA may be advised to have HLA typing for presymptomatic or prenatal diagnosis.

The spinocerebellar ataxias are a heterogeneous group of diseases characterized by a slowly progressive loss of neurons in the cerebellum. Friedrich's ataxia, an autosomal recessive trait, presents in childhood, whereas the autosomal dominant varieties of SCA, described by Marie, are usually distinguished by an onset in adult life.

In a clinical review of 20 childhood cases of Friedreich's ataxia at the Dept of Child Neurology, Aegean University, Bornova, Izmir, Turkey (Ulku A et al. *Acta Neurol Scan* June 1988; *77*:493-7), the mean age at onset was 6.1 years, a positive family history was present in 8 cases, ataxia was the main presenting symptom, and reflexes were depressed or absent in all cases. Electrophysiological studies, especially depressed or absent sensory nerve conduction velocities, were confirmatory of the diagnosis in 9 of 10 patients tested. The EKG was abnormal in 5 (25%). - Editor. *Ped Neur Briefs* July 1988.

Genetics Of Degenerative Diseases

Chromosome studies of four neurodegenerative diseases are described in current literature: Huntington disease cases in Finland show linkage disequilibrium of chromosome 4rflp haplotypes (Ikonen E et al. *Am J Hum Genet* Jan 1990; *46*:5-11). Hereditary Motor and Sensory Neuropathy Type I shows linkage to the pericentromeric region of chromosome 17. (Middleton-Price HR, Harding AE et al. *Am J Hum Genet* Jan 1990; *46*:92-94). Friedreich's ataxia gene has been assigned to chromosome 9q13-q21. (Hanauer A et al. *Am J Hum Genet* Jan 1990; *46*:133-137). The dystonia gene in Ashkenazi Jewish population has been located on chromosome 9q32-34. (Kramer PL, Fahn S et al. *Ann Neurol* Feb 1990; *27*:114-120). The same gene may be responsible for idiopathic torsion dystonia in non-Jewish kindred. Most familial forms of idiopathic torsion dystonia follow autosomal dominant transmission with reduced penetrance. The frequency in Ashkenazi Jewish population is 5-10 times greater than that in other groups. - Editor. *Ped Neur Briefs* February 1990.

Ataxia-Telangiectasia: T-Cell Antigen

The proportion of T-cell antigen receptors in ten patients with ataxia-telangiectasia were compared with normal subjects and patients with other immune deficits at the Departments of Clinical Immunology and Pediatrics, University of Rome, "la Sapienza" Rome, Italy. An increased ratio of gamma/delta bearing to alpha/beta bearing T-cells in ataxia-telangiectasia may reflect both a recombinational defect that interferes with T-cell and B-cell gene rearrangements and an inability to repair damage to the DNA. The criteria for the diagnosis of ataxia-telangiectasia included early cerebellar ataxia, chromosomal instability, and raised alpha fetoprotein levels. There were six boys and four girls ranging in age from 2-18 years. The diagnosis was confirmed by cytogenetic analysis which showed the typical increase in nonrandom chromosomal breaks and translocations. (Carbonari M et al. Relative increase of T cells expressing the gamma/delta rather than the alpha/beta receptor in ataxia-telangiectasia. *N Engl J Med* Jan 11, 1990; *322*:73-76).

COMMENT. In an editorial in the same issue Peterson RDA and Funkhouser JD of the University of South Alabama, Mobile, AL refer to their previously published proposal that essentially all clinical manifestations of ataxia-telangiectasia, including the degeneration of the CNS, are a consequence of a defect in genetic recombination. (*Immunol Today* 1989; *10*:313-5). Elucidation of the molecular abnormalities of the lymphocytes in patients with ataxia-telangiectasia may reveal molecular mechanisms responsible for the cellular differentiation of lymphocytes and other cell systems. The gene responsible for ataxia-telangiectasia has been localized to chromosome 11q22-23. These studies at the molecular level bring new insight in lymphocyte differentiation and the immune disorder that characterizes ataxia-telangiecasia. Absence of tonsils in a child with ataxia should prompt the determination of immunoglobulins. - Editor. *Ped Neur Briefs* January 1990.

Cerebellar Ataxia, Opsoclonus, And Neuroblastoma

A 20 month-old girl with cerebellar ataxia and opsoclonus associated with neuroblastoma is reported from the Pediatric Neurology Unit, Tel Aviv Medical Center, Israel. Ataxia, present since 1 year of age, and irregular, "jerky" eye movements, noted on admission, became worse over a 2 month observation period. An abdominal mass found at 20 months and removed at operation was a ganglioneuroblastoma. Following surgery, steroids for 3 weeks, and chemotherapy 1 year, blood pressure returned to normal immediately and the ataxia and opsoclonus disappeared within 6-7 weeks. At a 2 year follow-up, the neurological and general examinations were normal. (Harel S et al. Cerebellar ataxia and opsoclonus as the initial manifestations of myoclonic encephalopathy associate with neuroblastoma. *Child's Nerv Syst* 1987; 3:245-247).

> COMMENT. Opsomyoclonus or *dancing eye syndrome*, also known as myoclonic encephalopathy of infancy, is frequently of undetermined etiology. It may follow viral infection and it is sometimes associated with occult malignancies, notably neuroblastoma. Normal urinary catecholamines do not exclude the presence of tumor and repeat evaluations including radiographs of abdomen and chest are indicated. The acute stage of the dancing eye syndrome usually responds best to ACTH followed after a few weeks by prednisone. Steroids may need to be continued for several months. - Editor. *Ped Neur Briefs* December 1987.

Ataxia-Oculomotor Apraxia Syndrome

A new spinocerebellar degenerative syndrome has been described in 14 patients from 10 families and reported from the Hopital des Enfants Malades, Paris, France; Montreal Neurological Institute, Canada; Rashid Hospital, Dubai, UAE: Tokyo Women's Medical College, Japan; and University of Colorado Medical School, Boulder, CO. Six of the cases had been reported previously in the Japanese literature and in abstracts. The clinical features included onset between 2 and 7 years of age, ataxia, ocular motor apraxia, choreoathetosis, depressed or absent deep tendon reflexes, dysarthria, mask-like facies, intention tremor, and mildly subnormal intellectual function in one-half the patients. CT was normal in 6 and showed mild vermal atrophy in 1. None had conjunctival telangiectasis or abnormal immunoglobulins and a diagnosis of ataxia telangiectasia was considered unlikely. The syndrome was probably genetically determined with an autosomal mode of inheritance; it involved both sexes with consanguinity in 6 of 10 sibships. (Aicardi J, Barbosa C, Andermann E and F, Morcos R, Ghanem Q, Fukuyama Y, Awaya Y, Moe P. Ataxia - ocular motor apraxia; a syndrome mimicking ataxia - telangiectasia. *Ann Neurol* Oct 1988; *24*:497-502).

COMMENT. The differential diagnosis includes Cogan's ocular motor apraxia and ataxia telangiectasia. The authors, of whom 4 are already distinguished by eponymous syndromes (Aicardi J, Andermann E and F, and Fukuyama Y), report a specific neurodegenerative syndrome of genetic origin with patients originating from widely separate geographical areas and from different ethnic backgrounds. Ataxia, areflexia, and ocular muscle paralyses are also featured in the Fisher syndrome. - Editor. *Ped Neur Briefs* December 1988.

"Happy Puppet" Syndrome

The diagnostic features of 36 cases of Angelman's "happy puppet" syndrome are reported from the Hospital for Sick Children, Great Ormond Street, London. These include ataxia, developmental delay, paroxysmal laughter, seizures, and microcephaly. The facial appearance is characterized by a prominent jaw, wide mouth, and pointed chin. The ataxia of gait is associated with jerky limb movements and hand flapping. Muscle tone is variable, deep tendon reflexes normal, and plantar responses flexor. This series included 3 sibships of 3 affected sisters, 2 affected brothers, and 2 affected sisters, respectively. Males and females were equally affected. The electroencephalogram was abnormal in all cases and showed rhythmic slow waves at 4-6 Hz and runs of 2-3 Hz anteriorly. On closure of eyes, spikes and 2-4 Hz slow waves occurred posteriorly. CT showed mild cerebral atrophy in 8 of 23 patients tested. Chromosome deletions of 15q11-13 were detected in 5 patients. (Robb SA et al. The "happy puppet" syndrome of Angelman: review of the clinical features. *Arch Dis Child* Jan 1989; *64*:83-86).

COMMENT. Prior to this report, approximately 50 cases of Angelman's syndrome had been described in a period of 20 years. First considered to be sporadic it now appears to be genetic in nature. The authors stress the importance of the recognition of the syndrome so that genetic counseling can be offered. - Editor. *Ped Neur Briefs* December 1988.

Haw River Syndrome: Familial Ataxia Dementia

A newly defined familial disorder of progressive dementia, ataxia, chorea, and seizures is described from the Department of Neurology School of Medicine, the University of North Carolina at Chapel Hill and the Department of Pathology, Duke University Medical Center, Durham, NC. The first recorded member of the family was born in 1840 and lived at Haw River, NC. In 22 patients examined the initial symptoms were ataxia of gait, intention tremor and choreiform movements that developed usually between 15 and 30 years of age. Recurrent generalized tonic-clonic seizures and progressive dementia developed later, and 11 of the 22 died after 15-25 years of illness. Neuropathological findings in two deceased family members were: neuronal loss of the dentate nucleus, microcalcification of the globus pallidus, neuroaxonal dystrophy of the nucleus gracilis, and demyelination of the centrum semiovale. (Farmer TW et al. Ataxia, chorea, seizures and dementia. Pathologic features of a newly defined familial disorder. *Arch Neurol* July 1989; *46*:774-779).

COMMENT. The authors list in the differential diagnosis: Olivopontocerebellar atrophy, dentatorubropallidoluysian atrophy, Ramsay Hunt syndrome, familial idiopathic calcification of the basal ganglia, neuroaxonal dystrophy, Hallervorden-Spatz disease, Huntington's disease, Wilson's disease, and Gerstmann-Straussler syndrome (cerebellar ataxia, dementia, amyloid plaques). Farmer's syndrome appears to have distinctive features.

Dementia as defined by the American Psychiatric Association (1980) is a deterioration in cognitive abilities that exceeds the decline expected with normal aging and occurs in a state of clear consciousness. Classifications of the dementias have been based on etiology (degenerative, vascular, toxic metabolic, and infectious), pathology, and clinicopathological correlations. Cortical versus subcortical forms have been described and have been correlated with brain behavior relationships. In Alzheimer's disease corticopathology is prominent whereas in Parkinson's disease and Wilson's disease subcortical areas are the major sites of pathology. This dichotomy is probably an oversimplification. (See Chui HC. *Arch Neurol* July 1989; *46*:806). - Editor. *Ped Neur Briefs* August 1989.

PSYCHOGENIC ATAXIA

Hysterical Gait

In a study of the clinical features of conversion disorder in 52 children admitted to the Royal Alexandra Hospital for Children, Camperdown, New South Wales, Australia, hysterical gait disturbance was the main complaint in 71%, and pain, paresthesia or anesthesia in 77%. So-called classical conversion symptoms such as blindness and globus were relatively rare. The disorder was rare below 8 years of age and girls outnumbered boys three to one. Spring and summer (Sept-Nov and Jan-Mar in Australia) accounted for 75% of admissions, coinciding with the end of year exams and the beginning of the new school year. Only 6 children had organic disease before the hysterical episodes. Psychological features included a model (54%), stressful event (46%), separation or loss of relative (46%), previous hysterical symptoms (33%), la belle indifference (19%). Treatment consisted of stopping unwarranted investigation, PT and OT, and psychologic counseling. At discharge, 61% were completely recovered or had appreciably improved. A core group of 13 (21%) did not respond. (Grattan-Smith P et al. Clinical features of conversion disorder. *Arch Dis Child* Apr 1988; *63*:408-414).

> COMMENT. In all but 3 of the 36 children presenting with an abnormality of gait, pain, and less frequently, anesthesia were prominent features. These associated symptoms are helpful in the differentiation from a dystonic gait, frequently misdiagnosed as hysterical in nature. The infrequent occurrence of organic disease as a prelude to conversion symptoms in this study is unusual. Gait disturbances of an hysterical nature may be preceded by minor trauma and pseudoseizures are frequently accompanied by true seizures requiring treatment with anticonvulsant drugs. - Editor. *Ped Neur Briefs* May 1988.

Astasia-Abasia

Twenty-seven children and adolescents diagnosed as having conversion reaction manifested as an inability to stand or walk are reported from the Department of Pediatrics, Mayo Clinic, Rochester, MN. There were 9 males and 18 females, ages 8 to 16 years, and duration of the symptoms varied from 1 to 60 weeks. Precipitating events in 17 patients included minor illnesses, school and home related problems, and minor injuries. Onset of symptoms showed seasonal variation with maximal frequency in the winter months and none in the summer and at time of school vacation. The duration of symptoms, estimated at the time of follow-up some 5 to 22 years later, was from a few days to a maximum of 2.5 years. Twenty-two (80%) said they were healthy and the remainder had minor complaints. None had organic illnesses that might have explained the ataxia. Three had continued mental problems and one was in jail for having killed his parents. (Stickler GB, Cheung-Patton A. Astasia-abasia. A conversion reaction. Prognosis. *Clin Pediat* Jan 1989; *28*:12-16).

COMMENT. A prompt and firm diagnosis on the basis of positive in addition to exclusion criteria is advocated, and a neurologic examination and appropriate laboratory tests are essential as a reassurance for both patient and treating physician. Dystonia musculorum deformans can be a pitfall, a disorder frequently misdiagnosed as a conversion reaction initially. In a study of 7 children with neurological symptoms diagnosed as hysterical conversion reactions and reported from Duke University Medical Center (Bangash IH et al. *AJDC* Nov 1988; *142*:1203) all but one had been misdiagnosed as having organic diseases. When the correct diagnosis was made, all recovered and none relapsed after 3 to 11 months follow-up. - Editor. *Ped Neur Briefs* December 1988.

Cerebellar Ataxia Benefitted By 5-Hydroxytryptophan

Levoratatory 5-hydroxytryptophan (10 mg/kg/day) was found to benefit patients with various inherited or acquired cerebellar ataxias in a long-term randomized, double-blind study at the Hopital Neurologique, Alexis Carrel Faculty of Medicine, Lyon, France. Of 30 patients in test and placebo groups, 2 had Friedreich's ataxia, 8 had postsurgical ataxia, 6 multiple sclerosis, 2 brain stem infarction, and 12 cerebellar cortical atrophy. The majority were adults, and the degree of ataxia was measured by four semiquantitative subtests. The treatment continued initially for four months, was extended in five patients without controls for a further eight months. Levo-5-hydroxytryptophan significantly improved the ataxia score and modified the time of standing upright, the speed of walking, speaking, and writing. The process appears to be serotonin-dependent and provides benefit particularly in static cerebellar disturbances and speech dysarthria caused by lesions of the anterior vermis. (Trouillas P et al. Improvement of cerebellar ataxia with levorotatory form of 5-hydroxytryptophan. A double-blind study with quantified data processing. *Arch Neurol* Nov 1988; *45*:1217-1222).

> COMMENT. The rationale for this treatment was the discovery of serotoninergic nerve terminals in the cortex of the cerebellum, and the induction of cerebellar tremor by the experimental depletion of serotonin. The treatment was well tolerated and should be considered for trial in children with Friedreich's ataxia and in static, postsurgical or post-viral cerebellar syndromes. - Editor. *Ped Neur Briefs* March 1989.

Thyrotropin-Releasing Hormone For Cerebellar Ataxia

A nine year old girl with cerebellar ataxia that responded to thyrotropin-releasing hormone is reported from the Department of Pediatrics, Kyoto Prefectero University of Medicine, Kyoto, Japan. Clinical improvement occurred 18 months after the onset of cerebellar ataxia and neurological deficits which included speech impairment, gait disturbance, ataxia of the extremities and positional nystagmus. CSF examination demonstrated that the concentrations of 5-HIAA and HVA increased and that the 5-HIAA/HVA ratio rose from 0.243 to 0.358 during TRH treatment. The levels of monoamine metabolites in the CSF reflect CNS biogenic amine turnover. The changes observed suggested that TRH influenced serotonin neurons rather than catecholamine neurons. The preparation of TRH was protireline tartrate: Takeda Co. Ltd., Japan and the dose injected intravenously was 1 mg per day for 20 days. Improvement in gait began immediately after the treatment was begun. (Takeuchi Y et al. Efficacy of thyrotropin-releasing hormone in the treatment of cerebellar ataxia. *Pediatr Neurol* Mar-Apr 1989; *5*:107-110).

> COMMENT. Thyrotropin-releasing hormone (TRH) therapy has been used in several neurologic disorders, including spinocerebellar degeneration, amyotrophic lateral sclerosis, and infantile spasms with hypsarrhythmia (see *Ped*

Neur Briefs June 1987; *1*:3). The present patient had an acute cerebellar ataxia following an infection of unknown origin and persisting for 18 months before treatment with TRH was begun. - Editor. *Ped Neur Briefs* March 1989.

Progressive Spastic Cerebellar Ataxia And Histiocytosis

A syndrome of diabetes insipidus followed by progressive spastic cerebellar ataxia is reported in four boys from the Departments of Neurology, Pediatrics and Psychiatry, UCLA School of Medicine, Los Angeles, CA. In two patients central nervous system histiocytosis was detected. CT scan showed bilateral calcification of the cerebellar dentate nuclei and multiple hypodense areas in the skull; a biopsy confirmed the diagnosis of histiocytosis. A trial of Prednisone was beneficial. (Birnbaum DC et al. Idiopathic central diabetes insipidus followed by progressive spastic cerebellar ataxia. *Arch Neurol* Sept 1989; *46*:1001-1003).

COMMENT. Each of these patients developed idiopathic central diabetes insipidus between the ages of two and six years and all responded to intranasal Desmopressin. Spastic cerebellar ataxia developed eight to ten years later. Histiocytosis accounts for 8-16% of cases of diabetes insipidus in children. Patients with this syndrome may benefit from treatment with corticosteroids. - Editor. *Ped Neur Briefs* September 1989.

Hereditary Progressive Dystonia

Four cases of hereditary progressive dystonia with diurnal fluctuation were treated at the Sackler School of Medicine, Tel-Aviv University and the Technion-Israel Institute of Technology, Haifa, Israel. All were sporadic, 3 presented as spastic diplegia or were misdiagnosed as spinocerebellar degeneration, two resembled torsion dystonia, and one had been diagnosed previously as Huntington's chorea and tics. The correct diagnosis was determined by the marked diurnal fluctuation of signs and symptoms, which worsened toward evening, and a prompt, pronounced, and sustained response to levodopa in moderate doses (100-375 mg). Treatment had been continued for 2 to 7 years. Polysomnographic studies were useful in diagnosis and showed increased body movements during REM sleep. Close relatives had increased leg movements in sleep. (Costeff H et al. Fluctuating dystonia responsive to levodopa. *Arch Dis Childhood* 1987; *6*:801-804).

COMMENT. This syndrome was first described by Segawa M et al in Japan (*Therapy* 1971; *24*:667) and should correctly be referred to as *Segawa Syndrome*. Diurnal fluctuation of the dystonia is not invariably present and a trial of levodopa is worthwhile in possible variants of this dystonic syndrome. Emotional disturbance is a feature in some cases and may lead to a diagnosis of psychogenic etiology. In fact, in all cases of dystonia musculorum deformans (torsion dystonia) that I have treated, a diagnosis of conversion hysteria had previously been entertained and psychotherapy prescribed. - Editor. *Ped Neur Briefs* September 1987.

MITOCHONDRIAL CYTOPATHIES

Melas Syndrome

MELAS syndrome consists of mitochondrial myopathy, encephalopathy, lactic acidosis, and stroke. Three familial cases are described by members of the Departments of Neurology and Pediatrics, University of Texas Health Science center, San Antonio, TX. In these three cases, the onset was in adulthood whereas the majority of previously described patients developed symptoms at 4 to 11 years of age. Early development is usually normal except for short stature. Other features include sensorineural hearing loss, headache, nausea and vomiting, seizures, and basal ganglia calcifications by CT. The absence of ophthalmoplegia, heart block, retinal pigmentation, myoclonus, and cerebellar ataxia, seen in other mitochondrial myopathies, is noteworthy. The pathologic findings of MELAS are ragged red fibers, and lactic acidosis. Some have increased carnitine acetyl transferase activity in skeletal muscle.

The assessment of proposed treatments such as methyl-prednisolone and chlorpromazine is difficult because the course of MELAS is variable. The proband with the full syndrome in this report improved spontaneously and had remained stable for 16 months without therapy. (Driscoll PF, Larsen PD, Gruber AB. MELAS syndrome involving mother and two children. *Arch Neurol* 1987; *44*:971-973).

COMMENT. MELAS is familial and inheritance is almost exclusively by maternal transmission. Egger J and Wilson J at the Hospital for Sick Children, Great Ormond Street, London, report a high ratio of affected to unaffected siblings with mitochondrial cytopathy, making Mendelian inheritance unlikely (*N Engl J Med* 1983; *309*:142). Two other disorders associated with mitochondrial myopathy and cerebral disease are Kearns-Sayre syndrome and MERRF (myoclonus epilepsy and ragged red fibers). All 3 syndromes are characterized also by dementia, seizures, short stature, hearing loss and a positive family history. K-S syndrome includes ophthalmoplegia, retinal degeneration and cerebellar ataxia. MERRF includes myoclonus and ataxia. MELAS has cortical blindness and hemiparesis as distinctive features. - Editor. *Ped Neur Briefs* September 1987.

Leigh Syndrome And Cytochrome Oxidase Deficiency

Mitochondrial enzymes were studied in 5 unrelated children with neuropathologically proven subacute necrotizing encephalomyelopathy (Leigh syndrome) at the College of Physicians and Surgeons, NY. Four patients showed psychomotor regression, ophthalmoparesis, nystagmus, optic atrophy, hypotonia, areflexia, ataxia, and abnormal breathing beginning in the second year and died after three to four years of an intermittently progressive course. The fifth child was floppy at birth, regressed at 5 mos, and died of congestive heart failure at 7-1/2 mos. All had lactic acidosis and autopsies showed typical symmetrical necrotic and cystic lesions in the brain stem and cerebellum. Muscle biopsy was normal by light microscopy but showed mitochondrial changes on ultrastructural examination. A decrease in cytochrome c oxidase (COX) activity was found in brain, muscle, kidney, heart, liver and in cultured fibroblasts. The authors conclude that COX deficiency is an important cause of Leigh syndrome (DiMauro S et al. Cytochrome c oxidase deficiency in Leigh syndrome. *Ann Neurol* 1987; *22*:498-506).

COMMENT. The family history was negative in these patients but previous reports of autosomal recessive inheritance and occurrence in siblings are common. In one family from Quebec, 7 members in two generations had a mitochondrial encephalopathy and COX deficiency. Diverse clinical and pathological expressions of Leigh's disease in this family was explained by maternal transmission of varying proportions of mutant mitochondrial DNA. (Berkovic SF et al. *Neurology* 1987; *37 (suppl 1)*;233).

Leigh syndrome, previously termed Leigh's disease and first described in 1951, appears to be nonspecific biochemically as well as clinically. In addition to the COX deficiency described above, defects of the pyruvate dehydrogenase multienzyme complex and pyruvate carboxylase have been reported. An inhibitor of the brain enzyme that catalyzes the formation of the thiamine triphosphate has been found in the urine but the test is not diagnostic. Consistent early clinical features in the infantile cases are a quiet immobility with lack of crying and hypotonia. - Editor. *Ped Neur Briefs* November 1987.

Cytochrome C Oxidase
Deficiency And Respiratory Distress

A newborn male presenting with severe respiratory insufficiency, generalized muscle weakness, and lactic acidemia is reported from the Department of Pediatrics, Nagasaki University

School of Medicine, Japan. Within 27 hours after birth he was markedly hypotonic; spontaneous movements and the Moro reflex were almost absent. A respirator was necessary because of respiratory arrest and he died 75 hours after birth. At autopsy there was variation in muscle fiber size and an increased number of Type 2C fibers but no ragged-red fibers by Gomori trichrome staining. Biochemical and histochemical studies showed cytochrome c oxidase activity was decreased in skeletal muscle but not in cardiac muscle. (Takayanagi, T et al. Infantile cytochromic c oxidase deficiency with neonatal death. *Pediatr Neurol* May/June 1989; 5:179-81).

> COMMENT. The differential diagnosis of neonatal respiratory distress syndrome should include mitochondrial myopathy. The diagnosis should still be considered even in the absence of ragged-red fibers in skeletal muscle.

Two further papers concerning mitochondrial myopathy appeared in the June 1989 issue of the *Annals of Neurology*. Shimozumi H et al established cultured myogenic cell lines that were defective in cytochrome c oxidase enzyme from a patient with mitochondrial encephalomyelopathy. Two kinds of myogenic cell lines, one with and one without defective enzymatic activity were demonstrated showing that a partial enzyme defect is the result of the cellular mosaicism in the tissue. The authors comment that these cloned cell lines provide an excellent system for clarifying the cause of mitochondrial myopathy and for investigating the genetic factors.

Sakuta R and Nonaka I examined muscle taken at biopsy in six patients with complex I deficiency and one patient with the clinical characteristics of mitochondrial myopathy, encephalopathy, lactic acidosis and stroke-like episodes (MELAS). Striking abnormalities in the blood vessels were shown by electron microscopy in five patients. The authors considered that these abnormalities in small arteries might be responsible for the occasional occurence of transient cerebral ischemia causing stroke-like episodes and progressive mental deterioration in patients with mitochondrial myopathy. - Editor. *Ped Neur Briefs* June 1989.

Infantile Mitochondrial Disease

A detailed clinical, pathologic, biochemical, and genetic analysis of a case of lethal infantile mitochondrial disease is reported from the Departments of Biochemistry, Pediatrics, Neurology and Nephrology, Emory University School of Medicine, Atlanta, GA. During the first three months of life the child showed increasing lethargy, hypotonia, difficulty in feeding and growth retardation. On admission at three months of age there was respiratory failure, bradycardia, hypotension, and severe lactic acidosis. Over the next 21 days the condition rapidly deteriorated with a progressive hypertrophic cardiomyopathy, hepatic dysfunction, and generalized seizure activity. The patient died with bradycardia and hypotension at four months of age. There were abnormalities in the striated muscles, smooth muscle, heart and liver but not in the central nervous system. Biochemical analysis revealed a combined complex I and IV deficiency in skeletal muscle, heart and liver but not in kidney and brain. There was no abnormality in mitochondrial DNA. The disease was thought to result from a nuclear oxidative phosphorylation gene mutation. (Zheng X et al. Evidence in a lethal infantile mitochondrial disease for a nuclear mutation affecting respiratory complexes I and IV. *Neurology* Sept 1988; *39*:1203-1209).

COMMENT. Mitochondrial encephalomyopathies attributed to mutations in the mitochondrial DNA include MERRF and Kearns-Sayre syndrome with onset in childhood through adulthood. In the neonatal period some mitochondrial myopathies have a benign course and some are lethal and a variety of oxidative phosphorylation deficiencies have been associated with these disorders. - Editor. *Ped Neur Briefs* September 1989.

Menkes Disease With "Ragged Red" Fibers

Subsarcolemmal aggregates of mitochondria ("ragged red" fibers) in skeletal muscle were found at autopsy in a 30-month-old male infant with Menkes kinky-hair disease reported from the New York Hospital- Cornell University Medical Center, NY. At birth, the infant had multiple depressed skull fractures and a cephalhematoma. At 5 days, he developed vertical nystagmus and staring episodes; at 2 months, generalized seizures; at 4 months, multifocal myoclonic twitches; and by 6 months, he had hypotonia, poor head control, and visual inattention. His height, weight, and head circumference were at the 3rd percentile. His hair was sparse, poorly pigmented, and showed pili torti (twisted), monilethrix (bead-like) and trichorrhexic nodosa (fractured nodes) on microscopic examination. The plasma copper was 16 mcg/100ml (normal: approximately 100 mcg/100 ml), and ceruloplasmin 12 mg/dl (normal: 15-50 mg/dl). He was treated with sodium valproate for seizures, and he had multiple episodes of vomiting, weight loss and dehydration, and respiratory infections. The immediate cause of death was bronchopneumonia. The brain weighed 500 g (normal: 1100 g) and showed diffuse cerebral and cerebellar atrophy, with focal polymicrogyria. Electronmicroscopy demonstrated numerous mitochondria within Purkinje cell cytoplasm. This report, "the first to describe "ragged red" fibers in Menkes disease," supports the concept that Menkes disease may be due in part to a mitochondrial enzyme deficiency. (Morgello S et al. Menkes kinky hair disease with "ragged red" fibers. *Dev Med Child Neurol* Dec 1988; *30*:812-816).

COMMENT. Menkes kinky hair disease is an X-chromosome linked disorder of copper malabsorption characterized by low serum ceruloplasmin and copper levels, seizures, CNS degeneration, and pili torti (Menkes JH et al. *Pediatrics* 1962; *29*:764) (Menkes JH. *Textbook of Child Neurology* 3rd Edition 1985, Lea & Febiger, Philadelphia). Parenterally administered copper corrects the hepatic copper deficiency and restores serum copper and ceruloplasmin levels to normal but may not arrest the progressive cerebral degeneration. Nonetheless, Menkes advises initiation of copper therapy early since the clinical course of the disease is variable. - Editor. *Ped Neur Briefs* January 1989.

Alpers' Progressive Neuronal Degeneration

Reporting from the Hospital for Sick Children, Great Ormond Street, London WC1, the authors have selected 13 cases, 10 boys and 3 girls, with progressive neuronal degeneration of childhood (PNDC) that was complicated by liver disease and confirmed at postmortem in 11. During life, PNDC may be suspected by a characteristic clinical course, abnormal liver function tests, and abnormalities of EEG (grossly asymmetric, very slow activity of high amplitude mixed with polyspikes), VER, and CAT (cortical and central atrophy and areas of low density of the white matter). It is proposed that the term PNDC be reserved for a distinct syndrome characterized by normal initial development followed by developmental retardation and later onset of intractable seizures and liver degeneration, and by autosomal recessive inheritance.

Four patients received sodium valproate; 2 may have died from valproate toxicity although both had abnormal liver enzymes prior to treatment. Phenytoin was probably blameless; 8 patients never received it and the liver pathology of fatty degeneration, necrosis, and cirrhosis was not that expected in phenytoin toxicity.

Brain pathology revealed cortical atrophy with predilection for the calcarine cortex, astrocytic proliferation, and spongy degeneration also involving the thalamus, basal ganglia, and brainstem. Hippocampal sclerosis and cerebellar infarcts resembled epileptic anoxic changes in some patients. (Egger J, Hardin BN, Boyd SG, Wilson J, Erdohazi M. *Clinical Pediatrics* 1987; 26:167-173).

COMMENT. The syndrome of diffuse progressive degeneration of the cerebral gray matter was first described by Alpers in 1931. Ford (1951) differentiated infantile and juvenile types and reported familial cases. Huttenlocher et al (1976) emphasized a coincident hepatic cirrhosis. The cause is unknown. The cerebral pathology resembles anoxic encephalopathy secondary to status epilepticus in some reported cases and the liver disease might be the result of anticonvulsant toxicity, notably sodium valproate. In the author's cases, however, these causative factors were not generally accepted as primary, and a genetically determined metabolic explanation was preferred. - Editor. *Ped Neur Briefs* July 1987.

Carnitine Deficiency Syndromes

Carnitine deficiency syndromes manifested as metabolic encephalopathy, lipid storage myopathy, or cardiomyopathy are reviewed from the Department of Pediatrics, Park Nicollet Medical Center, Minneapolis, MN. Carnitine deficiency may be primary and caused by impaired renal conservation, or secondary to various inborn errors of metabolism that promote excretion of carnitine as acylcarnitine. The genetic defects of intermediary metabolism with secondary systemic carnitine deficiency include: 1) Acyl-CoA dehydrogenase deficiencies; 2) organic acidemias; 3) mitochondrial respiratory disorders; and 4) carnitine octanoyltransferase deficiency. Other disorders with secondary carnitine deficiency include Reye syndrome, valproate-induced, renal Fanconi, chronic renal failure with hemodialysis, parenteral nutrition in premature infants, Kwashiorkor, cirrhosis, severe myopathies, myxedema, adrenal insufficiency, hypopituitarism and pregnancy.

Systemic carnitine deficiency was first described in an 11 year old male with recurrent attacks resembling Reye syndrome from the age of three, and progressive muscle weakness from the age of ten. Metabolic encephalopathy is a frequent mode of presentation and the acute encephalopathic crises of systemic carnitine deficiency present with vomiting, progressive deterioration of consciousness, hepatomegaly, hypoglycemia, hyperammonemia, increased transaminase and hypoprothrombinemia. Acute crises produced by carnitine deficiency are treated with intravenous glucose supplementation to correct hypoglycemia. When hyperammonemia is present protein intake is restricted. Organic acidemias are treated with dietary modifications and/or vitamin supplementation. Frequent meals of high carbohydrate content and a low fat diet are advisable in all patients with carnitine deficiency. Maintenance therapy consists of L-carnitine 100 mg/kg/daily in infants and children. There are no known serious side effects of L-carnitine. (Breningstall GN. Carnitine deficiency syndromes. *Pediatr Neurol* March 1990; 6:75-81).

COMMENT. Early diagnosis of carnitine deficiency syndromes and prompt supplementation with oral carnitine may reduce mortality since oral carnitine administration in recommended doses is free from adverse effects except for occasional diarrhea. Supplementation with carnitine is recommended in infants and children with acute or recurrent encephalopathies, myelopathies, or cardiomyopathies associated with proven or presumed carnitine deficiencies. Meat products, especially red meats and dairy products, are important dietary sources of carnitine which maintain tissue stores. - Editor. *Ped Neur Briefs* May 1990.

Metachromatic Leukodystrophy

A ten year old girl with metachromatic leukodystrophy in whom neurophysiologic function and sulfatide metabolism had improved after she received a bone marrow transplant five years before is reported from the Bone Marrow Transplantation Program, Department of Pediatrics and Division of Pediatric Neurology, University of Minnesota, MN and other centers. The diagnosis was confirmed by enzyme analysis at eight months of age after an older sister had been found to have the disease. Serial MRI of the head obtained before and after bone marrow transplantation showed no further deterioration of white matter.

Sural nerve specimens obtained by biopsy before and two years after transplantation showed less accumulation of lipid in the macrophages on electron microscopy. Sulfatide levels in the CSF were within normal limits at seven and ten years of age. Asymptomatic infants, children and young adolescents who are found to have the disease after it has been diagnosed in an older sibling should be considered for bone marrow transplantation. (Krivit W et al. Treatment of late infantile metachromatic leukodystrophy by bone marrow transplantation. *N Engl J Med* Jan 4, 1990; *322*:28-32).

> COMMENT. Dr. John Menkes gives an excellent overview of the leukodystrophies in an editorial in this issue (*N Engl J Med* Jan 4, 1990; *322*:34-35). Metachromatic leukodystrophy and adrenoleukodystrophy may be amenable to new experimental therapies. No treatment is available for globoid-cell, Canavan, Pelizaeus-Merzbacher, and Alexander varieties of leukodystrophy. - Editor. *Ped Neur Briefs* January 1990.

Infantile Gangliosidosis

Three sisters with infantile-onset 3 GM1 gangliosidosis are reported from the University of Siens, Italy, and the University of Louvain, Brussels, Belgium. The diagnosis was based on the clinical findings of progressive intellectual deterioration by age 6-8 years, ataxia, spastic tetraparesis, and athetoid-choreiform movements; lysosomal vacuoles in CSF, bone marrow, and conjunctiva; and on decreased activity of serum, leukocyte, and fibroblast B-D-galactosidase and abnormal urinary excretion of oligosaccharides. (Guazzi GC et al. Type 3 (chronic) GM1 gangliosidosis presenting as infanto-choreo-athetotic dementia, without epilepsy, in three sisters. *Neurology* July 1988; *38*:1124-27).

> COMMENT. Gangliosidosis occurs in three forms: 1) infantile, characterized by Hurler's facial features, bony abnormalities, hepatosplenomegaly, cherry-red spot, and progressive neurological signs; 2) late infantile-juvenile, with-

out skeletal changes or marked visceromegaly, but severe intellectual deterioration, ataxia, myoclonic seizures, and retinal degeneration; and 3) dystonic juvenile form. The clinical findings in the present report resembled those in the dystonic form except that the intellectual deterioration was more severe. - Editor. *Ped Neur Briefs* August 1988.

Multiple Sulfatase Deficiency

A 9-year-old girl with a phenotype similar to a mucopolysaccharidosis (MPS) and a clinical history characteristic of late infantile metachromatic leukodystrophy (MLD) is reported from the Department of Neurology, National Defense Medical Center, Taipei, Taiwan, Republic of China; the Developmental and Metabolic Neurology Branch, NIH, Bethesda, MD; and Department of Pediatrics (Dr. Horwitz), University of Chicago, Chicago, IL. The girl's early history and development were normal up to 18 months of age. Following a high fever with a flu-like illness, her gait became unsteady and broad-based. Gradually her speech became slurred and her vocabulary deteriorated. Examination at 7-1/2 years showed short stature and microcephaly. She was autistic and inattentive, with marked cognitive impairment. She had hyperreflexia, extensor plantar responses, dysmetria, and incoordination. Dysmorphic features suggested MPS but dysostosis multiplex and organomegaly were absent. Funduscopic examination revealed a cherry-red-like spot and yellowish-granular appearance of the retina. Deficient activities of arylsulfatase-A, arylsulfatase-B, iduronate sulfatase, and heparan N-sulfatase in the leukocytes established the diagnosis as MSD. The total urinary content of the glycosaminoglycans was normal, but the concentration of heparan sulfate was increased, stressing the need for qualitative estimations when MSD is suspected. (Soong B-W, Casamassima AC, Fink JK, Constantopoulos G, Horwitz AL. *Neurology* Aug 1988; *38*:1273-75).

COMMENT. Multiple sulfatase deficiency or mucosulfatidosis (MSD) is an autosomal recessive genetic disease affecting the expression of lysosomal sulfatases with consequent accumulation of sulfate-containing glycolipids, glycosaminoglycans, and steroid sulfates in tissues and body tissues. The clinical manifestations represent a combination of 2 diseases: late infantile MLD and MPS. The disorder is rare and the authors cite 20 previous reports of this phenotype. - Editor. *Ped Neur Briefs* August 1988.

Niemann-Pick Disease Type C

The neurologic symptomatology in 22 patients with Niemann-Pick disease type C have been analyzed and reported from the Developmental and Metabolic Neurology Branch, National Institute of Neurological Disorders and Strokes, National Institutes of Health, Bethesda, MD. Three phenotypes are described: 1) an early onset, rapidly progressive form associate with severe hepatic dysfunction and psychomotor delay during infancy and later with supranuclear vertical gaze paresis, ataxia, spasticity, and dementia; 2) a delayed onset, slowly progressive form beginning in early childhood with mild intellectual impairment, supranuclear vertical gaze paresis and ataxia, and later associated with dementia, seizures and extrapyramidal deficits; 3) a late onset slowly progressive form beginning in adolescence or adulthood. The classic supranuclear disorder of gaze, initially and predominantly affecting vertical eye movements, is nearly pathognomonic for NPC. The biochemical disorder is a marked deficiency in the ability of cultured fibroblasts to esterify exogenously supplied cholesterol. This deficiency may be assayed in confirmation of the diagnosis when presentation is atypical. (Fink JK et al. Clinical spectrum of Niemann-Pick disease type C. *Neurology* Aug 1989; *39*:1040-1049).

COMMENT. Mild intellectual impairment presenting as poor school performance was the most common initial neurologic abnormality. Additional presenting signs included ataxia, dysarthria, and impaired vertical gaze. Within three years of the initial deficit most of the patients had cognitive impairment, abnormal vertical gaze and ataxia.

Saccadic paresis was manifested by a complaint of difficulty in reading or in descending stairs. Hepatosplenomegaly was first noted at varying ages from birth to 24 years with a mean age of six years. It preceded neurological abnormalities in one-half the patients and was found only in the early onset rapidly progressive group. - Editor. *Ped Neur Briefs* September 1989.

Neuroaxonal Dystrophy: Lysosomal Deficiency

The clinical, pathological and biochemical findings in two brothers with a newly recognized form of infantile neuroaxonal dystrophy associated with alpha-N-acetylgalactosaminidase deficiency are reported from the Divisions of Medical and Molecular Genetics and Neuropathology, Mount Sinai School of Medicine, New York; Department of Chemistry, University of Alberta, Edmonton, Canada; Department of Physiological Chemistry, University of Bonn, Federal Republic of Germany; and Department of Human Genetics, University of Wurzburg, Federal Republic of Germany. The brothers were the offspring of fifth cousins of German descent and their early development was normal. In the older brother, the clinical onset of disease was signaled by poor coordination of gait, clumsiness, and episodes of falling at 12 months. In the younger brother, grand mal seizures began at eight months and occurred five times over the next six months. Each had a regressive course beginning after 15 months of age, with loss of all mental and motor skills acquired previously. Strabismus, nystagmus, visual impairment, muscular hypotonia, and frequent myoclonic movements developed in both. By three to four years of age, both brothers had profound psychomotor retardation and spasticity, and were immobile and incontinent. CT and MRI showed atrophy of the cerebellum, brain stem and cervical spinal cord, with lesser atrophic changes in the cerebral gray and white matter, optic tracts and cranial nerves. EEG revealed multifocal isolated spikes and spike wave complexes. The urinary oligosaccharide profile was abnormal, suggesting the possibility of a lysosomal disease. The activity of alpha-N-acetylgalactosaminidase was deficient whereas 21 other lysosomal enzymes were normal. (Schindler D et al. Neuroaxonal dystrophy due to lysosomal alpha-N-acetylgalactosaminidase deficiency. *N Engl J Med* June 29, 1989; *320*:1735-1740).

COMMENT. The neuroaxonal dystrophies include the infantile (Seitelberger's disease), late-infantile, and juvenile forms, neuroaxonal leukodystrophy, and Hallervorden-Spatz syndrome, and all are characterized by the spheroids in the terminal endings of axons in the central nervous system. The axonal dystrophy in alpha-N-acetylgalactosaminidase deficiency described in this article differs from that observed in other lysosomal storage diseases. The absence of identifiable lysosomal storage in this newly described disorder suggests a causal relation between the enzyme deficiency and the resultant axonal pathology.

A report from the Departments of Pediatrics, Radiology and Neurology, Kyoto, Japan, suggests that magnetic resonance imaging may be useful in the diagnosis and classification of infantile neuroaxonal dystrophy (Ito M et al. *Pediatr Neurol* 1989; 5:245-8). A six year old boy with typical clinical features of infantile neuroaxonal dystrophy showed increased metal deposition in the globus pallidus and MRI findings of Hallervorden-Spatz syndrome suggesting that these two disease entities overlap. The "eye of the tiger" sign was described in the MRI of two patients with Hallervorden-Spatz syndrome and dystonia. (See *Ped Neur Briefs* October 1988, 2:77). - Editor. *Ped Neur Briefs* June 1989.

DEMYELINATING DISEASES

Multiple Sclerosis

Nine MS clinics from the Canadian MS study group collaborated in a retrospective study employing questionnaires about the MS populations and with particular reference to cases with onset before age 16 years. Childhood MS was more frequent in girls and their overrepresentation was even greater in the following subgroups: those with sensory initial symptoms, complete recovery from initial episode, a nonprogressive clinical course, and lower disability scores. Conversely, boys were overrepresented in subgroups of patients with no recovery from the initial episode and progressive course.

MS in girls has an early onset, is usually heralded by sensory symptoms that frequently remit completely, has a relapsing-remitting course and a slow progression. Boys with MS have a poorer prognosis and progressive course, usually related to late onset of the disease. The familial incidence was 28%. CSF showed normal IgG levels in 59% and abnormal oligoclonal bands in 82%. (Duguette P, Murray TJ et al. Multiple sclerosis in childhood: Clinical profile in 125 patients. *J Pediatr* 1987; *111*:359-63).

> COMMENT. MS is probably more common in children than we suspect and the diagnosis should be considered especially in girls with initial sensory or visual symptoms that remit completely and later evolve in a relapsing-remitting manner. An onset at 2 years of age is the earliest case report (Bejar, Ziegler. *Arch Neurol* 1984; *41*:881). The abrupt rise in incidence that coincides with puberty may be related to hormonal factors. Analysis of data from a Faroe Island epidemic of MS suggested a 2-stage process in the pathogenesis of MS: 1) acquisition of an exogenous factor such as infection, and 2) the onset of host factors related to pubescence that allow the pathogenesis to proceed (Fischman HR. *Am J Epidemiol* 1981; *114*:244).

Oligoclonal bands in the CSF are the best single laboratory test for the presence of abnormal IgG in patients suspected of having MS. A combination of oligoclonal band and IgG synthesis tests is 97% sensitive for probable and definite MS. (Bloomer IC, Bray PF. *Clin Chem* 1981; 27:2011). NMR imaging differentiates between gray and white matter and is superior to CT in the diagnosis of MS. (Young IR et al. *Lancet* 1981; 2:1063). - Editor. *Ped Neur Briefs* September 1987.

Familial Incidence Of Multiple Sclerosis (MS)

Age-adjusted familial rates for MS were determined in children and siblings of patients studied at the MS Clinic and Dept of Genetics, Health Sciences Centre Hospital, Univ British Columbia, Vancouver, BC, Canada. The risk for these relatives to develop MS was 3 to 5%, which was 30-35 times the 0.1% rate for the general population in this relatively "high-risk" area. For female index patients with MS, the proportion of children affected was 5/797 or 0.6% (all girls) but the age-adjusted risk was 2.6%, four times the crude rate. The proportion of daughters affected was 5/386 (1.3%) with an age-adjusted risk of 5%. (Sadovnick AD, Baird PA. The familial nature of multiple sclerosis: age-corrected empiric recurrence risks for children and siblings of patients. *Neurology* June 1988; *38*:990-991).

COMMENT. The onset of MS in childhood is unusual, but the 50-fold increase in risk for daughters of female patients with MS should alert neurologists to this diagnosis in young children with suggestive symptoms. The concordance rate for MS among monozygotic twins is 26% compared to 2% for dizygotic twins (Ebers GC et al. *N Engl J Med* 1986; *315*:1638). - Editor. *Ped Neur Briefs* June 1988.

Juvenile Multiple Sclerosis

A young girl with recurrent episodes of CNS demyelination associated with defective mitochondrial beta oxidation is reported from the Departments of Pediatrics, Medical Genetics, Oregon Health Sciences University, Portland, and University of Iowa Hospitals, Iowa City, IA. The child was well until age 14 months when she began having episodes of ataxia with slurred speech and extreme irritability lasting hours to days. At 19 months she was admitted in coma and a CT revealed periventricular loss of white matter. She recovered within three weeks after treatment with immunoglobulins, Acyclovir, and corticosteroids. A similar episode occurred at 22 months of age and the MRI had increased signals in the periventricular and frontoparietal areas. Many episodes of ataxia, slurred speech, painful bright red hands and feet, furrowed tongue and extreme irritability occurred from age 22 to 38 months. The episodes lasted from hours to weeks and were associated with an acrid body odor. Urinary sarcosine was elevated and an increase in ethylmalonic acid in the urine pointed to a disorder affecting fatty acid metabolism. Metabolic evaluations and decreased oxidation of palmitate demonstrated defective mitochondrial beta oxidation. The patient was treated and remained stable for 30 months on a low fat high carbohydrate diet, L-Carnitine (100 mg/kg/d), and Riboflavin (20 mg/kg/d). (Powell BR et al. Juvenile multiple sclerosis-like episodes associated with a defect of mitochondrial beta oxidation. *Neurology* March 1990; *40*:487-491).

COMMENT. The present patient appears to represent a unique disorder of beta oxidation producing multiple sclerosis-like episodes. The youngest patient with classic multiple sclerosis previously reported was two years old. Duquette P et al reported the clinical profiles of 125 children with multiple sclerosis (*J Pediatr* 1987; 111; 359) (see *Ped Neur Briefs* September 1987; *1*:25-26). The diagnosis of MS should be considered especially in girls with initial sensory or visual symptoms that remit completely and later evolve in a relapsing-remitting manner. Oligoclonal bands in the CSF are the best single laboratory test for the presence of abnormal IgG in patients suspected of having MS. MRI is superior to CT in diagnosis. - Editor. *Ped Neur Briefs* March 1990.

Pelizaeus-Merzbacher Disease (PMD): MRI In Diagnosis

The value of the MRI in the diagnosis of PMD in a 14-year-old Japanese boy is reported from the Depts of Pediatrics and Radiology, Tokyo Children's Rehabilitation Hospital, Tokyo 190-12, Japan. The child presented with rotatory nystagmus at 2 weeks after birth, titubation at 6 months, spasticity at 1 year, and a mask-like facial expression at 3 years of age. He was markedly retarded at 14 years and examination revealed spasticity, intention tremor, joint contractures, nystagmus and normal fundi. Head circumference, nerve conduction studies, and lysosomal enzymes were normal. CT showed ventricular enlargement, cerebellar atrophy, but normal appearing white matter. MRI demonstrated diffuse changes in white matter with sparing of scattered small areas consistent with a "tigroid pattern" of myelin preservation characteristic of PMD. (Schimomura C et al. Magnetic resonance imaging in Pelizaeus-Merzbacher disease. *Pediatr Neurol* 1988; 4:124-5).

COMMENT. Described by Pelizaeus in 1885 and by Merzbacher in 1910, this heredofamilial disease transmitted as an X-linked recessive character and occurring chiefly in males is a slowly progressive leukodystrophy with a long course, patients not infrequently surviving into middle age. When the family history is negative, as in the above case, confirmation of the diagnosis during life is difficult but may be facilitated by the MRI findings and may permit appropriate genetic counseling. - Editor. *Ped Neur Briefs* June 1988.

CHAPTER 17

RETT SYNDROME

Rett Syndrome: Diagnostic Criteria

Diagnostic criteria for Rett Syndrome are proposed by the International Rett Syndrome Association and the Centers for Disease Control, Koger Center, F-37, Atlanta, GA. The criteria are separated into three categories: 1) necessary, 2) supportive, and 3) exclusion criteria. Female sex is not included as a necessary criterion because the possibility of undiagnosed male cases cannot be ruled out. Diagnosis is tentative until 2-5 years of age, and the presence of one or more of the exclusion criteria is against the diagnosis, regardless of whether all of the necessary criteria have been met.

Necessary criteria include the following: 1) normal pregnancy, birth and psychomotor development through the first 6 or 18 months; 2) normal head circumference at birth and deceleration of head growth between 5 months and 4 years; 3) loss of purposeful hand skills between 6 and 30 months; 4) impaired language and psychomotor development; 5) stereotypic hand movements such as hand wringing; and 6) gait apraxia and ataxia between 1 and 4 years. *Supportive criteria* include breathing irregularities, EEG abnormalities, seizures, spasticity, scoliosis, growth retardation and small feet. Evidence of intrauterine growth retardation or perinatal acquired brain damage, microcephaly at birth, identifiable metabolic, degenerative or storage diseases are listed as *exclusion criteria.*

The clinical characteristics of Rett Syndrome and differential diagnoses are listed according to stages and age at onset: 1) Early onset deceleration stage, 6-18 months; 2) rapid "destructive" stage, 1-3 years; 3) pseudostationary stage, 2-10 years; 4) late motor deterioration stage, 10+ years. (Trevathan E, Moser HW et al. The Rett Syndrome diagnostic criteria work group. Diagnostic criteria for Rett Syndrome. *Ann Neurol* April 1988; *23*:425-428).

COMMENT. Heller's dementia, an infantile dementia described in 1908, almost 60 years before the first description of Rett Syndrome, should be added to the differential diagnosis (Millichap JG. *Lancet* 1987; *1*:440; Rett A and Olsson B. *Dev Med & Child Neurol* 1987; *29*:835), especially as the female sex is no longer considered a necessary diagnostic criterion for Rett Syndrome. At this stage of our understanding, the diagnostic criteria of Rett Syndrome should not be too strict and too exclusive (Opitz J. *Am J Med Genet* 1986; *24*:27).

Partington MW (*Am J Med Genet* March 1988; *29*:633) describes Rett Syndrome in a pair of monozygotic twin girls, pointing out that their development was delayed from birth with no period of normal progress in infancy and subsequent regression, findings at variance with the necessary diagnostic criteria listed above. He states that the cause is not necessarily genetic but could be explained by prenatal toxic or slow viral factors.

Karet D et al. (*J Pediat Orthopaedics* March/April 1988; *8*:138) reports scoliosis in eight of 10 females with Rett Syndrome treated at the Alfred I. DuPont Institute,

Wilmington, Delaware. Curve progression occurred in four and posterior spinal fusion was performed in five. Scoliosis developed at an average age of 11 years and progression was rapid in adolescence. Early surgery is recommended to arrest curve progression and to obtain correction of the deformity. - Editor. *Ped Neur Briefs* April 1988.

Rett Syndrome: Formes Frustes

The clinical peculiarities and differential diagnosis of Rett syndrome are reviewed from the Department of Pediatrics Children's Clinics, East Hospital, Goteborg, Sweden. The four clinical stages of classic Rett syndrome are as follows. 1) Early onset stagnation, 2) rapid developmental regression, 3) pseudo-stationary period, 4) late motor deterioration. A variety of atypical variants have been described including some in boys. The development during the first few months of life is sometimes abnormal, rarely there is no subsequent deterioration phase, and occasionally seizures occur early as infantile spasms. The term "formes frustes" has been coined for these abortive variants. The differential diagnosis in Rett syndrome stage 2, which includes rapid developmental regression, increased irritability, screaming episodes and loss of acquired skills, is as follows: Infantile neuronal ceroid lipofuscinosis, encephalitis, toxic encephalopathies, epileptic encephalopathies, infantile autism, neurocutaneous syndromes, glutaric aciduria, amino acidopathy, and ataxic cerebral palsy. Biologic markers and effective screening procedures for an early diagnosis are lacking. A possible viral origin with a disorder similar to SSPE is now being suggested as an etiology of this syndrome. (Hagberg BA. Rett syndrome: Clinical peculiarities, diagnostic approach, and possible cause. *Pediatr Neurol* Mar/Apr 1989; 5:75-83).

COMMENT. As the author concludes, the Rett syndrome concept is broader than previously believed and atypical variants must be recognized. Autopsy findings have been surprisingly limited even in advanced stages of the disease and have included moderate cortical atrophy and general brain shrinking with increasing age. Microscopically, there was mild gliosis without evidence of storage, underpigmentation in certain nigral structures, and axonal changes suggestive of degeneration in ascending and descending tracts.

Biochemical findings have included a reduction of brain noradrenaline, dopamine and serotonin, but no consistent abnormalities have been found. A genetic basis for Rett syndrome has been suggested but not satisfactorily confirmed. - Editor. Ped Neur Briefs June 1989.

Rett Syndrome: Diagnosis And Pertussis Vaccine Coincidence

The case-histories of 7 girls and 1 woman, 2 to 25 years of age, are reported from the Clinical Genetics and Child Developmental Center, Department of Maternal and Child Health, Dartmouth Medical School, Hanover, NH. Diagnosis was made after 5 years of age in four of the patients when the characteristic hand wringing, hand washing movements were first noted. In addition to these stereotypic hand behaviors, other clinical features included loss of hand function, hyperventilation, bruxism, irritability or self-injury, sleep disturbance, strabismus, seizures, scoliosis, ataxia, and hypotonia in infancy. Head growth deceleration, short stature and retarded rate of growth occurred in almost all cases. Three were small for gestational age at birth and experienced neonatal feeding problems. Previous diagnoses included Angelman syndrome, encephalopathy, and encephalitis, and in one case the syndrome appeared to develop as a reaction to pertussis vaccine. Treatment was symptomatic and supportive. Music and motion such as rocking or riding in a car had a calming effect, particularly when screaming attacks and sleep disturbances were troublesome. The absence of a "biological marker" for Rett syndrome makes diagnosis difficult and may lead to confusion with other defined neurodegenerative disorders, such as leukodystrophies, spinocerebellar heredoataxias, neuronal ceroid lipofuscinosis, and ornithine transcarbamylase deficiency. (Moeschler JB et al. Rett Syndrome: natural history and management. (*Pediatrics* July 1988; *82*:1-10).

COMMENT. The diagnostic criteria for Rett syndrome proposed by the International Rett Syndrome Association (See *Ped Neur Briefs* 1988; *2*:29) in April 1988 were separated into 1) necessary, 2) supportive, and 3) exclusion categories. Normal development through the first 6 or 18 months was regarded as a necessary criterion and intrauterine growth retardation and microcephaly at birth were thought to exclude the diagnosis. By these criteria, 4 of the 8 cases described here would not be accepted as examples of Rett syndrome or, alternatively, a "Forme fruste" atypical variety of the syndrome might be recognized. Even the female sex is no longer considered a necessary diagnostic criterion and a less restrictive symptom complex is proposed by some. The occurrence of a similar history and syndrome in boys is not uncommon. A plethora of publications on Rett syndrome has appeared in the last 12 months but none has uncovered a specific cause. The present authors note that pertussis vaccine was considered causative in 7 of 19 girls with Rett syndrome reported from Scotland (*Br Med J* 1985; *219*:579), and the onset of regression heralded by inconsolable screaming attacks had followed recent pertussis immunization in 1 patient in their series of 8. - Editor. *Ped Neur Briefs* July 1988.

Monoamine Metabolites In Rett Syndrome

Cerebral metabolites of noradrenaline, dopamine and serotonin, y-aminobutyric acid, and 23 amino acids were present in normal concentration in the CSF of 5 girls with Rett syndrome studied in the Depts of Pharmacology and Therapeutics, and Dept of Paediatrics, University of British Columbia, Vancouver, Canada. The authors doubt that any biochemical abnormalities have been clearly established as characteristic of the syndrome. (Perry TL, Dunn HG et al. Cerebrospinal fluid values for monoamine metabolites, y-aminobutyric acid and other amino compounds in Rett syndrome. *J Pediatr* Feb 1988; *112*:234-8).

COMMENT. A previous report of low CSF levels of monoamine metabolites in patients with Rett syndrome (Zoghbi HY et al. *N Engl J Med* 1985; *313*:921) is not supported by the present study. Hyperammonemia reported originally by Rett is another suggested biochemical basis for the syndrome unconfirmed in subsequent reports. The lack of uniformity of these findings suggests that Rett syndrome is a nonspecific entity with more than one etiology. - Editor. *Ped Neur Briefs* March 1988.

CSF Biogenic Amines In Rett Syndrome

Significant reductions in CSF metabolites of norepinephrine, dopamine, and serotonin are reported in 32 female patients with suspected Rett syndrome from the Baylor College of Medicine, Houston, TX. CSF biopterin, an essential co-factor that may limit the synthesis of biogenic amines, was elevated in patients compared with controls. Diet, drugs, and nutritional status, that may affect monoamine metabolites, were thought to be unlikely explanations for these biochemical changes. (Zoghbi HY et al. Cerebrospinal fluid biogenic amines and biopterin in Rett syndrome. *Ann Neurol* Jan 1989; *25*:56-60).

COMMENT. Abnormal biochemical findings reported in Rett syndrome, including hyperammonemia, have not been substantiated. If specific and unexplained by anticonvulsant drugs or diet, this report is the first to suggest a metabolic disorder underlying the stereotypic hand movements and other neurologic signs of Rett syndrome. Abnormal CSF biogenic amines are also reported in Parkinson's disease, Huntington's chorea, and Lesch-Nyhan syndrome. - Editor. *Ped Neur Briefs* January 1989.

Brain Biogenic Amines In Rett Syndrome

The biogenic amines, dopamine, serotonin, and noradrenaline, and their metabolites, were measured in selected brain regions obtained at postmortem from four patients ages 12-30 years with Rett syndrome and are reported from the

Departments of Pediatrics, Psychiatry and Neurochemistry, Goteborg University, Goteborg, Sweden. The cause of death was sudden and unexpected in one, severe pneumonitis and pulmonary abscess in one, in association with an operation for scoliosis at 12 years of age in one, and was unrecorded in one. Three of the patients had epilepsy; two were receiving carbamazepine and one sodium valproate at the time of death.

Compared to determinations in two adults who had drowned in ice cold water and one killed in a traffic accident, the two older patients with Rett syndrome showed a 50% or greater reduction in biogenic amines in the substantia nigra whereas the youngest patient showed normal or nearly normal levels of biogenic amines in the substantia nigra. The levels were normal in the caudate nucleus, putamen and globus pallidus. The oldest patients had rigidity and dystonic posturing at the time of death whereas the younger 12 year old child was motor disabled secondary to weakness and wasting. The biogenic amine data reflect the clinical patterns of the patients and parallel the neuropathologic finding of reduced melanin content in the neurons of the substantia nigra. (Lekman A, Witt-Engerstrom I, Hagberg BA, Percy AK et al. Rett syndrome: Biogenic amines and metabolites in postmortem brain. *Pediatr Neurol* Nov-Dec 1989; 5:357-62). Dr. Percy is at the Department of Pediatrics, Baylor College of Medicine, Houston, TX.

COMMENT. Hagberg et al have previously reported a postmortem analysis of brain biogenic amines in an 11 year old Rett syndrome patient in whom the dopamine was markedly reduced in all regions of the brain except the cerebellum and parietal cortex. (*Ann Neurol* 1983; *14*:471). Motor dysfunction generally deteriorates steadily in Rett syndrome and Parkinson-like features predominate during adolescence and early adulthood, suggesting a progressive involvement of the nigrostriatal system.

Jellinger K, Percy AK et al. (*Acta Neuropathologica* 1988; *76*:142) have described the autopsy findings in nine girls with Rett syndrome, ages 4-17 years. All brains were smaller than normal, lipofuscin was deposited in neuronal cytoplasm, melanin was absent in substantia nigra, and indications of dopaminergic nigrostriatal dysfunction were suggested. The intensive search for a biological marker for Rett syndrome continues. - Editor. *Ped Neur Briefs* December 1989.

Mitochondrial Alterations In Rett Syndrome

Muscle biopsy findings in two patients with Rett syndrome are reported from the Departments of Obstetrics/Gynecology, Pediatrics, and Pathology, Medical College of Ohio, Toledo, OH. Muscle biopsy was performed at 32 months of age and at 3 years 7 months of age. Light microscopy revealed fibers of uniform size with normal histochemistry. Electron microscopic revealed mitochondrial alterations including distention, vacuolation, and membranous changes. (Ruch A. Mitochondrial alterations in Rett syndrome. *Pediatr Neurol* Sept/Oct 1989; *5*:320-3).

COMMENT. Abnormal mitochondria have been reported previously in the muscle biopsies of two patients with Rett syndrome (Eeg-Olofsson O et al. *Brain Dev* 1988; *10*:260). The findings presented in patients with Rett syndrome did not correspond to the typical "ragged red" fibers found in mitochondrial myopathies. There are no biochemical or pathologial findings specific to Rett syndrome but further studies of mitochondrial functioning in muscle may be warranted. - Editor. *Ped Neur Briefs* September 1989.

Rett Syndrome And Heller Dementia

Six girls with Rett syndrome and two boys with Heller dementia are reported and contrasted with children with classic autism from the Department of Neuroscience and Pediatrics, University of North Dakota School of Medicine, Grand Forks,

North Dakota, and the Kennedy Institute, Johns Hopkins Medical Institutions, Baltimore, MD. The study was performed in response to a report that Rett syndrome may be a form of Heller dementia with a predilection for girls. (Millichap JG. *Lancet* Feb 21, 1987; *1*:440).

All eight children differed from those with classic autism in that they had normal prenatal and perinatal periods, followed by marked developmental regression, after which they acquired few or no skills. The boys with a diagnosis of Heller dementia differed from the girls with Rett syndrome in terms of estimated prevalence, age at onset, stereotypic breathing patterns, midline hand stereotypies, hand and gait apraxia, and speech development. The authors found no stereotyped movements in their two patients with Heller dementia although these have been described in other studies. The patients showed similarities in the normal prenatal and perinatal periods, behavioral, social and psychomotor regression, and epilepsy. The authors suggested that these children should be distinguished from those with classic autism and should be classified as "pervasive disintegrative disorder, Heller type" and "pervasive disintegrative disorder, Rett type". (Burd L, Fisher W, Kerbeshian, J. Pervasive disintegrative disorder: Are Rett syndrome and Heller dementia infantilis subtypes? *Dev Med Child Neurol* October 1989; *31*:609-616).

COMMENT. In 1908, almost 60 years before the first description of Rett syndrome, Heller reported an infantile dementia with symptoms and a course similar in some respects to that of Rett syndrome. By 1930, Heller had collected 28 cases of dementia in young children who previously had been entirely normal in development. Without antecedent illness, a change in mood and behavior was noticed. The children became irritable, negativistic, and disobedient; they had outbursts of temper without provocation; they showed signs of anxiety; and a mental regression led to a complete loss of speech and deterioration within a few months. Motor restlessness and stereotyped repetitive movements and mannerisms with grimacing and tics were most conspicuous. Seizures and growth retardation were mentioned in later reports. The cause was unknown but a suspected organic lesion was confirmed in cases examined at necropsy. Diffuse lipoid cell degeneration of the cortical neurons, atrophy of the brain, small disorganized cortical neurons lacking in Nissl bodies, and marginal gliosis have been described, and abnormalities in plasma lipids.

Heller dementia is recognized as a syndrome in text books of pediatric neurology and child psychiatry although some have suggested that some examples of the syndrome may have been confused with childhood schizophrenia, and other degenerative brain diseases. Heller dementia occurs in both boys and girls and unlike Rett syndrome, the disorder was not restricted to girls. It is surprising that in publications on Rett syndrome Heller dementia seems to have been overlooked in the differential diagnosis. Drs. Rett and Olsson have now corrected this omission (*Dev Med Child Neurol* 1987; *29*:834) but believe that research will show Rett syndrome to be an independent disorder. They admit that the differentiation may be difficult in older children and that the range of variations of both syndromes cannot be determined until the etiology is known. The suggestion that most cases of Heller dementia were disintegrative psychoses (Stephenson JBP, Kerr AM. *Lancet* March 28, 1987; *1*:741) does not fit with published neuropathological findings, and the introduction of the term "pervasive disintegrative disorder, Heller type and Rett type", based on two patients in the present report, is probably not of value in the classification of these dementias. - Editor. *Ped Neur Briefs* December 1989.

Rett's Syndrome Respiratory Patterns

The sleep and respiratory patterns associated with this disorder have been studied in 11 females aged 2 through 15 years

at the Methodist Hospital, Houston, TX. Polygraphic recordings showed a pattern of disorganized breathing and compen-
satory hyperpnea during wakefulness with regular, continuous
breathing during sleep. The findings suggest an altered or
impaired voluntary/behavioral respiratory control system in
patients with Rett's Syndrome. (Glaze DG, Frost JD Jr, Zoghbi
HY, Percy AK. Rett's Syndrome: characterisation of respiratory
patterns and sleep. *Ann Neurol* 1987; *21*:377-382).

COMMENT. In 1966, Rett described a progressive
dementia in girls with onset in early childhood and associated with autistic behavior, apraxia of gait, and stereotyped
use of the hands. The cause of Rett's syndrome is
unknown. I have seen several atypical cases that fit the
description except for the absence of so-called pathognomonic hand wringing movements and hyperventilation,
and some were boys. Is Rett's syndrome a specific disorder
or nonspecific, with more than one etiology"? For a review
of Rett syndrome, refer to *Ann J Med Genet* 1986 (suppl).
- Editor. *Ped Neur Briefs* June 1987.

EEG In Rett's Syndrome

The electroencephalographic (EEG) characteristics of
Rett's syndrome were studied in 17 girls between the ages of 1
and 16 years at the Sections of Neurophysiology and Pediatric
Neurology, Baylor College of Medicine and The Methodist
Hospital, Houston, TX. The criteria for the diagnosis of Rett's
syndrome included: 1) normal prenatal and perinatal development; 2) normal neurological development for the first 7 to 18
months; 3) cessation of development between 1 and 4 years of
age and subsequent regression; 4) dementia and autistic features; 5) loss of purposeful use of the hands and development of
stereotypical movements; 6) ataxia; 7) acquired microcephaly,
and 8) seizures.

A specific diagnostic EEG pattern was not seen but serial
records were characterized by a progressive deterioration: 1)

slowing; 2) loss of vertex transients and spindles in sleep. 3) multifocal epileptiform abnormalities; and 4) almost continuous generalized slow spike-and-wave activity. These EEG patterns appeared to correlate with the clinical stages: 1) early onset stagnation; 2) rapid destructive; 3) pseudo-stationary; and 4) late motor deterioration. The EEG of 3 patients was not typical and the average age at onset of their symptoms was later than usual. The authors suggest that the EEG may help to identify variants or atypical cases of Rett's syndrome (Glaze DG et al. Rett's syndrome. Correlation of EEG abnormalities with clinical staging. *Arch Neurol* 1987; *44*:1053-1056).

COMMENT. Others have described similar age-related changes in the EEGs of patients with Rett's syndrome. This EEG classification correlated with clinical stages may be useful in diagnosis and prognosis. The imprecise nature of the clinical-EEG correlation, admitted by the authors, may be explained by the nonspecific character and frequency of atypical cases of Rett's syndrome of undetermined etiology. - Editor. *Ped Neur Briefs* December 1987.

Oral-Motor Function In Rett Syndrome

The communication skills, oral-motor function and respiration patterns of 20 girls with Rett syndrome were studied at the Crippled Childrens Division, Oregon Health Sciences University, Portland, OR. All patients showed a regression in speech and language function by the onset of Stage II Rett syndrome. Oral-motor tone of the cheeks, lips and tongue changed from hypotonicity in Stages I and III to hypertonicity in Stage IV in a direct relationship with postural tone. Three girls in Stage IV showed fasciculations of the tongue. Most girls in Stages III and IV showed tongue deviation to the left at rest. (Budden S et al. Communication and oral-motor function in Rett syndrome. *Dev Med Child Neurol* Jan 1990; *32*:51-55).

COMMENT. This study documents the differences in oral-motor function in the various stages of Rett syndrome.

The same author has described abnormal chewing associated with tongue thrusting and involuntary undulating tongue movements in 11 of 13 girls with Rett syndrome. (Budden S. *Am J Med Genet* 1986; *24*:99). Feeding problems included difficulty in chewing and swallowing, choking and regurgitation.

An EEG study in 52 girls with Rett syndrome (Robb SA, Harden A., Boyd SG. *Neurol Ped* Nov 1989; *20*:192-195) showed that seizure discharges occurred in 43 patients and were not related to the onset of clinical seizures. They consisted of sharp waves or spikes, focal or multifocal, mainly limited to the central and midtemporal regions of one or both hemispheres. Light sleep enhanced the presence of discharges. Periodical hyperventilation seen frequently during EEG recordings in this study was not associated with any consistent EEG change. Sleep spindles were conspicuously absent in all records. The authors find the EEG features helpful in confirmation of the diagnosis of Rett syndrome in the appropriate clinical setting. - Editor. *Ped Neur Briefs* February 1990.

Motor Disorders In Rett Syndrome

The motor and behavioral findings in 32 patients with Rett syndrome aged 21 months to 30 years, are reported from the Departments of Neurology and Pediatrics, Baylor College of Medicine, Houston, TX. Hand stereotypies and gait abnormalities were present in all patients. Clapping, wringing, and clenching were the most common, followed by washing, patting, and rubbing movements. Gait ataxia was present in 31%, a broad based gait in 13%, and inability to walk in 28%. Bruxism was the next most common involuntary movement (97%) and occurred only when awake. Drooling occurred in 75%. Other motor disturbances included ocular deviations (63%), parkinsonian rigidity (44%), bradykinesia (41%), dystonia (59%), sometimes focal and sometimes associated with scoliosis (50%). Myoclonus, choreoathetosis and intention tremor also occurred.

Hyperkinetic disorders were prominent in younger patients and bradykinetic disorders occurred more frequently in older patients. (FitzGerald PM et al. Extrapyramidal involvement in Rett's syndrome. *Neurology* Feb 1990; *40*:293-295).

COMMENT. The number of cases and the plethora of published reports on Rett syndrome add credence to the viral infectious cause postulated by Hagberg (see *Ped Neur Briefs* 1989; *3*:44). A toxic environmental cause might also be considered and pursued further. - Editor. *Ped Neur Briefs* February 1990.

Cerebral Blood Flow In Rett Syndrome

Cerebral blood flow was studied with single photon emission computed tomography in seven girls with Rett syndrome at the John F. Kennedy Institute, Glostrup, Denmark and the Department of Clinical Physiology and Nuclear Medicine, Bispebjerg Hospital, Copenhagen, Denmark. Compared to results in an age matched control group of nine normal children, global cerebral blood flow was significantly lower in patients with Rett syndrome (54 vs 69 mL/100 g per minute). The blood flows in prefrontal and temporoparietal association regions of the telencephalon were markedly reduced, whereas the primary sensorimotor regions were relatively spared. The cerebral blood flow distribution in Rett syndrome was similar to the distribution of brain metabolic activity in infants of a few months of age. The most striking difference between the Rett syndrome and control groups was the pronounced frontal hypoperfusion in the Rett syndrome group; patients had a 30% lower anteroposterior flow ratio than the control group. These changes were not reflected in CT scans which showed cortical and central atrophy only in two of the seven patients. The age range of the patients was between 6.7 and 17.9 years with a median of 10.1 years. (Nielsen JB et al. Immature pattern of brain activity in Rett syndrome. *Arch Neurol* Sept 1990; *47*:982-986).

COMMENT. PET studies of human brain functional development have shown that the prefrontal and temporoparietal regions are relatively inactive before the sixth month of life and an adult pattern is seen at one year of age. (Chugani HT et al. *Ann Neurol* 1987; *22*:487-497). The theory of developmental arrest in infants with Rett syndrome is supported by the finding of an immature pattern of cerebral blood flow. However, the results of the present study conflict with those of Naidu et al who found an increase in the metabolism in the frontal region and a lower metabolism in the occipital region of two patients with Rett syndrome studied with PET (*J Child Neurol* 1988; *3* (suppl): S78-S86). - Editor. *Ped Neur Briefs* December 1990.

Sural Nerve Axonopathy And Rett Syndrome

The histopathologic findings of three sural nerve biopsies and one muscle biopsy from three patients with Rett syndrome are described from the Department of Pediatrics, National Sanatorium Yakumo Hospital, Yakumo, Hokkaido, Japan. The biopsies demonstrated mitochondrial changes in the cytoplasm of Schwann cells, occasional onion bulb formations, and mitochondrial alterations in myelinated axons with reduction in the number of large myelinated fibers. The muscle showed small dark angulated fibers with NADH-TR staining and dumbbell-shaped mitochondria. (Wakai S et al. Rett syndrome: Findings suggesting axonopathy and mitochondrial abnormalities. *Pediatr Neurol* Sept/Oct 1990; *6*:339-343).

COMMENT. These findings suggest peripheral nerve involvement and mitochondrial abnormalities in Rett syndrome. An additional article describes cerebellar pathology at autopsy of five patients with Rett syndrome (Oldfors A et al. Rett syndrome: Cerebellar pathology. *Pediatr Neurol* Sept/Oct 1990; *6*:310-314). Patients ranged in age from 7 to 30 years. All had reduced brain weights with small cerebella. There was loss of Purkinje cells, atrophy, astrocytic gliosis of molecular and granular cell layers, and gliosis and loss of myelin in the white matter. The cerebellar atrophy was greater in two patients treated with phenytoin. The pathology of Rett syndrome appears to involve the cerebellum, cerebral hemispheres, basal ganglia, especially substantia nigra, spinal cord, peripheral nerve, and muscle. - Editor. *Ped Neur Briefs* December 1990.

CHAPTER **18**

NUTRITION, DIET AND NERVOUS SYSTEM DISORDERS

Sucrose, Motor Activity, And Learning

The effects of sugar (sucrose) on the behavior of 30 preschool children (20 boys and 10 girls, mean age 5 years 4 mos) and 15 elementary school children (6 boys and 9 girls, mean age 7 yrs 2 mos) were investigated by psychologists from Colorado State University, Fort Collins, CO, and the Univ of Mississippi Med Centr, Jackson, MS. Parents and teachers questioned before the study complained that the child was behaviorally sensitive to sugar in approximately 50% of subjects. Two preschool children had been considered hyperactive by the school director. A basic breakfast included a 4 oz orange flavored drink of high sucrose content (50 g), low-sugar (6.25 g) or aspartame (122 mg), randomly selected, five days on each, using a double-blind control design. The mean sucrose intakes for the high, low, and "control" aspartame conditions were

2.26, 0.28, and 0.00 g/kg, respectively, and the total carbohydrate contents of breakfast averaged 3.95, 1.88, and 1.54 g/kg, respectively.

On cognitive measures, girls made significantly more errors on a paired-associate learning task performed 20-30 min following a high-sugar content breakfast when compared to a low-sugar meal, whereas boys were unaffected. On global ratings, younger preschool children were affected differently than older children. On an Abbreviated Conners Teacher Rating Scale completed before lunch, both boys and girls were more active in behavior after the high sugar meal than that of low sugar content. Measures of behavior by observation for fidgetiness, change in activity, running, vocalization and aggressiveness, and other cognitive measures involving matching and academic tasks failed to demonstrate changes after sugar ingestion. (Rosen LA et al. Effects of sugar (sucrose) on children's behavior. *J Consulting Clin Psychol* 1988; 56(4):583-589).

COMMENT. Evidently, the effects of sugar on children's behavior is not yet resolved. This study demonstrates significant adverse effects although the authors conclude that these are minimal in degree. Certain limitations of the study design are admitted: 1) The sugar challenge dose was the same for all subjects and younger and smaller children, affected differently, received larger amounts than did older and larger children. The design was not adequate to pinpoint the amount of sugar that may cause deleterious effects. 2) The prior dietary history of the subjects was unknown, and those accustomed to consuming large amounts of sugar may have reacted differently from children who usually ate low sugar meals. 3) The assumption that aspartame used as a control is innocuous may not be correct (see *Ped Neur Briefs* Nov 1987; 1:45). Further work on possible behavioral effects of sucrose is clearly indicated. The only proven contraindication to excess sugar in a child's diet is that emphasized by the dental profession. - Editor. *Ped Neur Briefs* September 1988.

Sugar, Aspartame, And Behavior

The effects of glucose, sucrose, saccharin, and aspartame on aggression and motor activity in 30 boys, ages 2-6 years, were studied at the Child Psychiatry Branch and Laboratory of Developmental Psychology, NIMH, Bethesda, MD. Eighteen boys were recruited or selected as "sugar responders" and 12 male playmates were "non responders". Single doses of sucrose, 1.75 g/kg; glucose, 1.75 g/kg; aspartame, 30 mg/kg; or saccharine administered in a randomized, double-blind design produced no significant effect on aggression or on teacher ratings of behavior. Actometer counts for two hours after ingestion of aspartame were lower than those following other sweeteners. Parent ratings of activity and aggression after home challenges with sweeteners failed to show differences between substances for either the alleged "responders" or "non responders". Consistent with baseline measures, parents rated responders more hyperactive than playmates who were not believed to be sugar reactive. No parent differentiated between sugar and non-sugar trials. Mean daily sucrose intake and total sugar consumption correlated with duration of aggression against property for the alleged sugar responsive group but acute sugar loading did not increase aggression or activity in preschool children. (Krnesi MJP et al. Effects of sugar and aspartame on aggression and activity in children. *Am J Psychiatry* 1987; *144*:1487-1490).

COMMENT. Conners CK at the Children's Hospital, Washington, D.C. reports that deleterious effects of sugar on children with attention deficit may be demonstrated if the challenge follows a high carbohydrate breakfast but the effects are blocked or reversed by a protein load. The beneficial and protective effects of a protein diet are correlated with neuroendocrine changes and the prevention of the serotonergic effects of sugar on behavior and attention (personal communication and in *Diet and Behavior*, Lubbock, Texas Tech Univ Press). Diets low in protein and high in carbohydrates might be expected to cause increases in spontaneous activity, as demonstrated in animal studies, but these effects are not necessarily related to swings in blood sugar concentrations. For recent reviews of the effects of dietary nutrients and deficiencies on brain biochemistry and behavior see Yehuda S. *Intern J Neuroscience* 1987; *35*:21-36; and *Nutrition Reviews/ Supplement* May 1986; *44*:1-250. - Editor. *Ped Neur Briefs* November 1987.

Aspartame And Learning And Behavior

The effects of aspartame on learning, behavior and mood of 9-10-year-old normal children were examined in the Department of Nutritional Sciences, University of Toronto, Ontario, Canada. Measures of associative learning, arithmetic calculation, activity level, social interaction and mood were unaffected by treatment with Kool-Aid containing 1.76 gram/kg of carbohydrate (polycose) plus either aspartame (34 mg/kg) or the equivalent sweetness as sodium cyclamate and amino acids as alanine. In a second experiment in which children received a drink of cold, unsweetened strawberry Kool-Aid containing either 1.75 gram/kg of sucrose or 9.7 mg/kg of aspartame, the frequency of minor and gross motor behaviors was significantly less after the consumption of sucrose than after aspartame treatment. (Saravis S et al. Aspartame: effects on learning, behavior and mood, *Pediatrics* July 1990; *86*: 75-83).

COMMENT. The authors concluded that the effects of aspartame on short-term behavior were more likely due to an "absence of metabolic consequences of providing sweetness rather than to neurochemical consequences related to its amino acid composition". The observed reduction in activity following sucrose ingestion is in agreement with some previous reports and adds to the controversy concerning hyperactivity and sugar. The tests in the above study that failed to show significant effects of aspartame included the Conditional Associative Learning Task, the Canadian Tests of Basic Skills, the Children's Depression Inventory and the State-Trait Anxiety Inventory for

Children. The minor and gross motor behaviors which showed significant improvement with sucrose included the actometer measure, a modified self-winding wrist watch, and a video taped observation of behavior. The children in this study were normal and different responses may occur in patients with ADHD. - Editor. *Ped Neur Briefs* August 1990.

Serum Fatty Acids And Hyperactivity

Serum essential fatty acids (EFA) levels were measured in 44 hyperactive children and 45 age-and-sex-matched controls at the Dept. of Pediatrics and Psychiatry and Behavioral Science, Univ. of Auckland, New Zealand. Docasahexaenoic, dihomo-grammalmolenic, and arachidonic acid levels were significantly lower in hyperactive children than controls. The hyperactive group of children had significantly lower birth weights than controls (3,058 and 3,410 g respectively; $p < 0.01$), a greater incidence of learning difficulties and dyslexia, but no increase in asthma, eczema, or other allergies. In a double-blind placebo controlled, crossover study of evening primose oil in 31 hyperactive children, effects on behavior were modest and equivocal. (Mitchell EA et al. Clinical characteristics and serum essential fatty acid levels in hyperactive children. *Clin Pediat* 1987; *26*:406-411).

COMMENT. The search for dietary related causes and treatments for hyperactive behavior continues and now involves fats in addition to food allergies, additives, preservatives, sugar and megavitamins. In support of fats, a beneficial effect of the ketogenic diet on the behavior of the epileptic child often complements its anticonvulsant properties in my experience. The present paper did not confirm previous reports of a high prevalence of allergy among hyperactive children and tends to minimize the possible importance of food allergy as an etiologic factor. - Editor. *Ped Neur Briefs* September 1987.

Adverse Reactions To Food Additives

As part of a multicentre study of food additive intolerance commissioned by the UK Ministry of Agriculture, Fisheries and Food, the prevalence of reactions to food additive was studied in a survey population by the Depts of Dermatology and Community Medicine, Wycombe General Hospital, High Wycombe, Bucks, and St. Thomas' Campus, London University. Of 18,582 respondents to questionnaires, 7.4% had reactions to food additives, 15.6% had problems with foods, and 10% had symptoms related to aspirin. The incidence of a personal history of atopy reported in 28% of all respondents was significantly higher in those reacting to additives, food, and aspirin (50%, 47.5%, and 36% respectively). A preponderance of reactions occurred in children, boys more than girls. Older patients were affected less often and with a female preponderance.

Abnormal behavior and mood changes were mainly related to additives whereas headache was associated with foods more frequently than additives. Of 44 individuals (7% of 649 interviewed) who reported monosodium glutamate sensitivity, 13 (30%) suffered headache, and 8 (18%) had behavioral or mood changes. Headache was related to food intolerance in 14% of those interviewed but had not previously been regarded as migrainous in nature. Of 81 reactive subjects who completed an additive challenge with annatto or azo dye, only 3 showed consistent reactions. The authors estimated the prevalence of food additive intolerance in the study population at 0.01-0.23%. (Young E et al. *J Roy Coll Physicians London* 1987; *21*:241-247).

COMMENT. The debate in the UK on food additives and behavior waxes while in the USA interest wanes, with more attention being given to sugar and the effectiveness of stimulants in therapy (see *Ped Neur Briefs* 1987; *1*:5,22,38). In the same issue of the JRCP London, Pollock L and Warner JO at the Brompton Hospital report a follow-up of children with food additive intolerance showing that symptoms were mainly transient, 76% showing no reaction on rechallenge studies, and Lessof MH at Guy's Hospital reviews the literature and concludes that more reliable diagnostic tests and toxicological screening methods are needed. A food intolerance databank has been compiled at the Leatherhead Food Research Association, UK, that will provide constantly updated information on food product composition and brands free from ingredients most commonly associated with food intolerance (milk, egg, wheat, soya bean, cocoa, BHA and BHT, sulfur dioxide, benzoate, glutamate and azo colors). - Editor. *Ped Neur Briefs* November 1987.

Food Additives And Hyperactivity

Of 220 children referred to the Dept of Paediatrics, Royal Children's Hospital, Parkville, Victoria, Australia, because of suspected hyperactivity, 55 were included in a six week open trial of the Feingold Diet, 26 (47%) showed a placebo response, and 14 were identified as likely reactors. Of eight who subsequently completed a double-blind crossover study (utilizing each child as his own control), two demonstrated a significant dependent relationship between the challenge and ingestion of azo dye colorings (tartrazine and carmoisine 50 mg) and behavioral change. Extreme irritability, restlessness and sleep disturbance rather than attention deficit were the common behavioral patterns associated with the ingestion of food colorings, as described by the parents in this study. The authors conclude that the inclusion of children in trials on the basis of attention deficit alone may miss some reactors, and there is little place for use of a coloring-free diet in children with ADD unless the other behavioral features of irritability, restlessness and sleep disturbance are present. (Rowe KS. Synthetic food colourings and 'hyperactivity': A double-blind crossover study. *Aust Pediatr J* April 1988; *24*:143-147).

COMMENT. The phoenix of the Feingold Diet rises again with the suggestion that the treatment has been erroneously discarded because of inappropriate behavioral rating instruments and failure to identify specific reactors to food additives. In England, where the avoidance of all foods containing additives is widespread, the major problem is the level of public misinformation, occasionally leading to handicapping dietary restriction. (David TJ. *Arch Dis Child* 1988; *63*:582). - Editor. *Ped Neur Briefs* June 1988.

Elimination Diets In
Pre-School-Aged Hyperactive Boys

The effect of an experimental elimination diet was examined in 24 hyperactive boys aged 3.5 to 6 years at the Alberta Children's Hospital, and the Learning Center, Calgary, Alberta, Canada. The diet was broader than those studied previously in that it eliminated not only artificial colors and flavors but also chocolate, monosodium glutamate, preservatives, caffeine, and any substance that the families reported might affect the child. It was low in simple sugar (mono- and disaccharides) and dairy-free if an allergy to milk was suspected. A within-subject cross-over design was divided into 3 periods: a baseline of three weeks, a placebo-control period of three weeks, and an experimental diet period of four weeks.

Approximately 42% (10) of the children showed 50% improvement in behavior on the elimination diet; an additional 16% (4) had lesser degrees of improvement (12%) with no placebo effect. Headache was less frequently reported during the diet period compared to placebo but not less than the baseline phase. Other nonbehavioral variables such as night awakenings and halitosis tended to improve during the dietary treatment phase. (Kaplan BJ et al. Dietary replacement in preschool-aged hyperactive boys. *Pediatrics* Jan 1989; *83*:7-17).

COMMENT. These results of replacement diets indicate larger response rates than challenge studies with specific items. Further studies of additive-free and hypoallergenic-sugar-restricted diets are warranted in the management of attention deficit disorders with hyperactivity, and headache and sleep disorders, particularly in preschool children. - Editor. *Ped Neur Briefs* March 1989.

Ketogenic Diets In Epilepsy

The classical ketogenic diet, the medium chain triglyceride (MCT) diet, and a modified MCT diet were used in the treatment of 55 children and 4 adults with intractable epilepsy at the University and Clinical Departments of Paediatrics, John Radcliffe Hospital, Oxford, England. The main types of seizures were drop attacks (24), infantile spasms (7), tonic-clonic (6), partial complex (5), primary absence (2), myoclonic absence (2), complex absence (4), and partial simple (4). Forty-five of the patients were under ten years of age. Cooperation and compliance were good and 57 patients completed at least six weeks dietary management and some continued for periods up to four years. Fifty-six had significantly elevated blood ketones bodies and all were reported to have ketonuria.

Eighty-one percent showed greater than 50% reduction in seizure frequency. The response was independent of the type of diet used; all three diets appeared to be equally effective in children under the age of 15 years. The high fat diet was found to be palatable by all of the children but the adults found the restrictions unacceptable. Large quantities of MCT oil were also found to be unpalatable by all age groups. No patient found the cream and butter content of the classical diet to be unacceptable. Analysis of variance failed to show any significant difference between the type of seizure and the success of treatment. The EEG showed improvement in 14 cases, 9 while the children were on the MCT diet and 5 while on the classical diet. Nausea, vomiting or abdominal discomfort occurred in approximately one-half the patients taking the MCT diet; drowsiness occurred in 25% at the introduction of the diet. Loss of ketosis occurred during the prodromal phase of an intercurrent illness and was often accompanied by an increase in the frequency of seizures. Two children under one year of age showed no increase in weight, length or head circumference during a six month period on the diet. (Schwartz R H et al. Ketogenic diets in the treatment of epilepsy: Short term clinical effects. *Dev Med Child Neurol* April 1989; *31*:145-151).

Metabolic Effects Of Ketogenic Diets

The results of 24 metabolic profiles performed on 55 epileptic children receiving the classical ketogenic diet, the MCT diet, a modified MCT diet, and normal diets are reported from the University Department of Paediatrics, John Radcliffe Hospital, Oxford, England. The clinical effects of the diets are reported in the previous paper. All three therapeutic diets improved the control of epilepsy and induced a significant increase in the concentrations of blood aceto-acetate and 3-hydroxybutyrate, the greatest elevation being seen in patients on the classical diet (4:1). The pre- and post-prandial blood ketone levels with the classical diet reached a mean of 2.6 mmol/L before breakfast and 4 mmol/L before supper. The three ketogenic diets led to a buildup of ketone body concentrations during the day, reaching maximum levels in the afternoon. This was in contrast to the normal diet which led to slightly higher levels in the morning fasting samples. The Ketostix reagent strip test for urinary ketone bodies reflected these changes and showed higher levels in the afternoon and lower levels in morning samples. Children between 5 and 10 years of age showed the highest blood ketone levels. Levels of blood glycerol were highest while fasting and lowest after meals. Despite the high fat content of the diets none of the concentrations of plasma cholesterol, high density lipoproteins, low density and very low density lipoproteins was significantly raised in any of the therapeutic diet groups. Hypoglycemia was not documented in any patient at any time but blood concentrations of pyruvate were significantly lower. Lower blood levels of alanine occurred on all three diets, the most marked difference being in children receiving the classical diet. The remaining plasma amino acid concentrations tended to be lowest on the classical diet but other than alanine values, the mean concentrations of individual amino acids on the three diets failed to show any significant change. Plasma insulin concentrations corresponded to the blood glucose profiles, showing elevations after each meal, the highest levels occurring with the normal and modified MCT diet and the lowest responses occurring with the classical ketogenic diet. The mean plasma concentrations of sodium, potassium, chloride and bicarbonate did not differ significantly between the four diets, and plasma urea, creatinine, calcium, phosphate, total protein, albumin and bilirubin levels were also similar. Plasma uric acid levels were higher on all three ketogenic diets with the highest increase on the MCT diet. The mechanism of action of the ketogenic diet was not determined. (Schwartz R M et al. Metabolic effects of three ketogenic diets in the treatment of severe epilepsy. *Dev Med Child Neurol* April 1989; *31*:152-160).

COMMENT. The above two studies performed at the John Radcliffe Hospital in Oxford and including patients from the pediatric practice of Dr. B.D. Bower have reconfirmed the efficacy of the ketogenic diet in the management of intractable epilepsy in children under 15 years. The classical diet was more acceptable than the MCT diet, being equally effective and better tolerated by most patients. The authors were unable to document any significant changes in blood lipid profiles in the short term study, and the theoretical risks of inducing ischemic heart disease appeared to be outweighed by the benefit of the diets in controlling disabling seizures. With the increasing concern and attention to cholesterol and heart disease, however, this aspect of treatment must be followed carefully and patients with a family history of hypercholesterolemia or ischemic heart disease should probably be excluded from the ketogenic treatment program.

Balance studies are needed to determine the effect of the ketogenic diet on body water and electrolytes. In a balance study performed at the Mayo Clinic (Millichap JG, Jones JD. Acid-base, electrolyte, and amino-acid metabolism in children with petit mal. Etiologic significance and modification by anticonvulsant drugs and the ketogenic diet. *Epilepsia* 1964; 5:239-255) we found a decrease in the blood pH, PCO2, and standard bicarbonate during short ketogenic periods. The urinary excretion of electrolytes was increased and particularly that of calcium, magnesium and sodium, and the balance of sodium, potassium, calcium, magnesium, phosphorus and nitrogen were negative. The excretion of alphaaminonitrogen was reduced, the excretion of free amino acids was variable, and the level of leucine in the serum was elevated. Fluid intake and urine output were reduced and the fall in body weight was rapid and marked in the initial week of treatment. The total lipids, fatty acid and cholesterol in the serum were increased but not significantly during the ketogenic diet period; they became elevated significantly when carbohydrates and the antiketogenic diet were reintroduced. The anticonvulsant action of the ketogenic diet was unrelated to diuresis, independent of acidosis and was correlated with an increased urinary excretion and a negative balance of sodium and potassium. Calcium supplements are usually advised with the ketogenic diet and in addition magnesium supplements should probably be included.

The ketogenic dietary therapy of childhood epilepsies deserves further attention from pediatric neurologists. Assurance of parental and patient cooperation is essential as well as skilled dietetic advice and follow-up. The classical diet is probably more acceptable and has less gastrointestinal side-effects than the MCT diet; a lower and more palatable ratio (3:1) than that used in the Oxford study is usually sufficient and effective. If the diet is continued for long periods, consultation with a specialist in lipid metabolism should be obtained and ultrasound of the liver ordered to exclude fatty infiltration of the liver. (See *Ped Neur Briefs*, April 1988; 2:28). - Editor. *Ped Neur Briefs* April 1989.

Corn Oil Ketogenic Diet

The successful substitution of corn oil for MCT oil in 6 children treated with the ketogenic diet for intractable seizures is reported from the Depts of Pediatrics, Neurology and Psychiatry, University of Arkansas for Medical Sciences and Arkansas Children's Hospital, 804 Wolfe Street, Little Rock, AR. Seizure types were mixed in all 6 patients, absence in 5, minor motor in 4, myoclonic in 3, and complex partial and generalized tonic-clonic in 1. All had been controlled with MCT oil diets but corn oil was the major advantage of being less expensive, more readily available without prescription, and better tolerated. Anticonvulsants were reduced in 5 patients and eliminated in 3, without deterioration in seizure control. (Woody RC et al. Corn oil ketogenic diet for children with intractable seizures. *J Child Neurol* Jan 1988; *3*:21-24).

COMMENT. The medium chain triglyceride (MCT) oil was advocated by Huttenlocher et al. (*Neurology* 1971; *21*:1097) as a substitute for dietary fats in the ketogenic diet. MCT's are more ketogenic and less restrictive of carbohydrates, they are more rapidly absorbed than dietary fat and may induce ketosis more quickly. A disadvantage of the MCT diet is the frequency of gastrointestinal side-effects, many patients suffering from bulky, loose stools, diarrhea, vomiting and abdominal pain. Perhaps the superiority and availability of corn oil will encourage a renewed interest in the ketogenic diet for the treatment of refractory seizures in children. - Editor. *Ped Neur Briefs* April 1988.

Fatty Liver And MCT Diet In Intractable Epilepsy

Fatty infiltration of the liver in 4 children treated with the medium chain triglyceride (MCT) diet is reported from the Depts of Paediatrics and Radiology, Leeds General Infirmary, Belmont Grove, Leeds, England. This was not associated with hepatic dysfunction and resolved after discontinuing the diet. The patients' ages ranged from 4 to 12 years. The seizures were astatic myoclonic in pattern and resistant to medications, including sodium valproate, clobazam, or carbamazepine. The duration of the diet was 2 to 3 years at time of diagnosis by ultrasound scan and, in one case, by liver biopsy. Triglyceride and cholesterol levels were normal in 2 and liver function tests normal in 3 patients tested. Seizure control was improved during treatment with the MCT diet. (Beverley D, Arthur R. Fatty liver and medium chain triglyceride (MCT) diet. *Arch Dis Child* July 1988; *63*:840-842).

> COMMENT. The mechanism of the fatty liver infiltration was undetermined. The standard ketogenic diet is not always associated with a significant increase in serum lipids but it is accompanied by a fall in blood pH, standard bicarbonate, and blood sugar. (Millichap JG et al. *Amer J Dis Child* 1964; *107*:593). The accumulation of excess hydrogen ion within the liver cell is cited as one possible mechanism of fatty change in the liver. The concomitant therapy with anticonvulsant drugs, particularly valproate, might also be contributory. - Editor. *Ped Neur Briefs* July 1988.

Oligoantigenic Diet For Migraine And Epilepsy

A diet low in antigenic items was used to treat 63 children with epilepsy refractory to medication at the Depts of Neurology, Immunology, and Dietetics, The Hospital for Sick Children, Great Ormond Street, and the Institute of Child Health, London, England. The authors had previously reported beneficial effects of the "oligoantigenic" diet in the treatment of migraine *(Lancet* 1983; *2*:865) and the hyperkinetic syndrome (*Lancet* 1985; *1*:940). The diet consisted of 2 meats (lamb and chicken), 2 carbohydrates (potatoes and rice), 2 fruits (banana and apple), vegetables (cabbage, sprouts, cauliflower, broccoli, cucumber, celery, carrots, parsnips), water, salt, pepper, pure herbs, and calcium and vitamins for 4 weeks. Patients who responded (no seizures or migraine for the last 2 weeks) were reintroduced to essential foods (e.g. milk, cheese, wheat) at the rate of one a week. If symptoms were provoked, soy-based or goat milk products, rye or oats were substituted. Setbacks were avoided by first giving foods least likely to be antigenic (e.g. beef, oats, peaches, or grapes).

Of 45 children who had epilepsy with recurrent headaches, abdominal symptoms, or hyperkinetic behavior, 25 had no seizures and 11 had fewer seizures during diet therapy. Foods most likely to provoke seizures when reintroduced were cow milk and cheese, citrus fruits, wheat, tartrazine and benzoic acid food additives, eggs, tomato, pork, and chocolate. In double-blind, placebo-controlled provocation studies introducing cow milk, orange juice, wheat, pork, egg, and benzoate, symptoms recurred in 15 of 16 children, including seizures in 8; none recurred with placebo. The oligoantigenic diet was unsuccessful in the treatment of 18 children who had epilepsy uncomplicated by migraine or hyperkinetic behavior. (Egger J, Wilson J, et al. Oligoantigenic diet treatment of children with epilepsy and migraine. *J Pediatr* Jan 1989; *114*:51-58).

COMMENT. If reproducible and sustained, these results are impressive and deserve further investigation in children with frequently recurrent seizures and headache resistant to anticonvulsant medication. The authors point out that the diets are socially disruptive and may cause malnutrition. In the US, pediatric allergists are not generally impressed with the theory of food hypersensitivity as a cause of neurological disease and their enthusiastic collaboration in studies of this type is not readily available. - Editor. *Ped Neur Briefs* December 1988.

Vitamin E And Epilepsy

The value of D-alpha-tocopheryl acetate (Vitamin E 400 IU/day) as an adjunct therapy for drug resistant epilepsy is reported from The Hospital for Sick Children and the University of Toronto Faculty of Medicine, Canada. In a randomized, double-blind, placebo-controlled trial, 10 of 12 children aged 6-17 years showed a greater than 60% reduction in seizure frequency whereas none in the control group showed a significant change. One-half of the responders had concomitant EEG improvements. The study period was 9 months: 3 month pre-trial, 3 month double-blind, and 3 month open-label trial in which patients receiving placebo initially changed to Vitamin E as their own controls. The majority had generalized tonic-clonic seizures and anticonvulsant drug levels showed no significant change during treatment with Vitamin E. Plasma Vitamin E levels increased from 5 to 37 mcM during the treatment phase, the variability dependent on body size. Improvement in seizure control was similar in the open-label phase and no clinically significant alterations of blood counts, SGOT, alkaline phosphatase, and amylase was noted. (Ogunmekan AO, Hwang PA. A randomized, double-blind, placebo-controlled, clinical trial of D-a-tocopheryl acetate (Vitamin E), as add-on therapy, for epilepsy in children. *Epilepsia* Jan/Feb 1989; *30*:84-89).

COMMENT. These authors and others have reported reduced plasma levels of Vitamin E in children taking antiepileptic drugs. Hyperbaric oxygen-induced seizures in rats are prevented by prior administration of Vitamin E. (Jerrett SA et al. *Aerospace Med* 1973; *44*:40-4). The clinical trial reported here and a previous uncontrolled study support the experimental findings in animals that Vitamin E may inhibit the effects of oxidation in brain tissue and act as a membrane stabilizer in epileptic cerebral cortex. Further trials of this adjunctive treatment for refractory epilepsies are certainly warranted. - Editor. *Ped Neur Briefs* December 1988.

Wernicke's Encephalopathy

Two cases of Wernicke's encephalopathy (WE) diagnosed at autopsy are reported from the Depts of Pediatrics and Pathology, British Columbia's Children's Hospital, and the University of British Columbia, Vancouver, Canada. A 5 year old child was persistently febrile due to repeated pulmonary infections and died of respiratory failure after nine weeks in coma following cold-water submersion. Her average daily nutritional

tional intake (1,200 calories, 2.2 mg thiamine) was deficient in calories and her thiamine intake, adequate for a healthy child, was apparently insufficient for a severely ill child with high carbohydrate intake.

In a nine month old infant with Zellweger syndrome who died of hemorrhage from esophageal varices due to cirrhosis of the liver, feeding was made difficult because of frequent seizures and no vitamin supplements had been given. The mammillary bodies and periventricular areas in the brainstem showed spongy change, persistence of neurons, and astrocytosis characteristic of WE. The diagnosis was not suspected during life. (Sear MD, Norman MG. Two cases of Wernicke's encephalopathy in children: An underdiagnosed complication of poor nutrition. *Ann Neurol* July 1988; *24*:85-87).

> COMMENT. WE in alcoholic adults classically presents with ataxia, confusion, ophthalmoplegia, and coma and death if untreated. The onset and course may be acute, subacute, or chronic. In 6 cases cited in infants, deterioration was rapid, with lethargy, apneic spells, hypertonia, and hypothermia. The authors emphasize that WE often occurs without alcoholism, it is preventable and treatable with thiamine supplements, and the diagnosis should be suspected in malnourished infants, especially those with persistent vomiting. - Editor. *Ped Neur Briefs* July 1988.

Vitamins And Neural Tube Defects

The use of vitamin supplements by women around the time of conception was examined and compared in those having babies with neural tube defects, those with still births or some other type of malformation, and in women who had normal babies. The study was performed at the National Institute of Child Health and Human Development, National Institutes of Health, Bethesda, Maryland; Northwestern University, Chicago; and the California Public Health Foundation, Berkley. The rate of periconceptional multivitamin use among mothers of infants with neural tube defects (15.8%) was not significantly different from the rate among mothers in either the abnormal or the normal control group (14.1% and 15.9%, respectively). There were no differences among the groups in the use of folate vitamin supplements. The authors conclude that the periconceptional use of multivamins or folate-containing supplements did not decrease the risk of having an infant with a neural tube defect. (Mills JL et al. The absence of a relation between the periconceptional use of vitamins and neural-tube defects. *N Engl J Med* Aug 17, 1989; *321*:430-5).

COMMENT. Several studies have suggested that women who take multivitamins or supplements of folic acid around the time of conception may have a reduced risk of delivering an infant with a neural tube defect such as myelomeningocele or spina bifida. British studies have reported that folic acid in a dose of 4 mg/day or multivitamins can reduce the risk of recurrence in women who have already delivered an infant with such a defect.

In a report published from the Atlanta Birth Defects Case Control Study, mothers of children with neural tube defects were significantly less likely to report vitamin use around the time of conception than were the mothers of infants with other malformations or normal control children. The results of the present study were strikingly different from those of the Atlanta Birth Defects Case Control Study in which 7% of mothers with affected babies and 50% of controls reported using multivitamin supplements at least three times a week in the periconceptional period. It is possible that the use of vitamins was not itself protective but was a marker for other health conscious behavior that prevented the malformations. Other explanations for the difference in the results might include the variation in the years studied and geographic differences. It should be noted that the Vitamin A analog Isotretinoin is teratogenic and should be avoided during pregnancy.

Further studies are obviously needed to confirm these results. In the meantime mothers might be advised to take vitamins in the recommended daily allowances but not to resort to megavitamin therapy with possible adverse effects. - Editor. *Ped Neur Briefs* August 1989.

Biotinidase Deficiency And Seizures

Preliminary experiences with screening of 24,300 newborns detected 1 infant with biotinidase deficiency at the Depts of Paediatrics, Univ of Verona, Policlinic Borgo Roma, Verona, Italy, and the Hosp for Sick Children, Toronto, Canada. The patient was a full-term baby girl with uncomplicated delivery and a positive family history for seizures in an aunt who had died at 8 months of age. At 2 months of life, the infant developed dermatitis and sparse scalp hair followed by multifocal motor seizures resistant to anticonvulsant drugs. Neurological exam showed hypertonia and hyperreflexia, the EEG revealed increased slow wave activity, and the CT finding was a mild cortical atrophy. Large amounts of 2-oxoglutarate and small amounts of 3-hydroxyisovalerate were found on chromatographic examination of the urine. Treatment with 10 mg/biotin daily resulted in complete recovery within two to three days. (Burlina AB et al. Neonatal screening for biotinidase deficiency in north eastern Italy. (*Eur J Pediatr* April 1988; *147*:317-318).

COMMENT. The authors consider that biotinidase deficiency is as common as other well-known metabolic disorders and satisfies all criteria for inclusion into neonatal mass screening programs for inborn errors of metabolism. The absence of the expected organic acidopathy noted in the present case-report confirms the need for biotinidase enzyme estimations in diagnosis. - Editor. *Ped Neur Briefs* June 1988.

Biotin Responsive Encephalopathy

A case of biotin responsive infantile encephalopathy is reported from the Department of Pediatrics and Child

Neuropsychiatry, University of Verona, Italy; and Hopital des Enfants Malades, Paris, France. At one month of age the infant developed dermatitis of the ears. At two months she began to have tonic clonic seizures occurring several times a day and refractory to treatment with carbamazepine, phenobarbital, phenytoin, clonazepam, nitrazepam, ACTH, and hydrocortisone. Seizure frequency increased up to ten per day. At three months, she became hypotonic and a CT scan showed enlargement of cortical sulci and lateral ventricles. At four months she was very lethargic and floppy, reflexes were hyperactive, and plantar responses were extensor. Her behavior was autistic-like and her scalp hair was sparse. The urine examination showed an increased excretion of 2-ketoglutaric acid and 3-hydroxy-isovaleric acid. Serum biotinidase activity was 0.15 nmol min-1 ml-1 (normal range 5.2). Father's biotinidase activity was 0.31 (8% of normal) and the mother's 0.42 (10% of normal). An electroencephalogram showed frequent independent spikes of variable amplitude prominent in the left posterior temporal region and numerous EEG seizures.

Within 36 hours of starting biotin therapy 5 mg BD there was dramatic clinical improvement; the infant became responsive to surrounding stimuli, seizures were controlled and antiepileptic treatment was reduced to only phenobarbital 15 mg BD. After ten days of treatment the urinary examination was normal and the EEG showed a well organized background activity and no paroxysmal abnormalities. At two years four months the neurological exam was normal, the CT scan and EEG normal, and the dose of biotin was at 7.5 mg a day. The authors suggest a therapeutic trial of biotin in all drug resistant infantile seizures. (Colamaria V et al. Biotin-responsive infantile encephalopathy: EEG-polygraphic study of a case. *Epilepsia* October 1989; *30*:573-578).

COMMENT. Two forms of biotin responsive encephalopathy are reported. 1) neonatal holocarboxalase synthetase deficiency (HCSD) and 2) late onset infantile or juvenile biotinidase deficiency (BD). HCSD patients have vomiting, lethargy, and hypotonia associated with metabolic ketoacidosis, hyperammonemia, and organic acidemia. BD infants present with seizures, ataxia, skin rash and alopecia. Seizures are reported in two of five HCSD cases and in 15 of 28 BD cases. The authors stress that the epileptic symptomatology may be the first clinical feature in BD cases. Myoclonias, auditory myoclonus, and repetitive startles documented in the present case were thought to be nonepileptic in nature. - Editor. *Ped Neur Briefs* November 1989.

Partial Biotinidase Deficiency

The symptoms, biochemical features and inheritance pattern of partial biotinidase deficiency have been studied at the Departments of Human Genetics and Pediatrics, Medical College of Virginia, Richmond, VA; the State Laboratory Institute, Massachusetts Department of Public Health; Massachusetts General Hospital, Boston; the Lincoln Clinic, NB; and the Division of Human Genetics, University of Maryland School of Medicine, Baltimore. Twelve boys and four girls identified by newborn screening had partial biotinidase deficiency, defined as 10% to 30% of the mean normal activity. Three siblings of these children also had partial deficiency. Fourteen children ascertained by neonatal screening had profound biotinidase deficiency (less than 10% mean normal activity). Two siblings with profound deficiency were found among older siblings of these children. In 24 children with symptoms biotinidase activity levels were less than 10% of the mean normal level. All children with partial deficiency were healthy at the time of diagnosis. One child not treated initially with biotin later developed hypotonia, hair loss and skin rash which resolved with biotin therapy. Delayed development of symptoms in some cases may depend on the interaction of reduced biotinidase activity with other factors. e.g. availability of exogenous biotin and alterations in metabolic demand for the vitamin. The need for biotin supplementation may be increased at times of infection and stress. (McVoy JRS, Wolf B et al. Partial biotinidase deficiency: Clinical and biochemical features. *J Pediatr* Jan 1990; *116*:78-83).

> COMMENT. Biotin responsive late onset multiple carboxylase deficiency is an autosomal recessive inherited disorder manifested by seizures, alopecia, skin rash, hypotonia, ataxia, hearing loss, and developmental delay. Lactic acidosis and organic aciduria are often present and if untreated the symptoms become progressively worse and coma and death may occur. Symptoms of biotinidase deficiency resolve rapidly after treatment with biotin 5-10 mg daily orally, but neurologic damage may be irreversible. Early diagnosis and treatment of partial biotinidase deficiency may prevent the development of potentially serious consequences. - Editor. *Ped Neur Briefs* January 1990.

Taurine And BAER Maturation

A blinded randomized trial of taurine supplementation of preterm infants was conducted at the Department of Pediatrics, University of Texas Southwestern Medical Center, Dallas, and Ross Laboratories, Columbus, Ohio. Infants who received taurine supplementation had more mature brainstem auditory evoked responses with a reduction in the interval between stimulus and response at two different stimulation rates. Neurobehavioral development was similar in the supplemented and nonsupplemented groups and there were no differences in weight, length and head circumference in the two groups. (Tyson JE et al. Randomized trial of taurine supplementation for infants less than 1300 gram birth weight: Effect on auditory brainstem evoked responses. *Pediatrics* Mar 1989; *83*:406-415).

> COMMENT. There had been reports in the literature that taurine deficiency retarded growth of primates and caused abnormalities in the electroretinograms in infants. The present study failed to show an effect of taurine deficiency or supplementation on weight gain, but maturation of audito-

ry brainstem evoked responses (BAER) was delayed in preterm infants who were fed taurine deficient diets. Nutritional needs of infants may be evaluated by methods other than clinical signs and growth measures. New approaches such as the BAER to studies of amino acid requirements may provide correlation between maturation of electrophysiological responses, diet and metabolism of the brain. - Editor. *Ped Neur Briefs* May 1989.

Familial Magnesium Deficiency Syndrome

Two sisters aged 4 and 8 years with convulsions and hypo-magnesemia are reported from the Depts of Pediatrics and Nuclear Medicine, Univ of Nijmegen, The Netherlands. Both began to have seizures in infancy, one with fever, and both were mentally retarded. One had cerebral atrophy on CT scan. EEG showed seizures discharges with photostimulation in the older child. Phenobarbital and valproate were necessary for the control of convulsions. A low serum magnesium, accompanied by normal calcium and parathormone levels, was not related to the seizures. Urinary excretion of magnesium was elevated and urinary calcium was normal. Parents were consanguineous and had normal magnesium metabolism. An autosomal recessive mode of inheritance was presumed. (Geven WB et al. Isolated autosomal recessive renal magnesium loss in two sisters. *Clinical Genetics* 1987; *32*:398-402).

COMMENT. The above case shows an association of low magnesium and seizures with CNS pathology. Magnesium deficiency syndromes occur in association with 1) primary hyperparathyroidism, 2) primary aldosteronism, 3) fatty diarrheas, and 4) malnutrition. - Editor. *Ped Neur Briefs* January 1988.

Soft Neurological Signs In Malnourished Children

The relation of abnormal soft neurologic signs and EEG abnormalities to the severity of malnutrition was investigated in 208, 8-10 year old male school children at the Nutrition Section,

Department of Paediatrics, and the Section of Neurology, Department of Medicine, Institute of Medical Sciences, Banaras Hindu University, Varanasi, India. No child had a history of birth anoxia, head injury, or drug ingestion. Seven motor tasks were tested for soft neurologic signs: 1) Finger tapping, 2) successive finger movements, 3) toe tapping, 4) heel toe tapping, 5) repetitive hand patting, 6) alternating hand pronation supination, 7) alternating hand flexion extension. Both dominant and nondominant limbs were evaluated. Choreoathetoid movements were examined as a child walked 20 steps on inverted feet (Fog test).

There was a strong correlation between nutritional status and performance of motor tasks in both hands and a progressive increase in abnormalities with increased severity of malnutrition. Of 71 children with normal nutritional status 4.2% were positive for soft neurological signs whereas in 79 children with moderate malnutrition 87.3% were positive for neurological abnormalities and 50% showed a positive Fog test with choreoathetoid movements. The EEG pattern in 16 children with soft neurological signs showed abnormalities in the form of slow and sharp waves, particularly in the frontal lobe, but also in the parietal and temporal lobes. Motor deficits were more marked on the contralateral side of the EEG abnormality. (Agarwal KN et al. Soft neurological signs and EEG pattern in rural malnourished children. *Acta Paediatr Scand* Nov 1989; *78*:873-878).

COMMENT. The same authors have shown that malnourished children are at risk for depressed cognitive function, learning disabilities, and poor achievement at school. In the present paper they emphasize the occurrence of soft neurologic signs and EEG abnormalities in relation to poor nutrition. The influence of early malnutrition on subsequent behavioral development, learning disabilities, and soft neurologic signs has also been stressed by other authors (Galler JR et al. *Pediatr Res* 1984; *18*:309 and 826).

Perhaps the term minimal brain dysfunction (MBD) in relation to hyperactive children with learning disabilities was discarded prematurely in favor of ADHD. The pediatric neurologist's role in the diagnosis and treatment of children with behavior and learning disabilities has been usurped to some extent by the increasing interests of the psychologists and developmental pediatricians. The importance of pediatric neurology and the recognition of symptoms and signs of brain dysfunction in these patients should receive more emphasis, and nutrition and diet in nervous system disorders of children is a field for further investigation (Millichap JG. *Nutrition, Diet, and Child Behavior.* Charles C. Thomas, Springfield 1986). - Editor. *Ped Neur Briefs* March 1990.

AUTHOR INDEX

SUBJECT INDEX

JOURNAL INDEX

B
Biochemical Medicine
Brain
Brain Development
Brain Nerve (Tokyo)
British Journal of Ophthalmology
British Medical Journal

C
Canadian Journal of Neurological Science
Cancer
Child's Brain
Child's Nervous System
Chinese Medical Journal
Cleveland Clinic Quarterly
Clinical Care Medicine
Clinical Chemistry
Clinical Electroencephalography
Clinical Genetics
Clinical Pediatrics
Clinical Orthopedics
Clinics in Developmental Medicine
Cognitive Neuropsychology
Contemporary Pediatrics
Contraception
Current Problems in Pediatrics

D
Deutsch Medizinische Wochenschrift
Developmental Medicine and Child Neurology

E
Electroencephalography and Clinical Neurophysiology
Epilepsia
European Journal of Pediatrics
European Neurology
Excerpta Medica

F
Federation of American Societies for Experimental Biology Journal

H
Headache
Helvet Paediatrica Acta

Neuropediatrics
Neuropsychologia
Neuroradiology
Neurosurgery
New England Journal of Medicine
New York Academy of Sciences
New York State Journal of Medicine
Nutrition Reviews

O
Ophthalmic Review
Ophthalmology

P
Pediatric Annals
Pediatric Clinics
Pediatric Clinics of North America
Pediatric Infectious Disease Journal
Pediatric Neurology
Pediatric Research
Postgraduate Medicine

Q
Quarterly Journal of Medicine

R
Revue Neurologique Paris

S
Science
Science of Total Environment
Sleep Research
Surgical Neurology

T
Therapy
Transactions of the Neurological Association